Origin and Development of Cerebral Vessels

Gianni Boris Bradac

Origin and Development of Cerebral Vessels

Springer

Gianni Boris Bradac
Department of Neuroscience
University of Turin
Turin, Italy

ISBN 978-3-031-78435-4 ISBN 978-3-031-78436-1 (eBook)
https://doi.org/10.1007/978-3-031-78436-1

This Springer imprint is published by the registered company Springer Nature Switzerland AG
The registered company address is: Gewerbestrasse 11, 6330 Cham, Switzerland

Acknowledgements

The author would like to express his gratitude to all colleagues, both neuroradiologists and neurologists in the stroke unit, who were involved in the investigations and treatments of the cases.

Special thanks are due to MSc Dr. M. Coriasco, technologist in the Neuroradiology Unit of the University of Turin, for the support in the technical structure of the manuscript and in the graphic preparation of the figures.

Finally, I would like to express my gratitude to all members of the Springer team in Paris and Chennai who were involved in this work.

Introduction

This work is based on extensive bibliographic research, starting with that of the pioneers involved in the studies of embryogenesis.

Also useful in this research were phylogenetic studies comparing the appearance and evolution of vessels in all vertebrates, including humans.

The study has been completed using cerebral angiograms, which have described the final configuration of the vessels in humans, including their typical pattern as well as less common deviations from normality.

The study of the various phases of the evolution of the cerebral vessels as well as a phylogenetic comparison was very useful in demonstrating the process that leads to the normal configuration as well as the phases in which anomalies develop and the possible causes responsible for these deviations.

Contents

1 Brain Formation and Development

An important point in the evolution of the brain is the relationship between brain parenchyma and cerebral vessels supplying it. This was definitely clarified in the early twentieth century following the fundamental studies of Streeter [15] and Shellshear [13]. These authors pointed out that brain parenchyma and cerebral vessels do not have an independent evolution. In their development brain parenchyma and vessels are tightly connected, what Streeter calls *Integrative Development*.

Other important considerations came through the phylogenetic studies [3–9, 12, 16] making a comparison of the developing brain in all vertebrates including the humans. They have shown a striking similarity in the evolution in all groups in the earlier phases. In the progressing phases, the evolution showed differences depending on the vital need and function related to the specific animal including the humans. These studies were also useful showing sometimes in which phases of the common evolution important changes of parenchyma and associated vessels occur which progressively differentiated the humans from other vertebrates.

The formation of the human brain has been already studied in details [5, 6, 8, 10, 14, 16]. In this chapter, only a short description is made, summarizing the most important points which are necessary to explain the associated evolution of the vessels.

The central nervous system (CNS) develops from a plate called the "neural plate" formed by a thickened ectoderm extending longitudinally on the dorsal surface of the embryo. The plate changes in a tubular structure called the "neural tube," composed by a few vesicles. The most cranial forms the future brain with prosencephalon (forebrain), mesencephalon (midbrain), and rhombencephalon (hindbrain). The vesicles continue caudally in a small channel from which develops the spinal cord. This is demonstrated in the left part of Fig. 1.1. The further evolution of the vesicles is shown in the same figure, in its central and right part.

At the embryo of 4.5 mm, the prosencephalon (1) divides in two vesicles corresponding respectively to the telencephalon (1a) and diencephalon (1b). From the telencephalon develop the future cerebral hemispheres, which expand greatly laterally forming two cavities (the future lateral ventricles). These are separated by an interhemispheric fissure. The two cavities communicate through a small channel (the future foramen of Monro). The wall of the vesicles is relatively thin, formed by three layers (the pallium). It will be the future cortex. Differently from the lateral wall, the base of the vesicles is thick. It is the subpallium from which develops the basal ganglia.

From the diencephalon (1b) develop the thalamus, hypothalamus, and optic vesicles. The wall is very thickened. This reduces the lumen of the

G. B. Bradac, *Origin and Development of Cerebral Vessels*,
https://doi.org/10.1007/978-3-031-78436-1_1

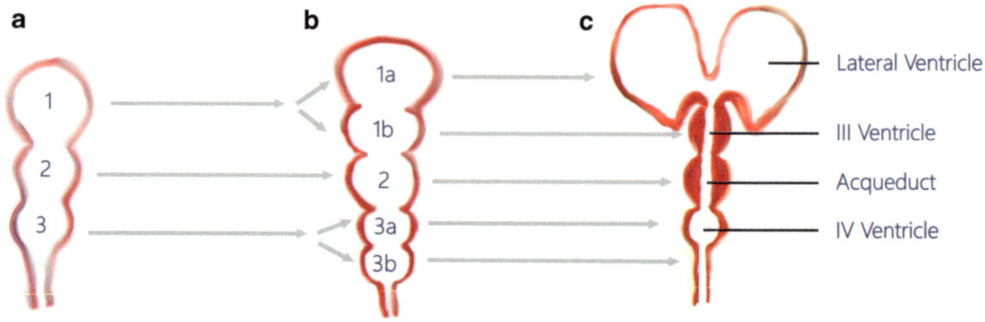

Fig. 1.1 Diagram showing the evolution of the central nervous system. (**a**) Formation of the "neural tube" with its primordial vesicles. (1) Prosencephalon, (2) Mesencephalon, (3) Rhombencephalon, continuing in the small canal (future spinal cord). (**b**) Formation of Telencephalon (1.a) and Diencephalon (1.b), Mesencephalon (2), Metencephalon (3a) and Myelencephalon (3b). (**c**) Great expansion of the Telencephalon (future cerebral hemisphere). Development of the Ventricles system with its components. (Simplified drawing modified from Kuntz [8] and Truex [16])

primary vesicles preparing the formation of the third ventricle.

The mesencephalon (2) undergoes little changes. From it will develop the quadrigeminal plate, the tegmentum and cerebral peduncles. The wall thickens greatly narrowing the lumen (the future aqueduct).

From the most caudal vesicles develop the metencephalon (3a) and the myelencephalon (3b). From Metencephalon arise pons and later cerebellum. The wall extends laterally causing enlargement of the vesicle which will be the fourth ventricle. As far as it concerns, the myelencephalon (the future medulla), it has the same structure of the spinal cord with which it is continuous. The wall is thick; the lumen of the vesicle is small continuing in the central canal.

Due to the different growth of the developing segments occurring in a confined space [10], flexures and curvature appear. The optic vescicle are already developed (Fig. 1.2).

In the further evolution, up to the embryo of 40–44 mm, aged of 52–56 days, the process is mainly characterized by growing of the telencephalon (the future cerebral hemispheres) which in the early phases is limited to the fronto-basal region forming the olfactory lobe. The cerebral hemispheres expand laterally and dorsally to the fronto-parietal regions leading to the formation of the frontal and then of the parietal lobes. The olfactory lobe is compressed and regresses. Following this process, the cerebral hemispheres cover progressively the diencephalon and partially the mesencephalon. Evolution of pons, medulla, and the cerebellar hemispheres is slow.

At the 18–20 mm embryo, appearing of the choroid plexus. It is first small limited to the region of the foramen of Monro, increasing in volume following the growth of the ventricles. This evolution is shown in Fig. 1.3. Slowly appearing also of the choroid plexus of the fourth ventricle.

The choroid plexus develops as a response to the increased metabolic demand.It is formed, from invagination from the roof of the lateral wall of telencephalon of a layer of ependymal cells associated with a layer of rich vascularized pia. The plexus develops first on the roof of the third ventricle extending later laterally through the foramen of Monro in the lateral ventricles. Figure 1.4 shows the appearing of the choroid plexus.

At the embryo of 40–44 mm (52–56 days of age), the first phase of the evolution which is called "Embryogenic Phase" can be considered concluded. The main components of the brain including the vessels (next chapter) typical in the adult can be identified. The evolution, however, continues in the next phase called "fetal phase" which extends up to the birth. Many changes of the brain parenchyma which influences the

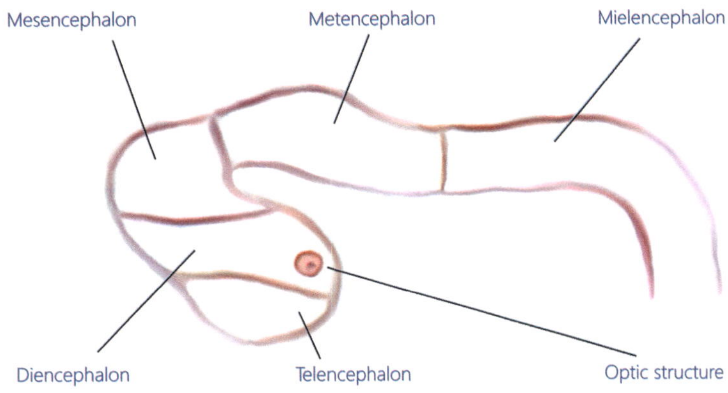

Fig. 1.2 Diagram (Lateral view). Appearing of the primordial flexures. Early development of the optic vesicles. (Simplified drawing modified from Kuntz [8] and Truex [16])

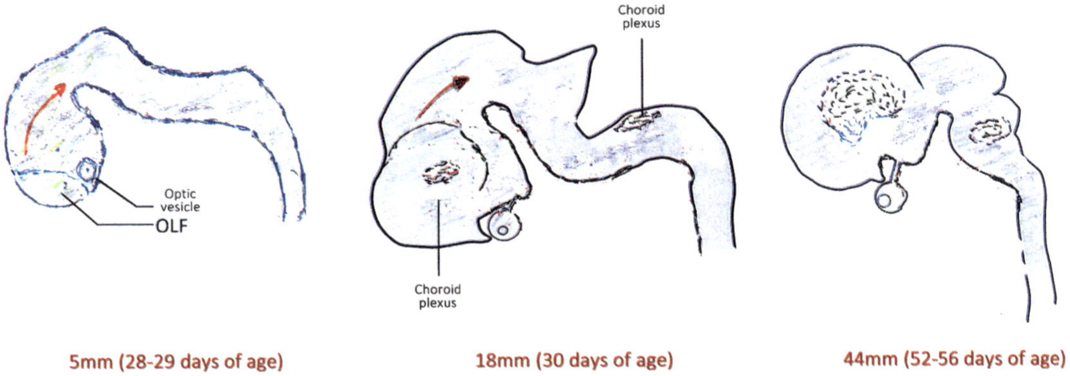

Fig. 1.3 Diagram showing the evolution of the Embryo from the Phase of 28–29 days to the embryo of 56 days. In the first phase, the Telencephalon is basic represented by the olfactory lobe (OLF). Later the Telencephalon extends dorsally (arrow), covering the Diencephalon an progressively the Mesencephalon. Early appearing of the Optic vesicle and the Choroid plexus. (Simplified drawing modified from Kuntz [8] and Truex [16])

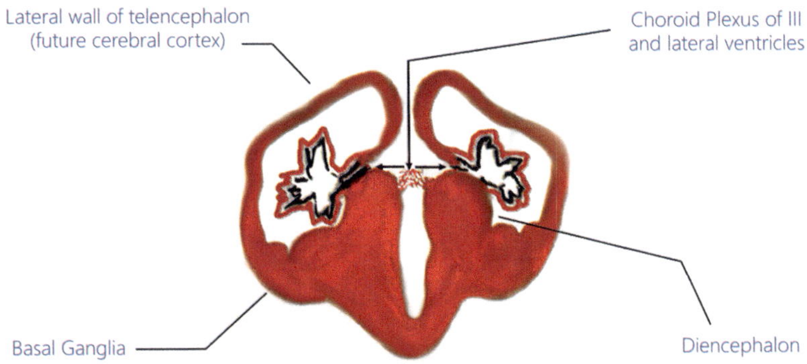

Fig. 1.4 Diagram showing the appearing of the Choroid plexus (coronal view) formed by layers of ependymal and vascularize pia migrate from the lateral roof of telencephalon to the third ventricle and later to the lateral ventricles. (Simplified drawing modified from Kuntz [8] and Truex [16])

evolution of the brain vessels occur. The most important are presented in the following list and demonstrated in Fig. 1.5.

1. The growth of the cerebral hemispheres continues extending from the fronto-parietal to the occipital area forming the corresponding

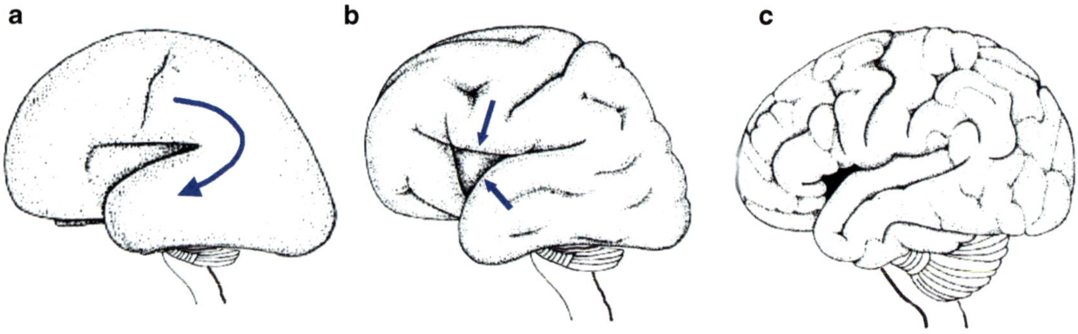

Fig. 1.5 Evolution of the cerebral hemispheres. (**a**) Formation of the Frontal-Parietal, then of the Occipital and Temporal lobes. There is a smooth cerebral convexity. (**b**) Formation of the insula and appearing of the first sulci and circumvolutions (**c**) Final development of circumvolutions and sulci. (**a–c**) Progressive evolution of Pons and Medulla. Slow growing of Cerebellum. (Simplified drawing modified from Kuntz [8] and Truex [16])

lobes. The hemispheres then bend downwards and extend anteriorly forming the temporal lobe. This evolution is accompanied with growing of the ventricles with the formation of the temporal horn associate with the extension of the choroid plexus.

2. The deep part of brain parenchyma adjacent to the basal ganglia is not involved in this growth. It will be covered by the growing of the adjacent lobes (the frontal, parietal, and temporal lobes). This deep part of parenchyma is called the "Insula" which communicates with the surface through a small fissure the "Sylvian insular fissure."
3. Developing of cortex: It begins at the fetus age of 150 days and it is completed at 190 days. This occurs through cells migration from two "Germinal Matrices." One located in the so-called Subventricular Zone and the other in the "Zones of the Basal Ganglia" (The lateral and medial ganglionic eminence). The migration occurs respectively through a radial and tangential process [1, 2, 11] and progressively shifts from smooth cerebral surface to cortex with gyri and sulci.
4. Following the formation of cortex appearing that of white matter.
5. Formation of corpus callosum.
6. There is a progressive evolution of the pons and medulla. The growth of the cerebellar hemisphere occurs later, beginning not before the fetus of 90–100 days of age, becoming more rapid in the following months.

References

1. Anderson SA, Marín O, Horn C, Jennings K, Rubenstein JLR. Distinct cortical migrations from the medial and lateral ganglionic eminences. Development. 2001;128(3):353–63.
2. Bayer SA (Shirley A. Atlas of human central nervous system development. CRC Press; Boca Raton 2002.
3. De Beer GR. Embryos and ancestors. Revised ed. Oxford: Oxford University Press; 1954.
4. Gillilan LA. A comparative study of the extrinsic and intrinsic arterial blood supply to brains of submammalian vertebrates [Internet]. J Comp Neurol. 1967;130:175–96.
5. Hamilton WJ, Boyd JD, Mossman HW. Hamilton, Boyd and Mossman's human embryology: prenatal development of form and function. London: Macmillan Press; 1972.
6. Hochstetter F. Beiträge zur Entwicklungsgeschichte der Kraniozerebralen Topographie des Menschen: Vorgelegt in der Sitzung am 17. Dezember 1942. Springer-Verlag; 2013.
7. Kier EL. Development of cerebral vessels. Radiology of the skull and brain. St Louis: Mosby; 1974. p. 1089–130.
8. Kuntz A. A textbook of neuroanatomy. Acad Med. 1950;25(2):158.
9. Larsell O. The development of the cerebellum in man in relation to its comparative anatomy. J Comp Neurol. 1947;87(2):85–129.
10. Patten BM. Human embryology. New York/Toronto/London: McGraw Hill; 1953. p. 523.

11. Rakic P. Neuronal migration and contact guidance in the primate telencephalon. Postgrad Med J. 1978;54(Suppl 1):25–40. PMID: 364453.
12. Romer AS, Parsons TS. The vertebrate body. 5th ed. Philadelphia: Saunders College; 1977.
13. Shellshear JL. The basal arteries of the forebrain and their functional significance. J Anat. 1920;55(Pt 1):27–35.
14. Streeter GL. Die Entwicklung des Nervensystems. In: Handbuch der Entwicklungsgeschichte des Menschen. Leipzig: Zweiter Band Hirzel; 1911. p. 1–156.
15. Streeter GL. The developmental alterations in the vascular system of the brain of the human embryo. Contrib Embryol Carneg Inst. 1918;8:5–38.
16. Truex RC. Human neuroanatomy. Acad Med. 1959;34(9):955.

2 Development of the Cerebral Vessels

At the beginning of the twentieth century, there was an increased interest for the Embryogenesis of the cerebral vessels. This is documented by the works of many authors, pioneers in this field [11, 19, 33]. An important contribution came from the studies of Streeter [31]. As already mentioned in the previous chapter, this author pointed out that the cerebral vessels do not have an anticipated development independent from that of parenchyma, instead both, parenchyma and vessels, grow and develop as a unity. This starts in the early phases of the embryogenesis where the primordial vessels are formed and continue in the further evolution with a process of adaptation of the vessels to the changes and growth of the parenchyma. The appearing and formation of the vessels will be described in the following chapters.

In this context very useful information came from the comparative studies performed in all vertebrates including the humans made by many authors [1, 2, 8, 14, 28, 29, 38]. These authors, as it has been already described for the parenchyma (Chap. 1), demonstrated that while the evolution of the cerebral vessels in the first phases was similar, progressively differences appear in the various groups, following the different evolution of the parenchyma.

2.1 Primordial Development of the Cerebral Vessels

In 1918, Streeter published a work about the development of the cerebral vessels. In this study, he followed basically the previous reports of Evans and Sabin [11, 25] made on embryos of chickens which presented an evolution similar to that of humans. Streeter distinguished two phases: pre-circulatory and circulatory phase.

2.1.1 Pre-circulatory Phase

In this phase, we are dealing with an embryo of 1–2 mm and an age of 15–20 days. The wall of the Neural Tube is covered by a dense mesenchymal tissue (mesoderm) called the "*Meninx Primitiva.*" In this tissue, develop angioblasts (vaso-formative cells) which rapidly increase in number forming cells cords grouped together in a plexus extending to the surface of the brain, especially around the forebrain and midbrain. From the outer cells of these cords develop endothelial cells, from the inner cells, through a process of "Liquefaction" develop plasma and the future blood cells. In this phase, there is no clear blood circulation (Fig. 2.1).

G. B. Bradac, *Origin and Development of Cerebral Vessels*,
https://doi.org/10.1007/978-3-031-78436-1_2

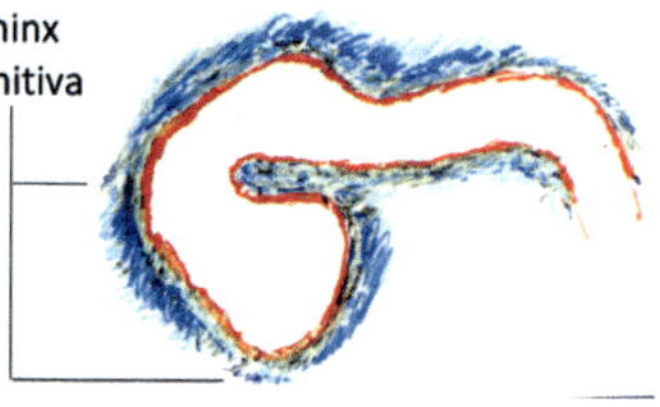

Fig. 2.1 Diagram showing the embryo of 1–2 mm. The superficial capillary network (red layer) on the surface of the brain is covered by the *Meninx Primitiva* (blue layer)

2.1.2 Circulatory Phase

In this phase at the embryo of 2–3 mm aged of 26–28 days, from the primary capillary plexus develop arteries, capillary, and veins. Three layers can be distinguished: In the *more superficial* layer, vessels progressively acquire the feature of arterial or venous trunks. These are connected with the deep capillary network through vessel branches running in an *intermediate layer*. A circuit develops in which from the superficial arterial trunks runs the supplying blood towards the deep network, from which a draining blood runs to the superficial veins. The superficial arterial and venous channels connect, respectively, with ascending vessels arising from the developed aortic arches and with descending trunks draining in the primordial venous part of the Heart.

2.1.3 Separation of Cerebral from Extra-Cerebral Vessels

According to the studies of Streeter, in the further phases of evolution about the Embryo of 12–14 mm, the *Meninx Primitiva* undergoes great changes leading to the formation of meninges, skull, and soft tissues. The consequences are the separation of the vessels in three different sectors: those of the brain, those of the meninges, and those of external structures.

2.2 Development of Aortic Arches

Independent from the formation of the primordial cerebral vessels, contemporaneously or preceding that, other vascular structures develop in the body of the embryo. From the surrounding mesoderm, arise angioblasts from which develops the paired dorsal aorta. This extends cranially, and at the level of the pharynx the vessel bends caudally connecting with the developed primordial heart, appearing as a double channel fusing rapidly in a unique tube. In the further evolution, the primordial heart develops and from it arises a trunk (aortic trunk) which continues cranially in a dilatation (aortic sac) from which arise the aortic arches.

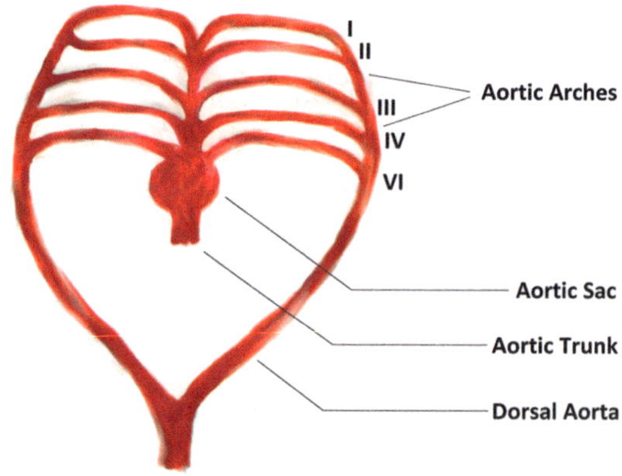

Fig. 2.2 Diagram showing the development of the dorsal aorta and of the aortic arches (I–VI) arising from the heart. Aortic trunk, aortic sac

According to the detailed studies of Congdon [7], six arches develop (Fig. 2.2). They are bilateral, having an ascending course towards the pharynx, then bend down connecting with the paired dorsal aorta. They do not appear all together, but separately in different phases of the evolution. The earlier appearing are the first and second arches, which regress rapidly replaced by the new arches, the third and fourth. These latter are the most important vascular structures from which develop the ascending vessels (basically the carotid arteries) connecting with the network developed at the surface of the brain. The arches appear first as a plexural structure evolving rapidly in tubular vessels. A far as the vertebral arteries are concerned, they are not developed in this first phase, appearing only later arising from the dorsal aorta.

As far as it concerns the fifth aortic arch, its presence is not accepted by all authors and anyway, if developed regresses rapidly. The sixth aortic arch is involved in the formation of the pulmonary arteries.

It should be remembered that the particular form and evolution of the arches is a consequence of their adaptation to the already present anatomy of the pharynx with its pouches reproducing the configuration present in the lower vertebrate precursors of the "Gill Apparatus." This pattern, temporary in the humans, has been called by Congdon the "Branchial Phase" lasting 30–32 days. It is followed by the "Post-branchial Phase" with a typical pattern in the human.

2.3 Development of Cerebral Vessels

Many authors have been involved in this study. Among them, the most comprehensive study is that of Padget [23], which remains still today a fundamental work even if Padget was mainly concentrated in the first phases of the evolution. Furthermore, due to the limited number of embryos studied, some aspects remained a little unclear. Further studies have followed adding progressively new information about the evolution characterized by a very complex process, occurring in different phases, in which vessels appear, then disappear, replaced by new vessels or sometimes the primordial vessels persist. The evolution can in some cases take an unexpected direction not always easily to be explained. Basically the complete evolution of the cerebral vessels can be divided in two phases. The one is the embryonic phase lasting from the embryo of 3 mm to the embryo of 40–44 mm. In this phase, the vessels acquire progressively a configuration comparable to that of the adult. This phase is followed by the so-called fetal phase ending at the birth. In this phase, the final configuration of the vessels is acquired. In this and in the following chapters, the phases of the normal and of the not so rare deviation of it are presented.

2.4 Primitive Vascular Structures at the Embryo of 3 mm, Aged of 24 Days

Appearing of the first and second aortic arches: From each first aortic arch develop the primitive internal carotid arteries (ICA), each extends cranially and loses itself in the superficial plexus at the base of brain. Another vessel arising from the first aortic arch appearing earlier is the Primitive Trigeminal Artery (TR).

In the early phases of evolution, the Superficial Vascular Plexus, which receives the blood from the above described ICA and TR *is the essential source of nutrition of the brain, through a process of diffusion. The nutrition through the intrinsic vascularization appears later following the development of the perforating branches*. Waiting for this, in an intermediate phase the nutrition through the process of diffusion occurs with the formation of the choroid plexus (see also Chap. 1).

The first and second aortic arches regress rapidly as a remnant appears, the mandibular and the hyoid arteries arising, respectively, from the first and second arch. As shown in the next phase, the above vessels are annexed by the new internal carotid artery which arises now from the developed third aortic arch.

2.5 Embryo at 4–6 mm, Aged of 29 Days

At the base of the cerebrum, each ICA divides in the anterior and posterior segments called by De Vriese [8] "The Cranial and Caudal Division." From the cranial division (CR) arises the olfactory artery supplying the basal part of the telencephalon contributing also to supply the optic vesicle. From the caudal division (CD) arises an irregular plexus (the future PcomA) supplying the developing diencephalon and mesencephalon. There are also minimal connections with the plexus on the surface of the hindbrain.

Along its course the ICA gives off many branches. These are the hyoid and the more cranial mandibular arteries, remnants of the second and first aortic arches, respectively. More cranially, opposite the mandibular artery at the level of the developed trigeminal ganglion arises the primitive trigeminal artery (TR) connected dorsally with the developed "bilateral longitudinal channel (BLC)." Close to the ICA cranial division a little more caudally located, arises the primary maxillary artery, involved in the vascularization of the basal telencephalon and maxillary process.

It also partially supplies the optic vesicle. This latter is also supplied by the early appeared dorsal ophthalmic artery. The Ophthalmic Artery, the Primary Maxillary Artery (PMA) and the Dorsal Ophthalmic Artery are connected on the surface of the optic vescicle (see also Chap. 6).

At this phase, the basilar (BA) and the vertebral arteries (VAs) are not developed.

As far as it concerns the vascularization of the brainstem, this occurs through the BLC from which develops later the BA. The BLC is not a single tubular channel, instead it is formed by an irregular plexus where vessels show dilatations, narrowing, interruptions. It extends bilaterally in a median, para-median position, on the anterior surface of the hindbrain which it supplies. The BLC receives the blood from the TR and the supply is reinforced caudally by other branches of ICA, the otic, and the hypoglossal arteries. More caudally, the BLC is connected with the artery called by padget the proatlantal artery, considering its course between the atlas and the occipital bone, arising from ductus caroticus (DC).

Paralleling to the BLC, lateral to it, there is another vascular structure "The Lateral Bilateral Channel" (LC). It has been described by Padget in the 1948, but has already been identified previously by Evans [11] and Schmeidel [26]. The LC connects with the BLC trough transverse anastomoses and caudally with the dorsal branch of the proatlantal artery and hypoglossal artery. The role of this latter connection is discussed in Chap. 5.

As far as it concerns the spinal cord, like the brain, its nutrition, in the first phases, is through a process of diffusion from superficial vascular plexus, receiving the blood from the segmental (also called "intersegmental") arteries arising from the dorsal aorta.

In the meantime, there is the appearing of the primitive external carotid artery (ECA) developing from the aortic sac, close to the origin of the third aortic arch. The artery has been called by Congdon [7] the "Ventral Pharyngeal Artery" (VPA). This has connections cranially with the mandibular artery.

The above described evolution is shown in the diagram in Fig. 2.3.

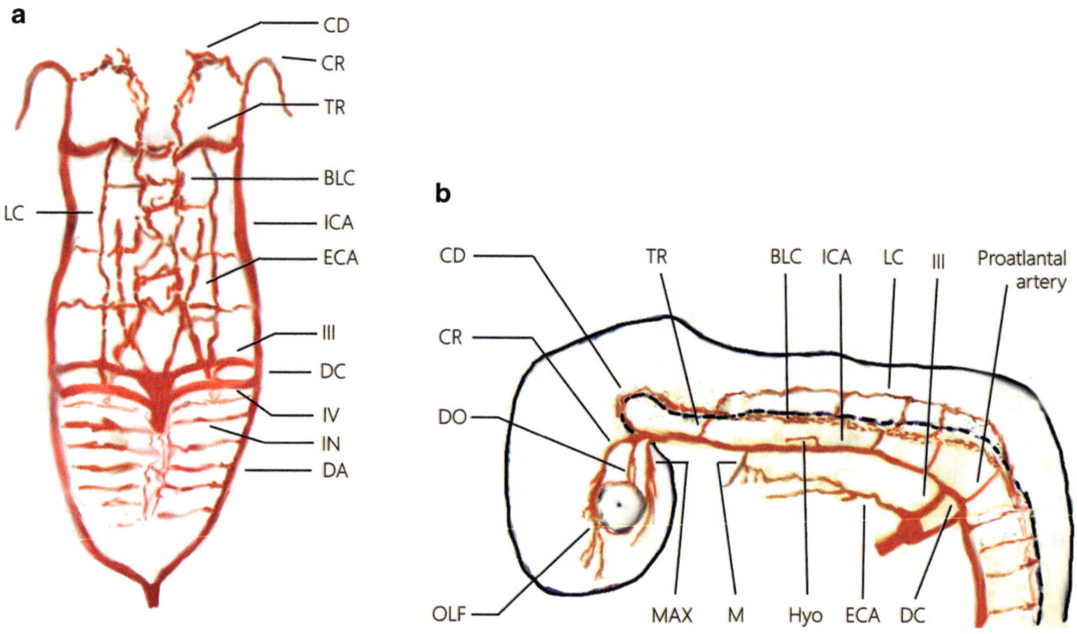

Fig. 2.3 Diagram (modified from Padget [23]) showing the evolution of the embryo of 4–6 mm, AP (**a**) and lateral (**b**) view. III, IV aortic arches connected through the *Ductus Caroticus* (DC). Internal carotid (ICA), external carotid (ECA) arteries, cranial (CR) and caudal (CD) division of ICA. Olfactory artery (OLF), primary maxillary artery (MAX). Dorsal ophthalmic artery (DOA), hyoid artery (HYO). Mandibular artery (M), primitive trigeminal artery (TR), bilateral longitudinal channel (BLC), lateral bilateral channel (LC), dorsal aorta (DA). Intersegmental arteries (IN)

2.6 Evolution of the Embryo from 9–10 mm to the Embryo of 40–44 mm (Aged of 50–56 Days)

This phase is characterized by great changes *of the aortic arches and their derivatives, as well as of the cerebral vessels*, which acquire progressively the configuration similar to that of the adult.

2.6.1 Aortic Arches

Their evolution has been described in details by Congdon [7]. Later Moffat et al. [20, 21] added interesting observations useful to explain the changes occurring in this area. In accordance to these authors, the process seems to be linked mainly with the displacement in the thorax area of the aortic arches, beginning at the embryo of 9–10 mm. In this evolution, the fourth arch descends more rapidly than the third causing stretching, narrowing, and finally regression of the *Ductus Caroticus* (DC) which is the segment of the dorsal aorta connecting the third and fourth arches. The evolution of the DC is associated with changes of the vessels connected directly or indirectly with it.

The third aortic arch is now "independent," no longer connected with the fourth arch. It acquires progressively one more upwards oblique course continuing directly in the ICA. In the further evolution about the embryo of 18 mm from the proximal part of the left third aortic arch with a contribution of the aortic sac develops the common carotid artery (CCA), which annexes the ECA arising also from the aortic sac. The ECA becomes the direct continuation of the growing CCA and migrates with it reaching distally the ICA, forming the carotid bifurcation. On the right, the distal part of the third aortic arch continues in the ICA, from his proximal part develops the innominate trunk from which arises the right CCA, which with a process similar to that described on the left annexes the ECA and together migrates to the ICA, forming the right carotid bifurcation. The process of formation of CCA and its migration cranially with the ECA can take an unexpected evolution explaining some variations of these vascular structures as described further in Chap. 3.

As far as it concerns the fourth aortic arch, from the left develops the final aortic arch which annexes the left CCA. On the right, the fourth arch contributes with the third arch to the formation of the innominate trunk, from which arise the CCA and the ECA.

As far as it concerns the proatlantal artery, the vessel following the changes of the aortic arches moves cranially from a position close to the dorsal end of the fourth aortic arch from which receives the main blood to the dorsal end of the third aortic arch The consequence is that the great flow from the fourth arch is reduced and that from the third is limited since this latter is mainly involved in the supply of the ICA. The proatlantal artery dwindles and eventually regresses accompanying the regression of the DC.

In the meantime, great changes involve the subclavian, vertebral, and the basilar arteries.

At the embryo of 10–12 mm between the cervical segmental arteries, longitudinal anastomosis develops, forming the primordial vertebral artery (VA). At the embryo of 14–18 mm, the cervical segmental arteries disappear, with exception of the artery from which develop in a common trunk the Vertebral and the the Subclavian Arteries.

In accordance to the description of Padget [24] used also in the present work, the persistent segmental artery is the sixth. *In this context, it is useful to recall that the indication of the persistent segmental artery reported in the literature is not unanimous. This occurs, probably, because by some authors the proatlantal artery is considered to be the first segmental artery, while by Padget the first segmental artery is that running between the first and second cervical segment. This explains the different numbering and the different indication of the persistent segmental artery.*

The Vertebral Artery takes an ascending course, joining cranially the Basilar Artery, formed at the embryo of 9–10 mm by the fusion on the midline of the BLC. As far as it concern the Subclavian Arteries from the primordial small trunk developed the final Subclavian Arteries, which join on the left the formed final Aortic Arch and on the right the innominate trunk. The Vertebral Arteries take now the final configuration arising from the Subclavian Arteries, which they have now their final position. *The vertebro-basilar system can be considered completed.*

It is interesting, as described by De Vriese in her comparative studies, to note that through the development of the vertebro-basilar system there is a new source of blood to the brain in addition to that of the carotid. This is a new acquirement typical in some mammals such as the apes and monkeys and is particularly well developed in Humans. In other mammals such as horse, zebra, giraffe, camel, … the ICA is the major supply, while the vertebro-basilar system is hypo-plastic or a-plastic.

The evolution of the vertebro-basilar system is associated with changes of other vessels. From the left intersegmental arteries distal to the sixth, develop the future intercostal and lumbar arteries, from which arise the radiculo-medullary arteries, involved in the supply of the spinal cord, in the thoracic-lumbar regions. The evolution of the intersegmental arteries in the cervical and sacral regions is different due to the development of the vertebral and ileo-sacral arteries.

As far as it concerns the right dorsal aorta, its segment, distal to the sixth intersegmental artery regresses. The proximal segment is involved in the formation of the innominate trunk.

Following the development of the vertebro-basilar system, the trigeminal artery and the other temporal arteries (see Chap. 5) loose their function as supplying artery of the brainstem, since the supplying is taken over by the new developed system. These arteries can sometimes persist in the adult (see Chap. 5). In these cases it is not completely absurd to think that the anomalous configuration reproduce in the human what in some mammals, as described above, is the normal evolution.

In addition to the above described evolution of the carotid and vertebro-basilar system, other changes in the embryonic phase occur, involving the aortic arches and the derivatives, basically following the shifting of the heart in his final thoracic position.

The aortic arches change the horizontal configuration in a more vertical one. The common carotid arteries and the innominate trunk are elongated. The proximal subclavian arteries are more caudally displaced, while the distal segment is more cranially located. The internal carotid and the vertebral arteries acquire the typically more vertical course.

Another important evolution, influencing the changes of the vessels, is the shifting of the head from his position close to the chest, to a more cranial vertical one.

The sixth aortic arches (pulmonary) undergoes also important changes. The distal portion of the right arch regresses while the proximal part is annexed by the left aortic arch from which arise the right and left pulmonary arteries. A connection (ductus arteriosus) with the dorsal aorta persists until the first week after the birth.

At the embryo of 40–44 mm the aortic arch and its derivatives have reached the configuration similar to that of the adult.

Diagram of the above described evolution in Fig. 2.4.

It is out of the scope of this work to analyze the evolution of the vascularization of the spinal cord, which has been already the subject of previous studies. These have been started with the works of Adamkiewicz [3] and Kadyi [13] followed by studies adding progressively more information [9–11, 18, 30, 36]. Later, an important contribution in the study of these complex evolution, came through the works of Thron [34], Lasjaunias and Berenstein [15] and, more recently, through the study of Thron and Stoeter et al. [35].

Only a few essential points of the evolution are summarized here and described in the following.

In the early phase, the antero-lateral surface of the spinal cord is covered by the primordial plexus arisen like the primordial plexus surrounding the brain from the meninx primitiva. It receives the blood from the segmental arteries arising from the dorsal aorta. In this phase, the

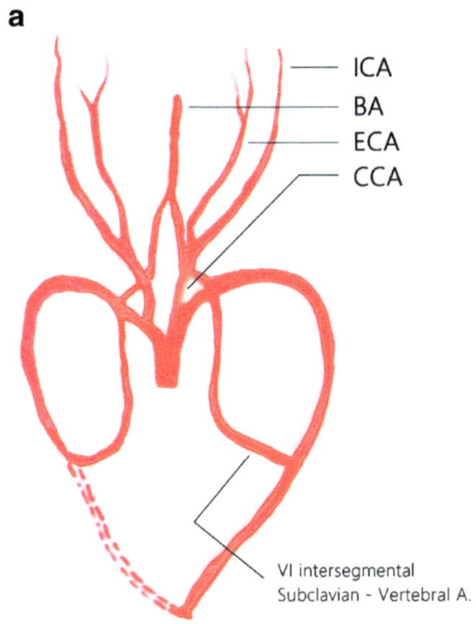

Fig. 2.4 (**a**) Diagram showing the evolution of the aortic arch and its tributaries. (**a**) Appearing of the common carotid artery (CCA), it annexes the external carotid artery (ECA). Both join the distal internal carotid artery (ICA). Longitudinal anastomoses between the intersegmental arteries lead to the formation of the VAs. Regression of the intersegmental arteries, with exception of the VI from which develop the subclavian and the VAs. The VAs connect cranially with the developed basilar artery (BA). (**b**) Diagram showing the aortic arch at the embryo of 44 mm, having acquired the configuration similar to that of the adult. The left CCA arises from the formed aortic arch. The right CCA arises from the innominate trunk. Internal carotid (ICA) and external carotid (ECA). VAs arise from the subclavian arteries. Basilar artery (BA)

plexus is the essential source of nutrition of the spinal cord, through a process of diffusion.

In the further evolution, capillary channels develop from which arise branches forming the primordial intrinsic vascularization of the cord.

About the end of the embryonic phase, the anterior spinal artery (ASA) appears as histological and micro-angiographic studies [9, 36] have shown.

The ASA appears first as a para-median paired channel, then as a unique longitudinal artery, running on the surface of the cord, along the formed anterior-medial fissure. From the ASA arise branches, running in the fissure, called *Sulcal-Sulco commissural* (Adamkiewicz), from which arise the most important branches supplying both emi-cord. Other branches run first on the antero-lateral surface of the cord, before entering it.

The process leading to the change from a paired to the unique vessel, is not completely clear. In accordance to the studies of Sterzi and Evans, this can be due to a fusion of the two channels, or only one vessel persists and the other regresses. The presence of transverse anastomosis guarantees the supply of both emi-cord, through the sulcal artery. Case of persistence of both channel can appear. This different evolution explains the variations of the ASA recognizable in the studies in the adult.

The ASA divides on the surface of the cord in ascending and descending branches, anastomosing with descending and ascending branches, respectively, of the superior and inferior segments of ASA, which therefore appear as a vessel formed by the connections of several segments.

Along its course, the ASA receives the blood from several segmental feeders (radiculo-medullary artery) which arise at every segment. In the evolution, these undergo a variable great reduction and so, in the adult angiogram, only a limited number of radiculo-medullary artery remains.

As far as it concerns the cervical region, from the formed vertebral artery, at the embryo of

14–18 mm [23] develops the primordial ASA, running caudally on the anterior surface of the spinal cord, reinforced by one or two remaining radiculo-medullary arteries.

As far as it concerns the posterior spinal artery, they appear a little later, running on the posterior surface of the spinal cord, with a more irregular pattern.

More about the spinal artery in Chap. 3.

2.7 Changes of the Cerebral Vessels Upto the End of the Embryonic Phase

Some changes are common to all cerebral vessels, which progressively appear with less plexiform pattern, acquiring a more typical tubular configuration. Other changes are more specific to each vessel which develop leading to the configuration at the end of the embryonic phase comparable to that of the adult.

2.7.1 Anterior Cerebral Artery (ACA)

The olfactory artery (OLF), appeared as the main branch of the cranial ICA division, begin to dwindle and regress at the embryo of 18–20 mm. From the same trunk, from which the OLF is arisen, more medially located, arises the ACA. The artery extends medially forming the A1 segment connecting at 18 mm embryo with the contralateral ACA. This connection (the future anterior communicating artery, AComA) appear first as a plexural structure. From the distal A1 develops with an ascending rectilinear course, the primordial peri-callosal artery. From the AcomA, as described by De Vriese [8] develops a branch the author called "*Median Artery of Corpus Callosum.*" The evolution and clinical significance of this artery is discussed later in Chap. 3.

From the regressed trunk of the OLF, in accordance to the study of Padget, has developed a branch which is considered its remnant. The branch or branches are annexed by the ACA. They are involved in the supply of the developed basal ganglia. Considering the medial position of the ACA the vessels are forced to reach the basal ganglia passing through, the more lateral APS, to take a recurrent course.

Other authors [4, 28] having identified the artery in their anatomic study called it the "Heubner Artery or Recurrent Artery of Heubner" in homage to Dr. Heubner [12], the German pathologist who first described the vessel in the 1872. Abbie [1, 2] and Alexander [5] suggested to call these branches the "Medial striate arteries" to distinguish them from the reciprocal appearing "Lateral Striate Arteries," arising from the M1 segment of the MCA.

2.7.2 Middle Cerebral Artery (MCA)

As far as it concerns the MCA, the artery develops at the embryo of 12 mm from the distal ICA, arising from many twigs developed from ICA and ACA. It grows rapidly. Its distal branches extend progressively to the frontal and parietal regions continuing its growth in the fetal phase. From its basal trunk, the future M1 develop as described above the "Lateral Striate Arteries" supplying the basal ganglia having passed through the APS.

2.7.3 Anterior Choroidal Artery (AChA)

At the 12 mm embryo from the cranial division of ICA, as the first and more prominent collateral, arises the AchA. At this phase, the artery is not involved in the supply of the choroid plexus. It gives off branches for the optic tract, mesencephalon and diencephalon (lateral geniculate body) structures devoted to the visual function. However, at the embryo of 18 mm following the appearing of the Choroid plexus, the AchA is involved in the supply of it. The plexus is first small (see also Fig. 1.3) limited to the area of the foramen of Monro. It expands rapidly in the lateral ventricle from the frontal of the parietal areas. The involvement of the AchA increases progressively associated with the involvement of the choroidal branches of the diencephalic arteries of the PcomA.

2.7.4 Posterior Cerebral Artery (PCA)

At the embryo of 18 mm, the posterior communicant artery (PcomA) arising from the primordial plexus of the earlier caudal division of ICA is a well-formed tubular vessel. From the PcomA arise two well developed groups of arteries: the diencephalic for diencephalon giving off also choroidal branches for the choroid plexus and the mesencephalic branches supplying at this phase the well-developed mesencephalon. Early anastomoses with the AchA are present.

Distally the PcomA becomes connected, through a short trunk with the formed basilar artery. This trunk which is the stem of the future posterior cerebral artery (PCA) has been called by De Vriese "Divisional PCA branch of the Ba" and can be considered what today is called the P1 segment of PCA. It is from the fusion of the proximal segment of the PcomA with its distal segment that in the fetal phase develops the PCA. At the present phase only the proximal part of the PCA can be identified, formed by the above described fusion with the important contribution of the diencephalic and especially mesencephalic branches from which arise later the thalamic perforates and the mesencephalic branches.

Comparing the above described evolution in human with that of lower vertebrate, as described by Abbie [1, 2] in his comparative studies, the presence of some similarities is evident. Indeed in this group of animals the mesencephalon in which the PCA ends, is well developed forming the "Optic Lobe" which is the visual center. In the human, the above described configuration is temporary. The PCA following the growth of the hemispheres extends dorsally to the occipital lobes where the visual centers develops.

2.7.5 Brainstem

As far as it concerns the vascularization of the brainstem, following the formation of BA and VA, the temporary arteries (trigeminal, hypoglossal, proatlantal) are no longer necessary and regress. From BA and VA arise branches which form a network of vessels on the surface of brainstem, which can be considered remnant of the disappeared BLC and LC.

This network is formed by many vessels supplying pons and medulla. At this phase, a few of these branches are particularly well-developed. These are the future anterior inferior cerebellar artery (AICA) and posterior inferior cerebellar artery (PICA), which, however, cannot be identified with certainty. Their typical configuration appears first in the advanced phase, linked to the late development of the cerebellar hemisphere, for which supply, the AICA and PICA are the essential tributaries. In this phase, the AICA and PICA are involved in the supply of pons and medulla and end their course in the formed choroid plexus. Differently is the evolution of the superior cerebellar artery (SCA), which already in this phase is well-developed, arising from the BA, supplying part of the primordial cerebellum (flocculus) and mainly involved in the supply of mesencephalon.

Figure 2.5 shows this evolution, in lateral and AP view.

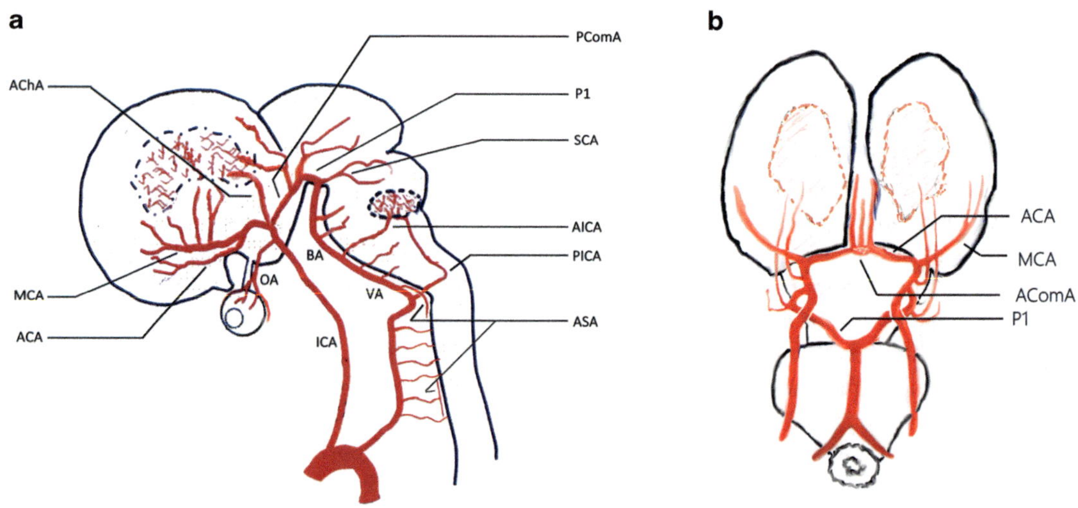

Fig. 2.5 Diagram (modified by Padget [23])). Lateral (**a**) and AP (**b**) view, showing the evolution towards the embryo of 44 mm. The olfactory artery is regressed. Appearing of the anterior cerebral artery (ACA) connected with the contro-lateral ACA through the AcomA from which develop the primordial peri-callosal artery and the median artery of corpus callosum. Development of MCA (MCA) and of the AchA. The primordial posterior communicating artery connects with the basilar artery through a short trunk (the future P1). From the fusion of this trunk, with the PcomA arises the primordial cerebral artery. The essential cerebral vessels are now present having a configuration similar to that of the adult. The circle of Willis is formed

2.8 Circle of Willis

At the end of the embryogenic phase, at the embryo of 40–44 mm, as identified by Padget, another important vascular structure is developed. As shown in Fig. 2.5 (right) and better in Fig. 2.6, following the connection of both ACA through the AcomA and the connection of ICA with the BA through the PcomA and the future P1, the anastomotic circle at the base of the brain, described by Dr. Willis in 1684 in an anatomic study in the adult, is formed. This is a natural-well-constructed security system. However, as shown in the further evolution, many anomalies occur due to hypo-aplasia of some segments of the circle. These appear progressively in the later fetal phases and continue after the birth and in the adult life as comparisons of the circle in the fetus and in the adult have shown.

The anomalies can involve both the anterior and the posterior segments, but the posterior is predominantly involved [8, 17].

To clarify the causes of some anomalies, explanations have been proposed. As far as it concerns the PCA, some authors [8, 27, 37] have suggested that the distal extent of the PCA occurring in the fetal phase, results in an increase distance of the artery from its origin. To compensate this, the origin is shifted from the ICA to the BA. The PcomA becomes hypo-aplastic, while

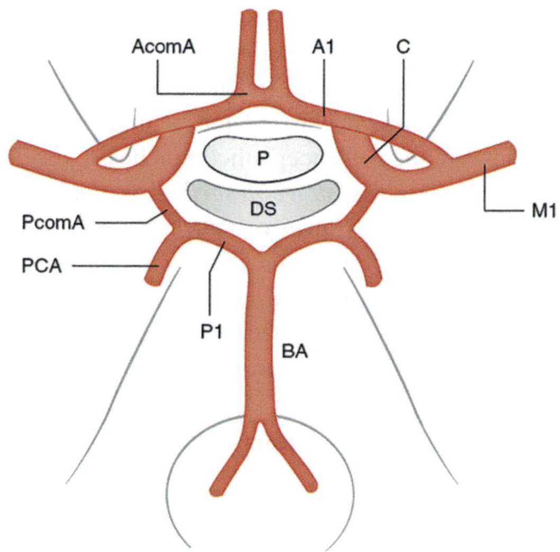

Fig. 2.6 Diagram showing the typical Circle of Willis. (Taken from Bradac [6])

the segment arising from the BA, the future P1 enlarges.

Other authors [16, 17], considering the anomalies of the circle in the adult life, have suggested that these could be due to many hemodynamic factors, among them especially important were the compression of the carotid and vertebral arteries by movements of the head and neck. These would cause changing of blood flow which leads progressively to permanent anatomic changes.

Interesting are also the studies of some authors [22, 32] who indicate that anomalies of the circle of Willis can be identified in the embryo in a phase where in accordance to previous studies [23], the circle is reported to be completed. This seems to indicate that further studies are necessary.

In conclusion, in its evolution the circle of Willis changes from a well-constructed security system, in many cases to an anomalous unfavorable configuration. Why this occurs is only partially explained. Fortunately, the present anomalies are frequently an incidental discovery in the routine angiographic studies. However, they can play an important role with clinical consequences if associated to pathological conditions.

References

1. Abbie AA. The blood supply of the lateral geniculate body, with a note on the morphology of the choroidal arteries. J Anat. 1933;67(Pt 4):491.
2. Abbie AA. The clinical significance of the anterior choroidal artery. Brain. 1933;56(3):233–46.
3. Adamkiewicz A. Die Blutgefäße des menschlichen Rückenmarks:DieGefäßederRückenmarksoberfläche. Sitzungsberichte der Akademie der Wissenschaften in Wein—Mathematisch-Naturwissenschaftliche Klasse—Abteilung 3. 1889;84:101–30.
4. Aitken HF. A report on the circulation of the lobar ganglia [Internet]. Fort Hill Press; 1909. Disponibile su: https://books.google.it/books?id=XxwTAAAAYAAJ.
5. Alexander L. The vascular supply of the stiopallidum. Res Publ Ass Res Nerv Ment Dis. 1942;21:77–132.
6. Bradac GB. Applied cerebral angiography. Normal anatomy and vascular pathology. Cham: Springer; 2017. https://doi.org/10.1007/978-3-319-57228-4. 497 pages, ISBN 978-3-319-57227-7.
7. Congdon ED. Transformation of the aortic-arch system during the development of the human embryo. Embryol Carneg Instn. 1922;14:47–110. Contributions to embryology.
8. De Vriese B. Sur la signification morphologique des artères. Arch biol (Liege). 1905;21:357.
9. Di Chiro G, Harrington T, Fried LC. Microangiography of human fetal spinal cord. Am J Roentgenol. 1973;118(1):193–9.
10. Djindjian R. L'angiographie de la moelle épinière. Paris: Angiography of the spinal cold, Masson et Cie; 1970.
11. Evans HM. On the development of the aortae, cardinal and umbilical veins, and the other blood vessels of vertebrate embryos from capillaries. Anat Rec. 1909;3(9):498–518.
12. Heubner A. Zur Topographie der Ernahrungsgebiete der einzelnen Hirnarterien. Zbl Med Wiss. 1872;52:817–21.
13. Kadyi H. Huber die blutgefaesse des menschlichen Rueckenmarks. Gubrynowicz & Schmidt. Lemberg, 1889. https://openlibrary.org/books/OL45630120M/%C3%9Cber_die_Blutgef%C3%A4sse_des_menschlichen_R%C3%BCckenmarkes.
14. Kier EL. Development of cerebral vessels. Radiology of the skull and brain. St Louis: Mosby; 1974. p. 1089–130.
15. Lasjaunias P, Berenstein A. Surgical neuroangiography. Vol 3: Functional anatomy of brain, spinal cord and spine. Berlin: Springer; 1990.
16. Lazorthes G. Vascularisation et circulation cérèbrale. Masson. Paris; 1961.
17. Lazorthes G, Gouazé A, Santini JJ, Lazorthes Y, Laffont J. Le modelage du polygone de Willis: rôle des compressions des vois arterielles d'apport dans les mouvements de la colonne cervicale et de l'extremité cephalique. Neuro-Chirurgie. 1971;17:361.
18. Lazorthes G, Gouazé A, Djindjian R. Vascularisation et circulation de la moelle épinière: anatomie, physiologie, pathologie, angiographie. Paris: Masson; 1973.
19. Mall FP. On the development of the blood-vessels of the brain in the human embryo. Am J Anat. 1905;4(1):1–18.
20. Moffat DB. Developmental changes in the aortic arch system of the rat. Am J Anat. 1959;105:1–35.
21. Moffat DB. The embryology of the arteries of the brain: Arris and Gale lecture delivered at the Royal College of Surgeons of England on 27th February 1962. Ann R Coll Surg Engl. 1962;30(6):368.
22. Okahara M, Kiyosue H, Mori H, Tanoue S, Sainou M, Nagatomi H. Anatomic variations of the cerebral arteries and their embryology: a pictorial review. Eur Radiol. 2002;12(10):2548–61.
23. Padget DH. The development of the cranial arteries in the human embryo. Carnegie Institution of Washington, Washington, DC; 1948. Contributions to embryology

24. Padget DH. Designation of the embryonic intersegmental arteries in reference to the vertebral artery and subclavian stem. Anat Rec. 1954;119(3):349–56.
25. Sabin FR. Origin and development of the primitive vessels of the chick and of the pig. Contrib Embryol. 1917;6:61–124.
26. Schmeidel G. Die entwicklung der arteria vertebralis des menschen. Gegenbaur Morph Jahrbuch. 1932;71:315–435.
27. Seydel HG. The diameters of the cerebral arteries of the human fetus. Anat Rec. 1964;150(1):79–88.
28. Shellshear JL. The basal arteries of the forebrain and their functional significance. J Anat. 1920;55(Pt 1):27–35.
29. Shellshear JL. The arteries of the brain of the Orang-utan. J Anat. 1927;61(Pt 2):167–97.
30. Sterzi G. Die Blutgefässe des Rückenmarks: Untersuchungen über ihre vergleichende Anatomie und Entwickelungsgeschichte, vol. 24. Bergmann; 1904.
31. Streeter GL. The developmental alterations in the vascular system of the brain of the human embryo. Contrib Embryol Carneg Inst. 1918;8:5–38.
32. Takakuwa T, Koike T, Muranaka T, Uwabe C, Yamada S. Formation of the circle of Willis during human embryonic development. Congenit Anom (Kyoto). 2016;56(5):233–6.
33. Tandler J. Zur entwicklungsgeschichte der kopfarterien bei den mammalian. Morphol Jahrb. 1902;30:275–373.
34. Thron AK. Vascular anatomy of the spinal cord: neuroradiological investigations and clinical syndromes. Berlin: Springer; 1988.
35. Thron A, Stoeter P, Schiessl J, Prescher A. Development of the arterial supply of the spinal cord tissue based on radioanatomical and histological studies in cattle. Clin Neuroradiology. 2022;32(2):325–43.
36. Torr JBD. The embryological development of the anterior spinal artery in man. J Anat. 1957;91:587.
37. Van Overbeeke JJ, Hillen B, Tulleken CA. A comparative study of the circle of Willis in fetal and adult life. The configuration of the posterior bifurcation of the posterior communicating artery. J Anat. 1991;176:45.
38. Watts JW. A comparative study of the anterior cerebral artery and the circle of Willis in primates. J Anat. 1934;68(Pt 4):534.

3 Further Evolution of Aortic Arches and Cerebral Vessels to the Adult Configuration

At the end of the embryonic phase, at the embryo of 40–44 mm aged of 50–56 days, the essential configuration of the Aortic arches and their derivative as well as of the cerebral vessels recognizable in the adult is present. The development, however, is far as to be completed. It still continues up to the birth in the Phase called the "Fetal Phase."

The changes involving the aortic arches and their derivative are minimal. They have already almost reached their final configuration at the end of the embryonic phase. Greater are those of the cerebral arteries, which continuously adapt to the many changes and growth of the brain, acquiring progressively the configuration typical in the Adult. This concerns their final course and progressively also the morphologic-histologic structure of their wall, which has a particular structure. It is composed of four layers: the adventitia, the media, internal elastic laminas, and intima. There is not external elastic lamina and the wall is thin.

Taken into consideration now the changes of the vessels described in the embryogenetic phase and those wich will presented in the final phase, it is clear that the evolution leading to the final configuration is not a simple and continuous, but a very complex process, occurring in several and separate phases. Therefore, is not surprising that some deviation, during the evolution can occur, leading to variations. These are probably favourized in the passage of transformation of two different configurations.

As it will be further described, some of these are so frequent, so that they are considered as "Normal Variations." In other rarer cases, the pattern of the vessels differs so greatly from the common typical configuration, so that it is considered as a real "Variation." In most of the cases, the variations are incidental discovery, but they can have clinical consequences when associated to pathological conditions.

The cause of these variations is not completely clear. In some cases, the type of the anomaly can indirectly indicate in which phase of the evolution the deviation has developed and which kind of deviated process can have been involved. In other cases, the phylogenetic study comparing the development of cerebral vessels in vertebrates including the humans, has shown similarities in the evolution between groups of animals and humans. In animals, these are typical common patterns, while in humans these are temporary, disappearing in the further evolution, but sometimes they can persist reproducing pattern typical in some group of animals.

G. B. Bradac, *Origin and Development of Cerebral Vessels*,
https://doi.org/10.1007/978-3-031-78436-1_3

3.1 Aortic Arches

As described in Chap. 2, the Aortic Arches and their derivatives undergo great changes which began at the embryo of 18–20 mm, following then they progressively have acquired a configuration which at the end of the embryogenic phase can basically be compared with that of the adult. In Fig. 3.1, the typical pattern of the aortic arch and its branches is shown.

During the evolution some anomalies can develop. Some of these have already been identified on autoptic studies by some authors [10, 116, 146]. Progressively reports about anomalies [7, 9] on the base of anatomic and radiographic studies have appeared in 43 years. A more detailed survey has been reported by Haughton and Rosenbaum [45] on angiographic studies. More recent examinations performed on conventional angiography [103] and on CT-angiography [99] have revealed the presence of anomalies in a rate of 17% and 13% respectively.

In accordance to these studies as well as to our experience, the most frequent anomaly is the origin of the left common carotid artery from the innominate trunk or close to it, called the "Bovin Trunk" (Fig. 3.2) since it resembles the typical aortic arch of cattle. This is followed by the "Bicarotid Trunk" in which the left and right common carotid arteries arise as avian common trunk.

The third frequent anomaly is the aberrant origin of the vertebral artery appearing commonly on the left (Fig. 3.3) with a frequency of 6%, described in many anatomic and angio-

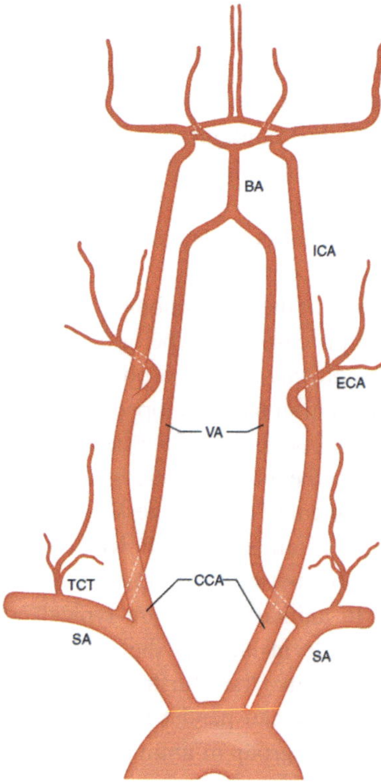

Fig. 3.1 Diagram showing the typical configuration of the aortic arch with its derivatives. Common Carotid Artery (CCA); Vertebral Artery (VA), Subclavian Artery (SA), Internal Carotid Artery (ICA), External Carotid Artery (ECA), Basilar Artery (BA), and Tyreo-Cervical Trunk (TCT). (Taken from Bradac [15])

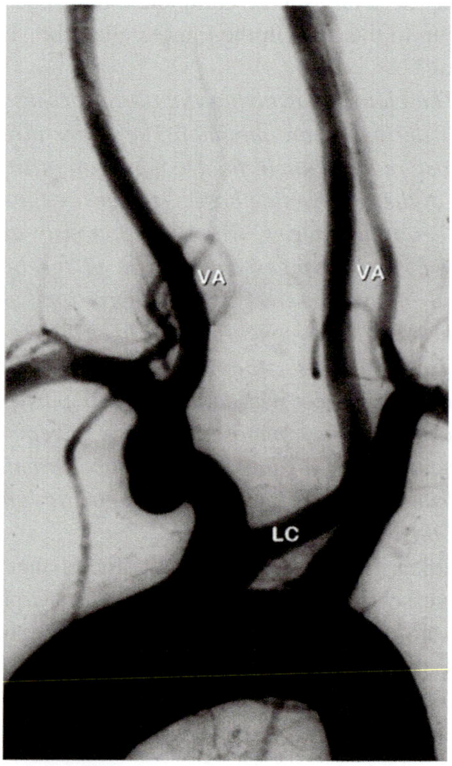

Fig. 3.2 Aortic arch angiogram. Origin of the Left Common Carotid Artery (LC) from the Innominate Trunk. (Taken from Bradac [15])

graphic studies [3, 14, 45, 104, 149]. The artery can arise from the aortic arch between the left common carotid artery and the left subclavian artery. In this condition, the artery enters the *foramen transversarium* at the fourth-fifth cervical vertebrae. The anomaly has been interpreted as due to the origin of the Vertebral artery from the fifth intersegmental artery instead of the sixth. The anomalous VA can also arise from the distal subclavian artery. In this case, the VA has taken its origin from the seventh intersegmental artery, entering the seventh foramen transversarium. Both the anomalous branch and the normal VA can be present giving the pattern of a duplicated VA (see in this chapter, section VA).

Other extremely rare conditions involving the VA, are the origin of the right VA from aortic arch distal to the left subclavian or proximal to it [45, 52, 53, 71, 77, 116, 134] and the origin of the VA from the common carotid artery commonly on the right [23, 45, 104, 116]. These conditions can appear alone or be associated with other anomalies.

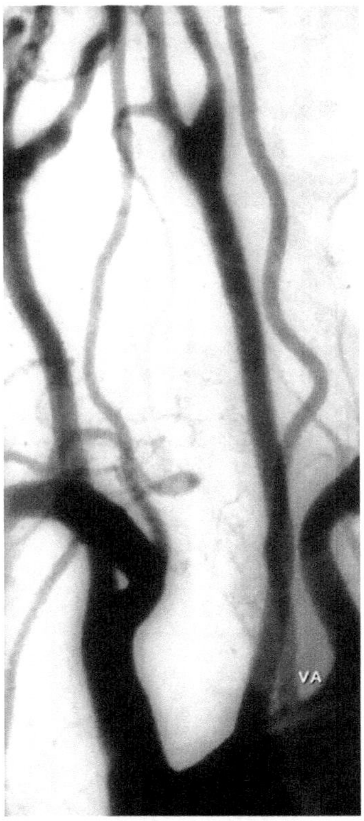

Fig. 3.3 Aortic arch angiogram. Anomalous origin of the left Vertebral Artery (VA) from aortic arch. (Taken from Bradac [15])

A rare, but a well-known anomaly reported with a frequency of 0.2–1.7% is the origin of the right subclavian artery distally to the left subclavian artery. The first case has been described by Bayford [10], who called it "Dysphagia Lusoria," term which is still used today. Many studies followed [14, 58, 59, 74, 75]. It is now considered as a persistence of the right distal dorsal aorta (see also Chap. 2), which in this case fuses together with the left dorsal aorta. From this fusion develops the anomalous right subclavian artery which runs left to right behind the esophagus. The proximal part of the right dorsal aorta does not develop resulting in the absence of the innominate trunk. The right VA has commonly a normal course (Fig. 3.4a, b). Frequent is the presence of other anomalies.

In 1936, Kommerell [59] described at the origin of the anomalous right subclavian a dilatation of the aorta, he called "Diverticulum" which is now known as "Kommerell Diverticulum." Later it has been shown that the diverticulum is not specific of the anomaly, but can be present in other anomalies especially in the right aortic arch.

There are other anomalies which, due to their rarity, are seldom reported. It can also occur that they can escape to the routine daily work performed to study other cerebral pathologies (Figs. 3.5 and 3.6).

Another rare anomaly is the right aortic arch. In this condition, which reproduces in the human a normal configuration typical in the birds, instead of the left fourth aortic arch is the right fourth arch which persists. The pattern is called "Mirror Imaging" of the normal aortic arch. In this anomaly, the origin of all the trunks is inverted, then the innominate trunk arise on the left, dividing in the left CCA and left Subclavian Artery and further, on the right, arise separately the right CCA and right Subclavian Artery. Further on the right arises separately the right CCA and the subclavian artery. The anomaly is frequently asymptomatic being an incidental dis-

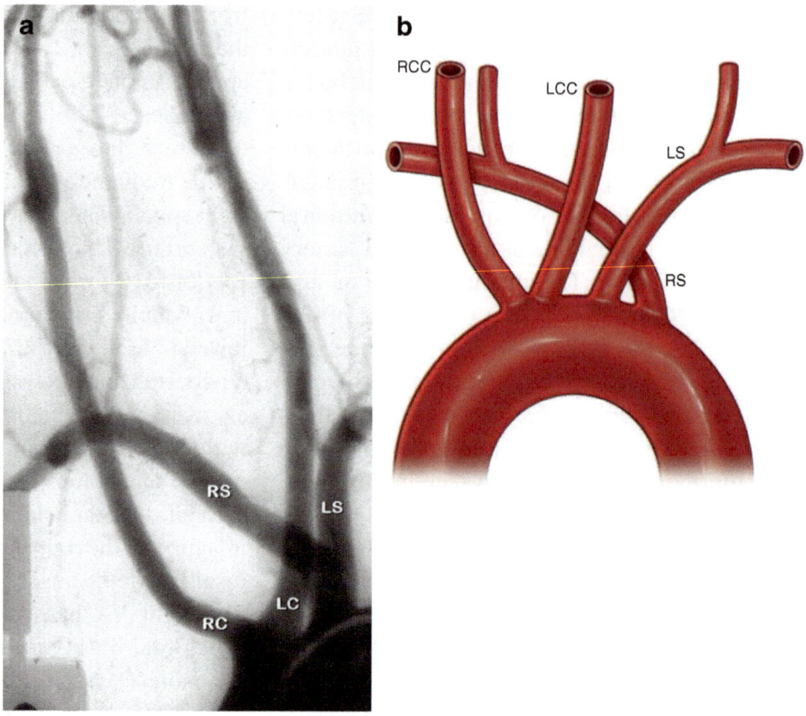

Fig. 3.4 Aortic arch angiogram and diagram. The Right Subclavian Artery (RS) arises distal to the Left Subclavian Artery (LS). There is a common origin of the Left and Right Common Carotid Arteries (LCC, RCC). (Taken from Bradac [15])

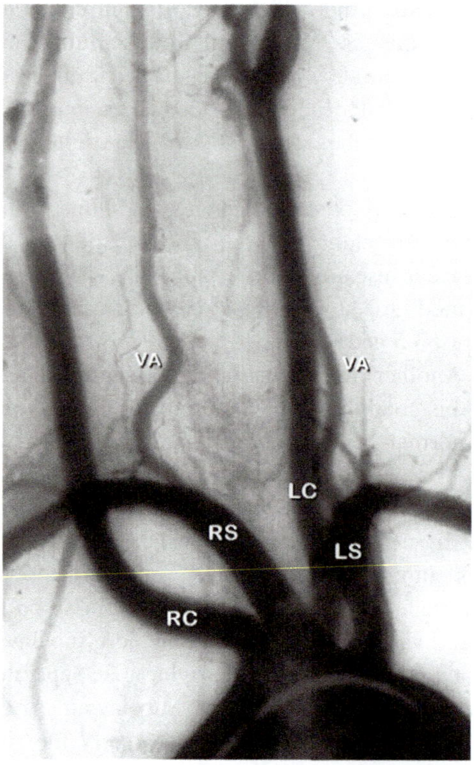

Fig. 3.5 The innominate trunk is not formed. Common origin of the Common Carotid and Right Subclavian Artery. (Taken from Bradac [15])

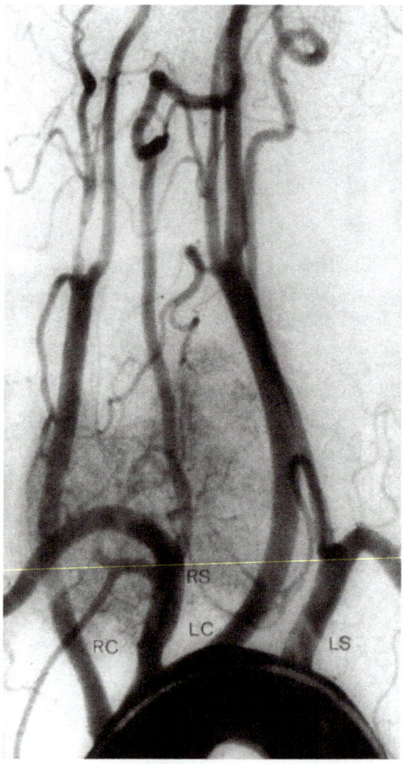

Fig. 3.6 Configuration similar to that of Fig. 3.5. The Right Common Carotid Artery (RC) has a proximal origin from aortic arch. Innominate trunk is not formed. (Taken from Bradac [15])

covery. It can be associated, however, with congenital heart diseases and other anomalies of the brachiocephalic vessels [45, 58, 133].

An extremely rare anomaly is the double arch [45, 58] which develops following the persistence of both the left and right fourth aortic arches.

3.2 Internal Carotid Artery (ICA)

ICA appears at the embryo of 4–5 mm arising from the third aortic arch. The artery runs cranially dividing at the base of the brain in the cranial and caudal division from which arise the main trunks for the brain. As described in detail in Chap. 2, the ICA undergoes many changes at the embryo of around 18 mm following that of the third aortic arch. From its distal part arises the ICA and from its proximal part develops the Common Carotid (CCA) annexing the External Carotid Artery (ECA). The complex CCA and ECA migrates cranially to join the ICA forming the Carotid Bifurcation (CB). Deviations in this evolution can explain anomalies involving the CB and origin of the ICA and ECA.

As far as it concerns the CB, it is commonly located at the level of the fourth cervical vertebra. Higher bifurcations at the C1–C2 as well as lower locations at C6–C7 have been reported in anatomic and angiographic studies [3, 74]. Also thoracic bifurcation can occur. The first reported case is that of Morgagni [94] in an autoptic case of a 50-year-old woman. Another case has been described by Von Kantor [51] in an autoptic study in an adult man. More recent cases have been reported by Lie [74] and Vitek and Reaves [152].

The cervical segment of ICA can maintain its rectilinear course or can develop tortuosity frequently in young children, disappearing later and appearing again in older atherosclerotic patients. The artery is accompanied by the Internal Jugular Vein, located postero-laterally, and portion of the cranial nerves IX, X, XI, and XII. It is surrounded by the sympathetic plexus. The ECA, first medially located, runs more cranially laterally. Near the skull base [44] the artery runs in the so-called Carotid Space surrounded by the parotid space laterally, the para-pharyngeal space, and the retro-pharyngeal space anteriorly and medially and the peri-vertebral space postero-medially (Fig. 3.7).

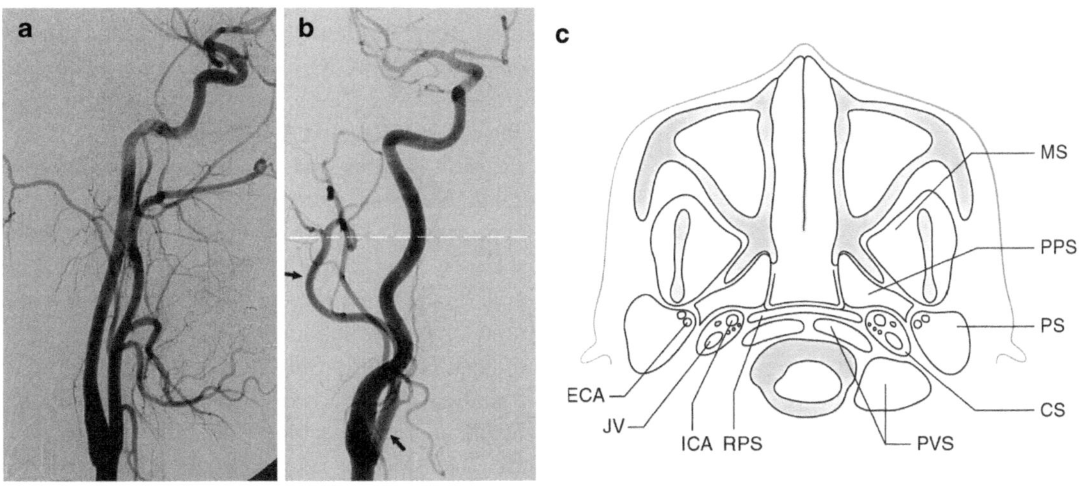

Fig. 3.7 Common carotid angiogram, showing the course of the internal and external carotid arteries. (**a**) AP view (**b**) Lateral view. The course of the ECA (arrows) first medial then lateral to ICA is shown. (**c**) Diagram showing the configuration of ICA running at the skull base in the Carotid Space accompanied by the dorsally located Internal Jugular Vein and by the IX, X, XI, XII cranial nerves. Parotid Space (PS) with ECA and Retromandibular vein. Para-Pharyngeal Space (PPS). Retro-Pharyngeal Space (RPS). Peri-Vertebral Space (PVS). Masticator Space (MS). (Taken from Bradac [15])

The ICA enters the skull base at the carotid foramen anteriorly to the jugular fossa and jugular vein. It runs then with a tortuous course with a few curves, through the skull base to reach the intracranial cavity (Figs. 3.8 and 3.9). *These curves probably have a protective function allowing the ICA to accommodate more easily to the movements of the head.*

The artery has first a vertically course in the petrous bone (Petrous Segment), then curves medially running horizontally being anterior to the cochlea. It emerges at the petrous apex running with a slight vertical short course above the Foramen Lacerum, entering then the cavernous space—formed by a division of the dura in two layers: the lateral separating the space from the middle crania fossa, the medial separating from Sella Turcica and Pituitary Gland. This segment if ICA is Called the Cavernous segment.

In this space, called "*space of the cavernous sinus*" [142], the ICA is directed first upwards, then curves anteriorly having a short horizontal course, making second curves directed posteriorly running medially to the anterior clinoid process. The Artery perforates the dura passing through a dural ring entering the subarachnoid space, continuing in the so-called Supraclinoid segment divided considering the arteries involved in:

- The ophthalmic segment is the one which arises from the ophthalmic artery. Other branches are those supplying the optic nerve and chiasm and those forming the Superior Hypophyseal arteries. These latter run on the surface of the pituitary stalk forming a capillary network connected with venules (Venous portal system) bringing the blood from Hypoyhalamus to the adenohypophysys.
- The PcomA arises from the communicating segment when it is present.
- The Choroidal segment gives off the Anterior Choroidal artery.

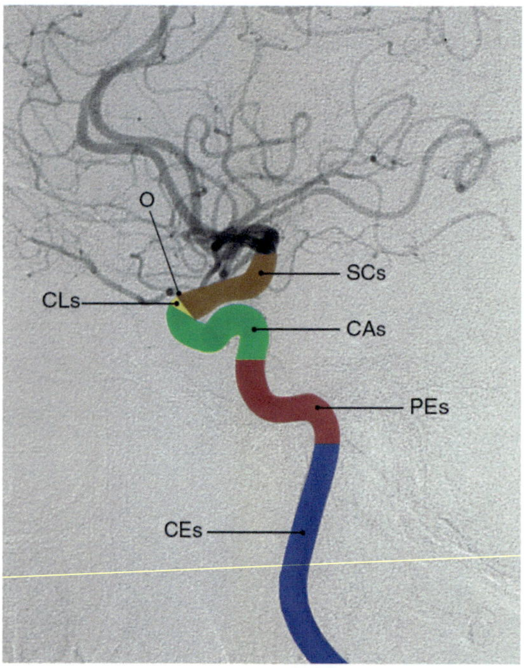

Fig. 3.8 Lateral carotid angiogram, showing the various segments of ICA. Cervical Segment (CES), Petrous segment (PES), Cavernous Segment (CAS), Clinoid Segment (CLS), Ophthalmic Segment (O), Supraclinoid Segment (SCS). (Taken from Bradac [15])

At the level of the anterior perforated substance, the ICA is divided in the Anterior and Middle cerebral arteries.

Along its petrous and cavernous course, the ICA is surrounded by the sympathetic fibers and the venous plexus. The latter will be described in more detail in Chap. 9. At the level of the cavernous sinus, the ICA has a close relationship with cranial nerves III, IV, and VI and with the first and second branch of the trigeminal nerve.

From petrous and cavernous segments arise small branches remnants of primordial arteries appearing in the embryo phase. From the petrous segment, occasionally identified in the adult angiogram, there are the Carotido-tympanic and more cranially the Mandibular Arteries, remnants of the Hyoid-Stapedial and Primordial Mandibular Arteries. From the Cavernous Segment, recognizable on the adult angiogram, are the Inferior lateral trunk (ILT) and the Meningo-Hypophyseal trunk (MHT) remnant of the Primary Maxillary Artery (see Chap. 5). *The appearing, development, and clinical significance of these branches have been described more in detail in Chaps. 2 and 5.*

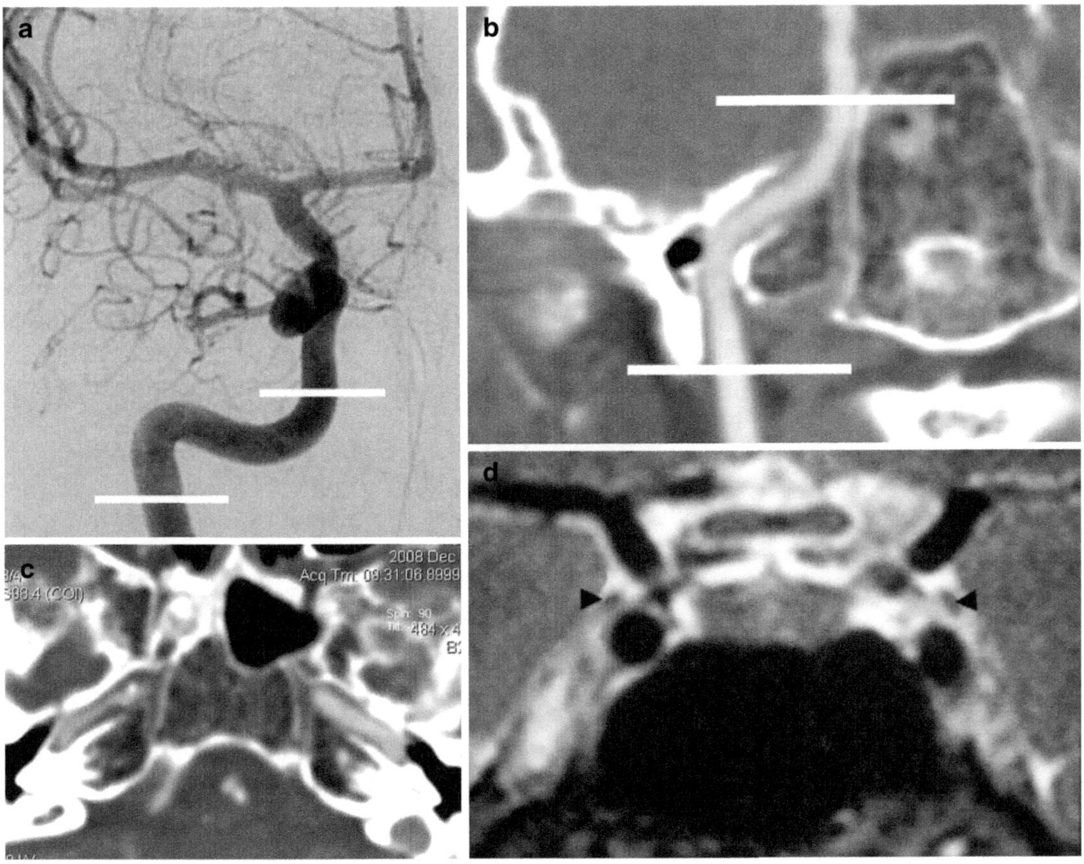

Fig. 3.9 (**a**) Carotid angiogram, AP view. (**b**) CT angiography showing the course of the petrous and partial of the cavernous segments of ICA. (**c**) CT angiography showing the horizontal part of the Petrous Segment of ICA running above the Foramen Lacerum. (**d**) MR image, coronal view: sellar and para-sellar area demonstrating the course of the ICA in the Cavernous Sinus. Third Cranial nerve (Arrowhead). (Taken from Bradac [15])

3.3 Anomalies of Internal Carotid Artery (ICA)

3.3.1 Aplasia of ICA

As described in Chap. 2, the ICA develops from third aortic arch. It runs cranially connecting with the plexus on the base of the embryo becoming the essential vessel for the supply of the brain in this phase. Why the artery regresses is not clear. It is conceivable, however, that the regression occurs in a phase in which cerebral vessels appear, allowing through the formation of collateral way to compensate the regression.

This anomaly has been described first by Tode [147]. Verbiest [151] and Lie [74] reported angiographic studies. It can be unilateral or bilateral and is commonly an incidental discovery. It appears frequently with other pathologies such as Phaces and Neurofibromatosis. It is associated with various type of collateral circulation. The most frequent is through the Circle of Willis, whose development begins at the embryo of 20–24 mm and it is certainly complete at the end of the embryonic phase at the embryo of 40–44 mm. Another important collateral circulation is that through the complex ophthalmic-external carotid arteries (Chaps. 6 and 7).

A particular form of collateral circulation is that through the Persistent Primary Maxillary Artery, identified in the adult in many angiographic studies [33, 39, 41, 57, 63, 74, 85, 131] (see also Chap. 5). In this condition, from the cavernous portion of ICA develops a large branch running on the floor of the sella, anastomosing with the contralateral ICA. This anomaly should be taken into consideration in patients in whom a trans-sphenoidal surgery for intra-sellar adenoma is planned (Fig. 3.10).

3.3.2 Segmental Aplasia of ICA

This anomaly can involve the extra-intracranial segment of ICA. To compensate this condition, vascular structures develop, with particular configuration.

3.3.2.1 Rete Mirabile

In this condition, the ICA can be normal in its cervical segment, the aplasia involves his distal

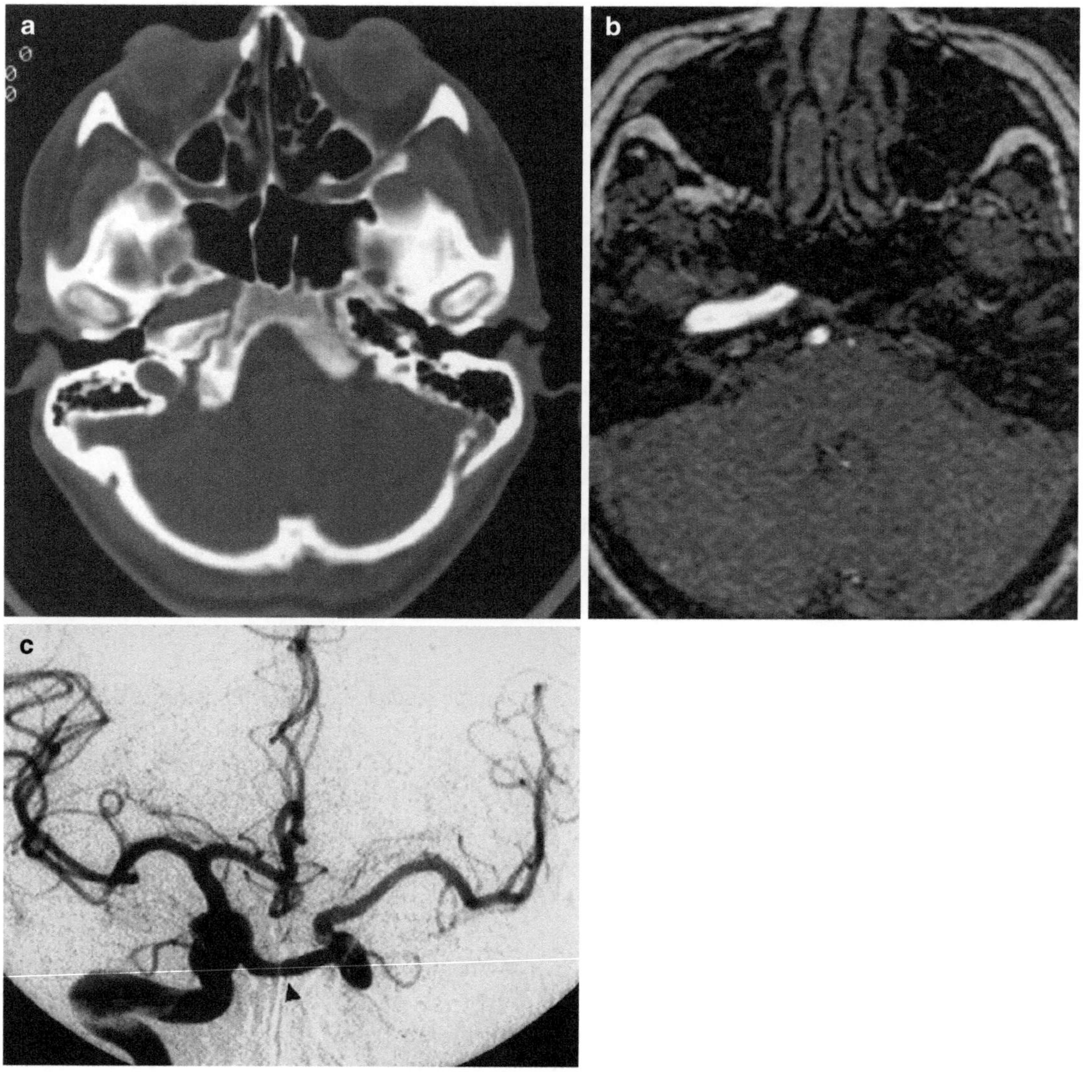

Fig. 3.10 Aplasia of ICA. (**a**) CT showing that the canal of the horizontal portion of the petrous segment of ICA on the left is absent. (**b**) MRI: there is no typical flow signal on the left. (**c**) Right carotid angiogram. AP view. There is filling of the cavernous portion of the left ICA through intra-sellar anastomosis (arrowhead). (Taken from Bradac [15])

petrous segment. In other cases, the ipo-aplasia extends from the cervical part up to the petrous segment. The reconstruction of the distal ICA occurs at the level of the distal petrous segment or at the level of the proximal cavernous sinus, through formation of a network involving branches of ECA (the internal maxillary artery and especially the AphA). The IMA is connected through its distal branches with branches remnant of the Primary Maxillary Artery (future ILT). The AphA can be involved with its tympanic branch, connected with the carotid tympanic branch of the petrous ICA, remnant of the Hyoid artery. Other connections can develop between the AphA and the MHT and ILT, through the Clival branches and the carotid ramus, respectively (see also Chap. 7).

Rete mirabile has been exceptionally demonstrated in the adult on the angiogram first by Minagi and Newton [89]. Later by Lie [74], Danziger [22], Mahadevan et al. [79]. It has been reported associated with similar pattern involving the vertebro-basilar sector [47, 79] and with other anomalies of the origin of the Carotid and Vertebral arteries from aortic arch [67]. A case associated with *Pseudoxhantoma Elasticum* has been also described [26]. An example is presented in Fig. 3.11.

It is interesting to mention that Rete Mirabile reproduces in the adult man the typical pattern present is some mammals (Cat, Pig, Goat, Sheep, Giraffe …) as described by some authors [4, 21, 29, 30] (see also Chap. 7).

3.3.2.2 Non Bifurcation Cervical Carotid Artery

Another form of segmental aplasia is that described and called by some authors [95, 102] "*Non Bifurcating Cervical Carotid Artery*" diagnosed on an adult angiogram. This study has been followed by other reports.

In this condition the proximal ICA is not present probably regressed. The Common carotid artery continues directly in the External carotid

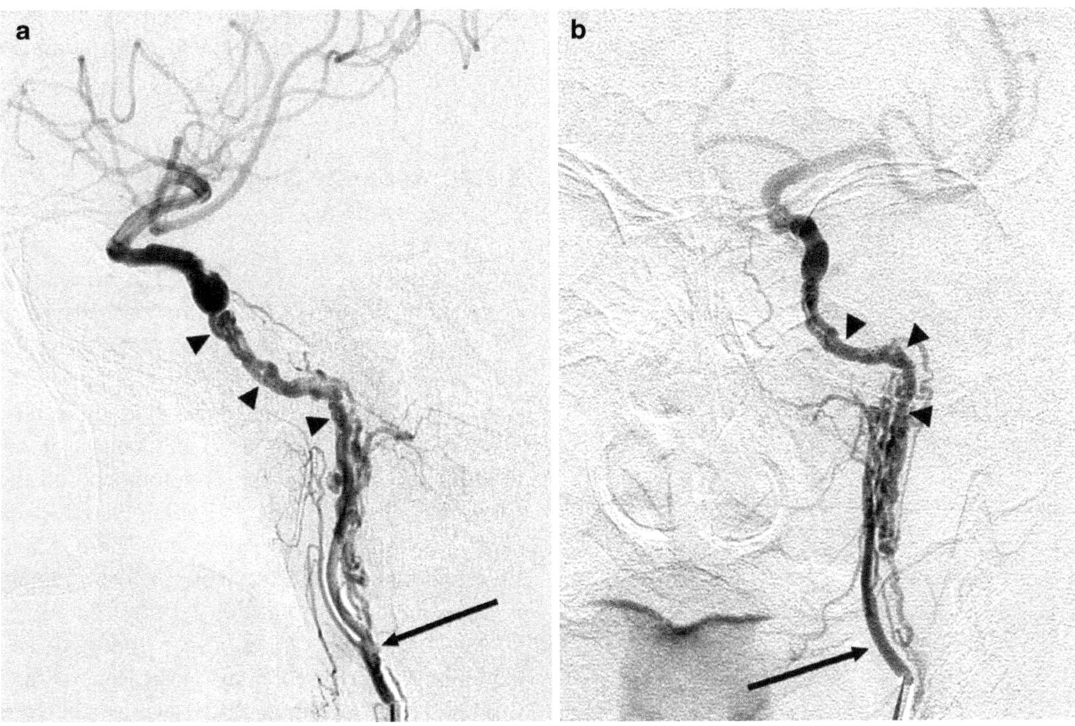

Fig. 3.11 Segmental aplasia of ICA in example of *rete mirabile*, involving its Cervical Segment and its proximal Petrous Segment (arrowhead). Reconstruction through branches of the AphA (arrow). (**a**) Angiogram in lateral view. (**b**) Angiogram in AP view. (Taken from Bradac [15])

artery which having given off its branches continues in the distal ICA which has distally a normal course. This is shown in the Diagram (Fig. 3.12).

Many hypotheses have been proposed to explain this anomaly. For this purpose, it is useful to consider the evolution of the third aortic arch and from it depends the development of the complex common carotid and external carotid arteries which migrate cranially to join the already developed ICA as it is described in the early phase of the embryogenesis in Chap. 2. Anomalous evolution in this phase especially the regression of the ICA could explain the anomaly.

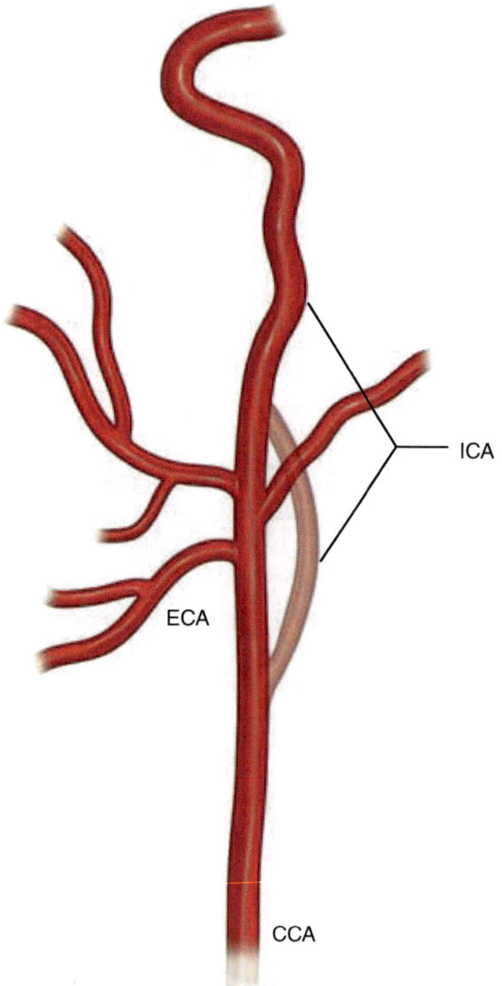

Fig. 3.12 Diagram showing an example of the so-called Non-bifurcating Cervical Carotid Artery. Common Carotid Artery (CCA), External Carotid Artery (ECA). ICA: distal segment normal, aplasia of the proximal segment

3.3.3 Aberrant Course of ICA

Another form of anomaly is also the consequence of partial agenesis of the cervical ICA. In this condition, the artery is located more posteriorly than in normal cases laterally to the jugular bulb. It enters the temporal bone through an enlarged inferior tympanic canaliculus. The vertical segment of the petrous ICA where it continues with its horizontal segment protrudes in the middle ear cavity.

This anomaly has been interpreted as an agenesis of the terminal part of the cervical ICA [44, 63, 78], with its recanalization formed by connection between the enlarged tympanic branch of the AphA and the Carotid-Tympanic branch of the petrous segment of ICA, remnant of the Hyoid-Stapedial artery.

It can be an important diagnosis in cases of suspect small tympanic para-ganglioma and generally in the presurgical diagnosis of the temporal bone, example in Fig. 3.13.

3.3.4 Separate Origin of ICA and ECA

In this condition, the ICA and ECA arise separately from the aortic arch if the anomaly is on the left. The vessels arise separately from the Innominate Trunk if the anomaly develops on the right. It has been interpreted as due to the persistence of *Ductus Caroticus*. The changes of the third aortic arch and the development of the Common Carotid Artery, which have been described in Chap. 2 do not occur. The ICA and ECA maintain their separate origin. The anomaly is shown in the diagram (Fig. 3.14a).

Angiographic studies are reported by Haughton and Rosenbaum [45], Roberts and Gerald [119], Dahn et al. [20].

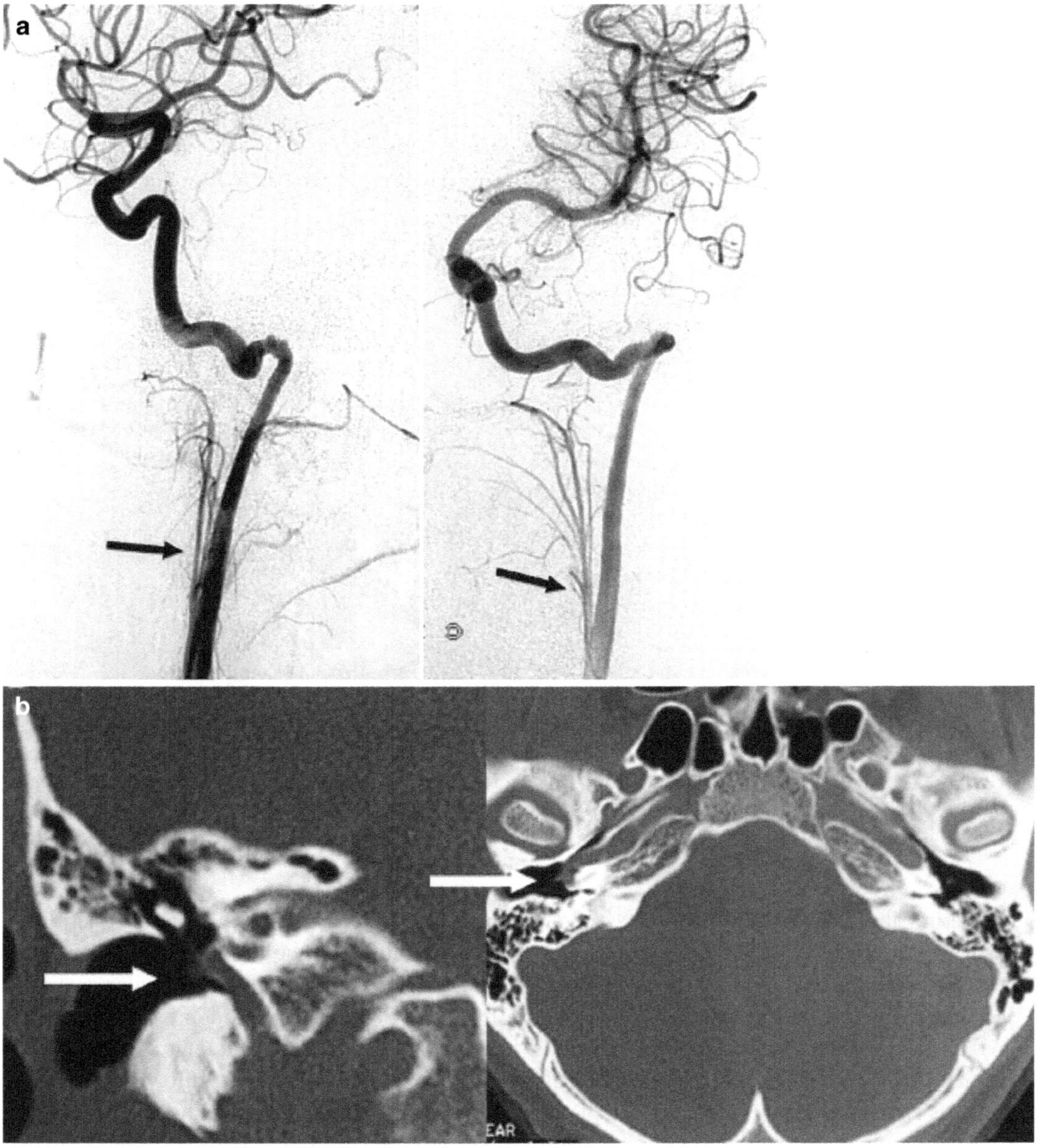

Fig. 3.13 Example of partial agenesis of ICA presenting with an anomalous course of the artery. (**a**) Angiogram in lateral and AP view: the artery is located more dorsally and laterally. Origin of AphA (arrow) from the ICA. (**b**) CT: the artery protrudes in the tympanic cavity (arrow). (Taken from Bradac [15])

3.3.5 Duplication of the Internal Carotid Artery (ICA)

This is a very rare anomaly reported in a few autoptic and angiographic studies [56, 60].

In this condition, in addition to the normal ICA, there is a second, commonly small vessel, running parallel to it. It takes its origin at the carotid bifurcation from Common Carotid artery or from proximal segment of ICA, joining the normal ICA at the level of its petrous segment.

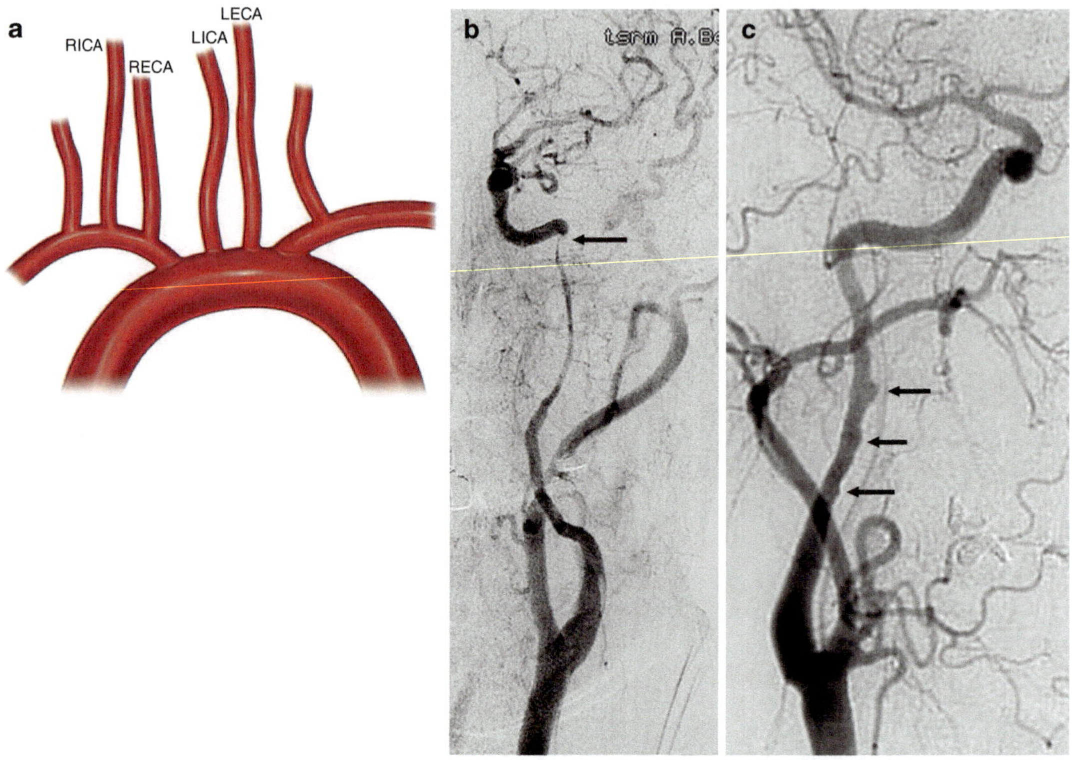

Fig. 3.14 (**a**) Diagram showing the separate origin of ICA and ECA, from the Aortic Arch on the left and from Innominate Trunk on the right. (**b**) ICA dissection. Severe stenosis which abruptly ends at the skull basis (arrow). (**c**) ICA dissection. Wall irregularity (arrows) with small aneurysmal dilatation. (Figs **b** and **c** taken from Bradac [15])

Considering the different origin of this second branch we prefer to use the definition of a "Complete duplication" (origin from CCA) or "Segmental duplication" (origin from proximal ICA). It is conceivable that the anomaly develops early in the evolution in a phase in which the ICA appears as a plexural structure. Part of the plexus can take an anomalous separate evolution leading to the formation of a second branch. This anomaly will be further described in this chapter involving other vascular territories. More about the definition of this anomaly is presented in the section "Vertebral artery."

3.3.6 Dissection

I think that it is useful to mention here, even shortly, this condition which is not an anomalous evolution indeed, it is real acquired pathology, involving not only the ICA and his branches, but also the vessel in the vertebro-basilar sector, as described further in the section.

It is a hemorrhagic pathologic process, affecting the wall of the artery, following trauma or occurring spontaneous, in patient with connective disease: fibromuscular dysplasia, Ehlers-Danlos syndrome, Marfan syndrome, alpha-glucosidase deficiency, polycystic kidney disease, osteogenesis imperfecta, and lupus erythematous. It can be present with small irregularity of the wall, stenosis extending for various length, double lumen with sometimes an aneurysmatic dilatation or occlusion.

Differently from anomalies linked to evolution, which are commonly an incidental discovery, the dissection is an acute syndrome, with clinical symptoms.

It has been first described by Jentzer [49]. This has been followed by many studies [6, 15, 16, 90, 92, 93, 117, 125, 126] who have progressively identified the dissection as a specific pathological entity (Fig. 3.14b, c).

3.4 Anterior Cerebral Artery (ACA)

At the end of the embryonic phase, the Aca has acquired the configuration which is basically similar to that of the adult. The A1 segment and the AcomA are formed. The perforators arising from these segments have already appeared (see also Chap. 2). The sub-callosal artery and the primordial peri-callosal arteries are already present, developed respectively from AcomA and each A1. Great changes involve the peri-callosal artery, relate to the growth of the cerebral hemispheres and especially to the formation of the Corpus Callosum (CC).

The CC begins to develop in the fetal phase at the embryo aged of 60–70 days [61, 158]. It is the most important and greater of the cerebral commissures. These are made up of the fibers which interconnect the cerebral hemispheres. The first appearing is the Anterior Commissure and the anterior part of CC at the level of the Genu. Whereas the Anterior Commissure is present in all vertebrates, the CC is typical in the Mammalian and reaches the best development in the humans. The CC grows rapidly extending dorsally forming the body running in the peri-callosal cistern continuing in the more dorsal segment called the splenium. Around the age of the fetus of 120–150 days, the formation of the CC can be considered as completed. This evolution has great influence on the peri-callosal artery which has been well shown by Kier [54, 55] in the study of injected fetus before and after the formation of the CC.

The peri-callosal artery which has a vertical, rectilinear, and relatively short course before the appearing of the CC, acquires its typical configuration following its development. The artery curves around the genu, runs around the body of CC ending with a curve around the Splenium (Fig. 3.15a, b). In cases of agenesis of corpus callosum, the artery maintains his primordial anomalous course. This condition is commonly asymptomatic, but can have clinical consequences if associated with other anomalies.

It is interesting to mention that in this phase from the distal peri-callosal artery develops small vessels described first by Bremer and later by Padget [109]. This is a branch directed to the choroid plexus at the level of the foramen of Monro. Following the evolution of the above described peri-callosal artery the small choroid branch commonly regresses. According to Padget, the disappearing of the artery is due to a hemodynamic unfavorable condition. The branch which has accompanied the distal peri-callosal artery is now constraint to reach the choroid plexus to make a long detour running around the splenium,

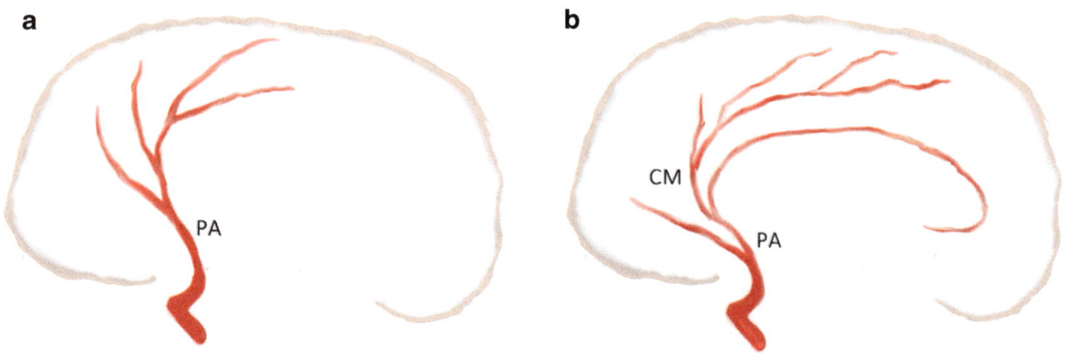

Fig. 3.15 Diagram showing the configuration of ACA, Peri-callosal (PA), and Calloso-Marginal (CM) arteries. (**a**) Before the appearing of the Corpus Callosum. (**b**) After the appearing of the Corpus Callosum

continuing on the floor of the third ventricle. Exceptionally, the artery can persist. It has been demonstrated in the advanced fetus by Kier [54, 55] and in the adult by a few authors [50, 115, 132]. This pattern has been reported by Shellshear [128] as a normal condition in the adult chimpanzee. It is typically involved in the Galen Vein Malformation (see Chap. 9).

From the peri-callosal artery (PA) develops the Calloso-Marginal Artery (CM, Fig. 3.16). This runs in the cingulate sulcus above the cingulate gyrus. PA and CM can be considered as the basic arteries from which arise all other distal branches, as it will be demonstrated further in the section.

At the end of the fetal phase, the ACA acquires the typical adult configuration which has been described in many anatomic-angiographic studies [76, 97, 115, 124].

The course of the ACA can be divided in a few segments. The first is the A1 arising from distal ICA at the level of the Anterior Perforate Substance (APS). It runs medially over the optic chiasma and nerve joining the contro-lateral A1 at the interhemispheric fissure through the AcomA.

From A1 arise perforators involved in the supply of the optic nerve, chiasma and supra-chiasmatic area. Other branches enter the Anterior Perforated Substance (APS), contributing to supply part of the Basal Ganglia together with the Heubner Artery. These branches are more abundant on the medial part of A1 and, as it is described in the Section MCA, can replace part of the perforator of M1. Another important branch, arising from the distal A1 sometimes from AcomA, is the Heubner Artery, already described in Chap. 2. The artery runs with rectilinear or undulating recurrent course, back to the APS, dividing distally frequently in several branches. It supplies the infero-medial part of head of nucleus caudatus; anterior limb of Internal Capsule and the anterior-inferior part of Pallidum and Putamen [28].

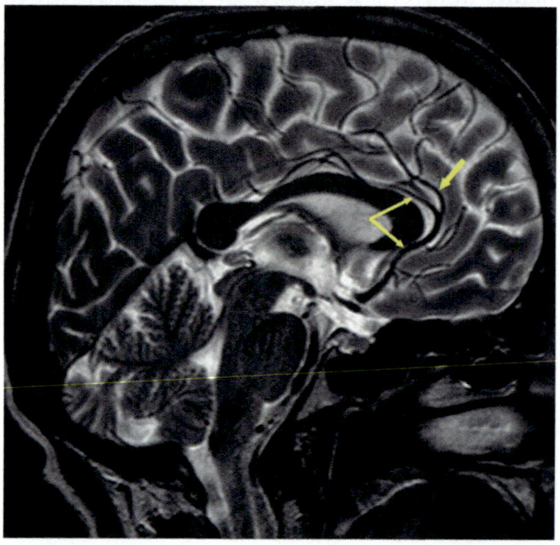

Fig. 3.16 MR showing the course of the Peri-callosal (arrow with angle) and Calloso-marginal (white arrow) Arteries

The final configuration of the ACA is shown in Fig. 3.17a–c.

As far as it concerns the distal cortical branches, these are better demonstrated on the lateral carotid angiogram (Fig. 3.18a, b).

In Fig. 3.19, the more frequent various origins of the branches are demonstrated. The first branch is the Orbito-frontal Artery (Infero-orbital Artery), arising commonly from PA as a single or common trunk with the Fronto-polar Artery. It supplies the inferior surface of the frontal lobe including the olfactory tract and the gyrus rectus. It anastomoses with the Orbito-frontal branch of MCA. The second branch is the Fronto-polar, arising from PA or CM. It supplies the inferior part of the superior frontal lobe. It can share a common trunk with the Heubner Artery.

Further branches are the frontal arteries, ascending vessels arising from PA or CM. They extend to and supply the internal surface of the superior frontal lobe. They are named frontal branches divided in anterior, middle, and posterior. They can appear as separate vessels or a common trunk dividing distally.

A further posterior ascending branch is the Para-central Artery arising from PA or CM, sometimes as a common trunk with the posterior frontal branch or the Superior and Inferior Parietal artery (SP, IP). It supplies the Paracentral lobe.

The last ascending branches of the ACA are the Superior and Inferior Internal Parietal arteries

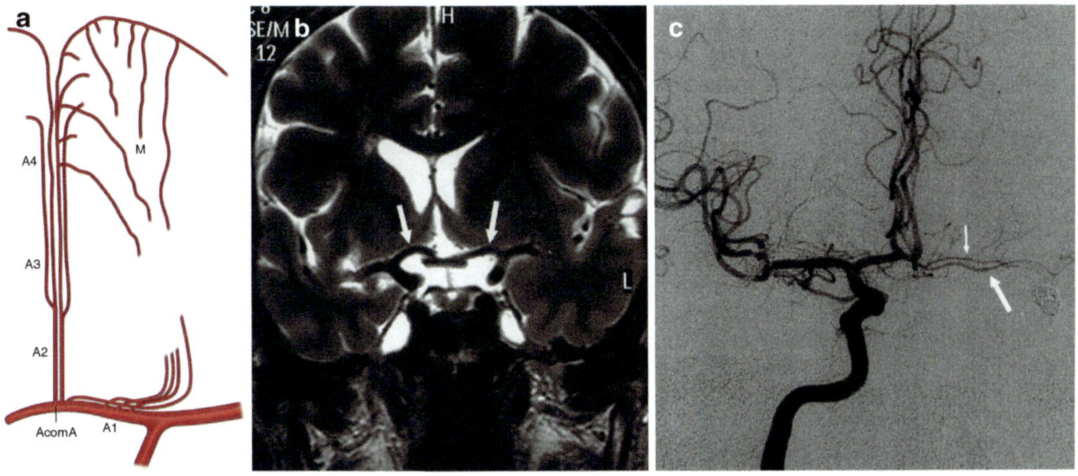

Fig. 3.17 (**a**) Diagram showing the A1, A2, A3, A4 segments of the ACA. Perforators of A1, with Heubner Artery. Anterior Communicating Artery (AcomA) from which arise the Peri-callosal Arteries. Medullary arteries (M). (**b**) MR showing the course of the A1 (arrow). (**c**) Carotid angiogram in a patient treated with coils for an MCA aneurysm. There is a well-developed right A1. Hypoplastic left A1 (arrow). Heubner Artery (small arrow). (Figs **b** and **c** taken from Bradac [15])

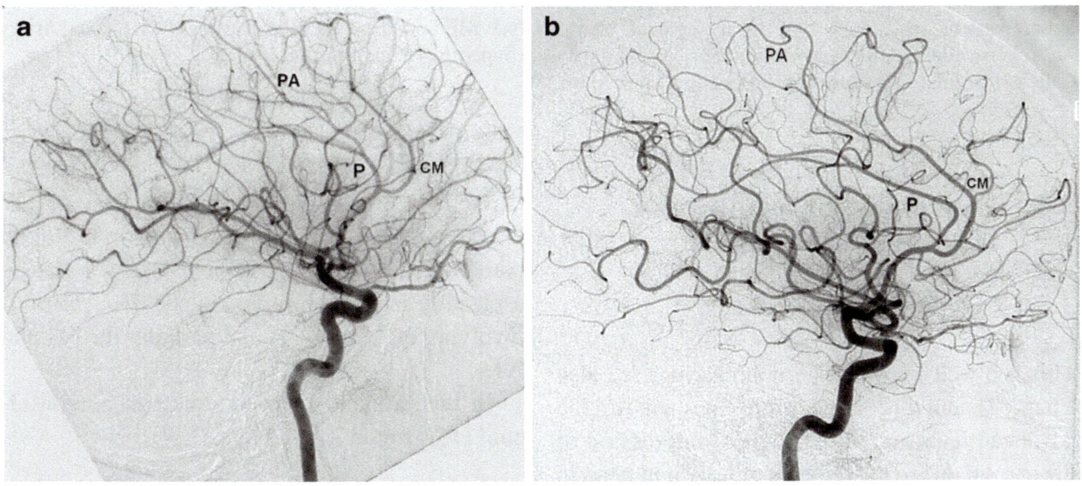

Fig. 3.18 Lateral carotid angiograms showing the course of the Peri-callosal (P) and Calloso-marginal (CM) arteries. Different origin of the Paracentral artery (PA). (**a**) From the Peri-callosal artery. (**b**) From the Calloso-marginal artery

arising commonly from the PA. The superior is the larger. It supplies the greater part of the precuneus, while the inferior is a small inferior portion of this lobe.

All ascending branches continue running on the lateral convexity for about 2–3 cm anastomosing with the ascending branches of the MCA.

The peri-callosal artery ends in the splenial artery anastomosing with the splenial branch of the PCA.

A meningeal branch can occasionally be present arising from the first segment of the peri-callosal artery. The artery runs cranially along the surface of the falx, anastomosing with descending meningeal branches of the middle meningeal artery. The artery is a typical pattern in the dog.

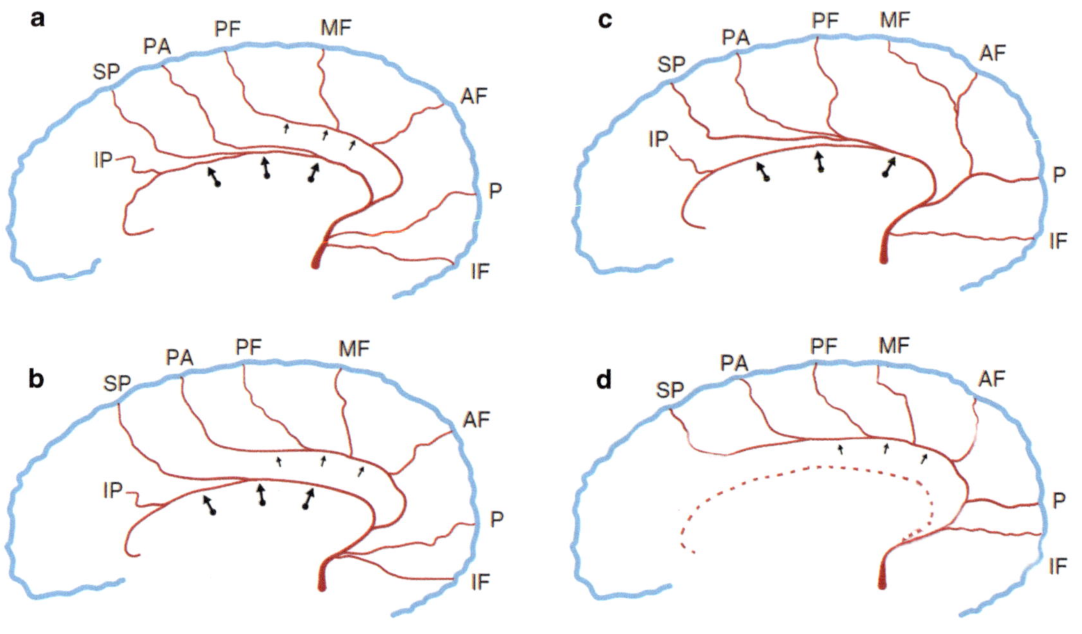

Fig. 3.19 Diagram (**a**–**d**) showing some examples of different patterns concerning the distal segment of the ACA. Peri-callosal Artery (arrow with dot) absent in (**d**). Calloso-marginal artery (arrow). Absent as a trunk in (**c**). Infero-Orbital (IF), Fronto-Polar (P), Frontal branches (AF, MF, and PF), Para-central artery (PA), Parietal Artery (Superior, SP and Inferior, IP)

3.5 Anomalies of the Anterior Cerebral Artery (ACA)

3.5.1 Hypo-Aplasia of A1

This is a well-known pattern appearing (see also Chap. 2) and becoming more frequent in the advanced fetus and in the adult. Compression of the carotid due to movements of neck and head in the adult has been proposed as the cause by some authors. The hypoplasia of A1 (diameter less than 1 mm) is reported in 10% and aplasia in 2% of the cases [114, 141].

Hypo-Aplasia of A1 is incidental discovery, without clinical consequences. It can, however, be unfavorable pattern, in pathological conditions, such as in cases of AcomA aneurysms (Fig. 3.20).

Furthermore, it should be taken into consideration, that the complex A1-AcomA is part of Circle of Willis and so an important way of collateral circulation. This can be very useful in pathological conditions such in case of stroke, especially in the condition called *"T-occlusion,"* involving the distal ICA and partially the M1 and A1.

In this context three patterns can be considered [15] (Fig. 3.21a–c).

- The distal ICA is occluded as well as the proximal M1 and proximal A1. The distal A1 is not involved and so it can be filled through the contralateral A1-AcomA. A collateral circulation towards M1 can develop. Some perforators, especially the Heubner's Artery are also spared (Fig. 3.21a).
- The proximal and the distal A1 are occluded. A collateral circulation from the contralateral A1-AcomA cannot develop. No collateral circulation towards M1 is possible. The

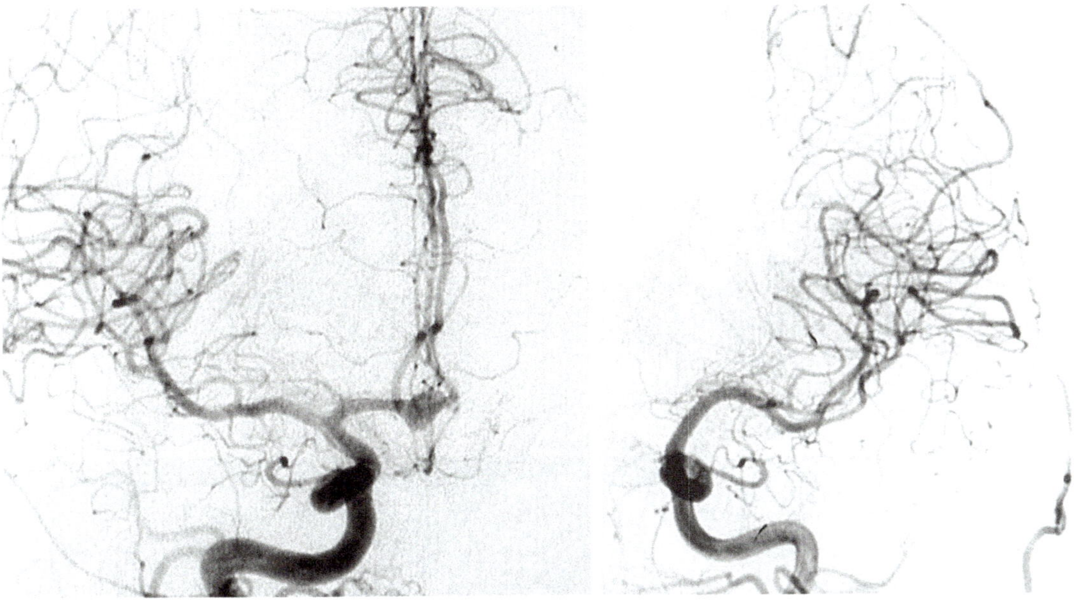

Fig. 3.20 Right and Left Carotid Angiograms. Well-developed Right A1. Aplastic left A1. (Taken from Bradac [15])

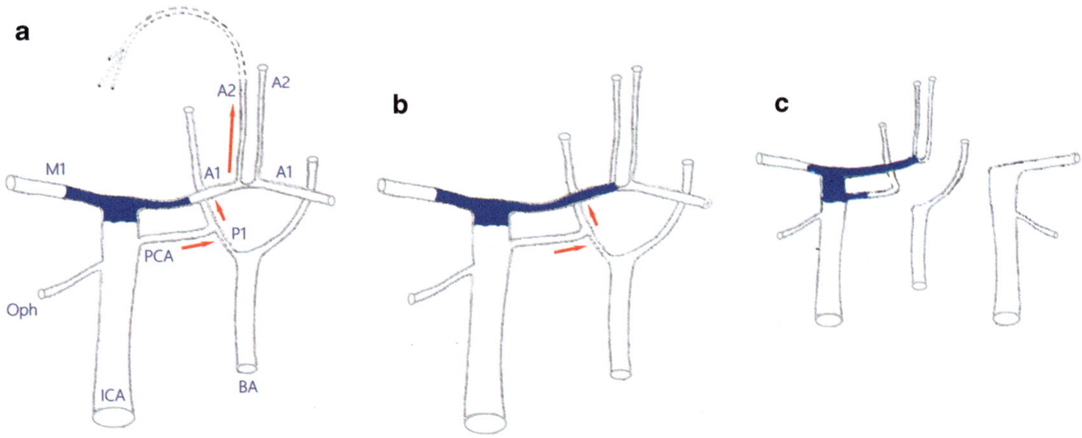

Fig. 3.21 Different pattern of involvement of A1, in patients with stroke due to occlusion of the distal ICA. See text

contribution of the medial striate perforators is lacking (Fig. 3.21b).

- The contralateral A1 is aplastic. The collateral flow is greatly affected since the flow of both A2 depends on the occluded A1 (Fig. 3.21c).

In both conditions (B-C), the collateral way to the MCA can develop from the PCA, provided that the artery does no arise from the occluded ICA and so involved in the occlusion (Figs. 3.22 and 3.23).

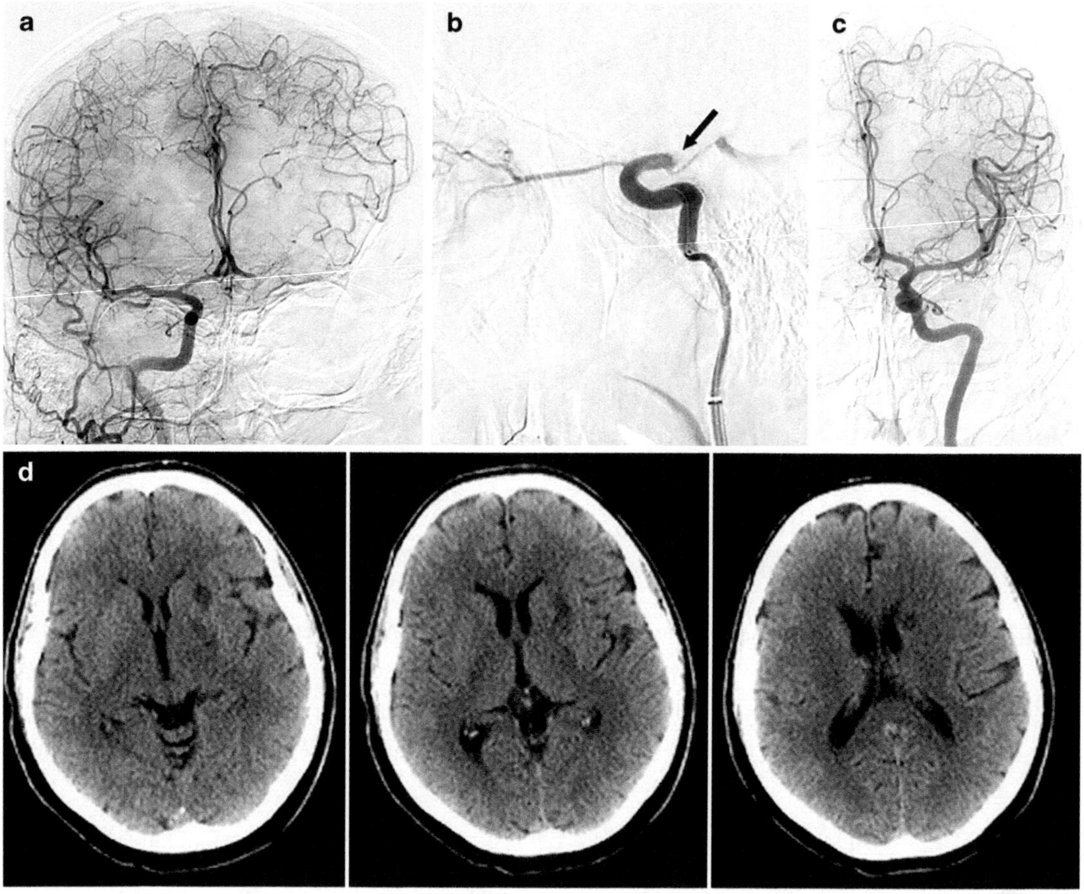

Fig. 3.22 Distal occlusion of the left ICA. (**a**) Right carotid angiogram partial filling of the left A1. There is a good collateral circulation from distal left ACA to the left MCA. (**b**) Occluded left ICA. (**c**) Recanalization of the occluded left ICA. (**d**) Post-treatment CT showing only a small infarct in the putamen

3.5.2 Duplication/Fenestration of A1

3.5.2.1 Duplication/Fenestration of A1. Plexural Pattern of AcomA

The A1 segment appears at the 10–12 mm embryo as a plexural vascular structure. This extends medially forming the AcomA connecting both A1 at the embryo of 20–24 mm. In the further evolution, the plexus changes becoming a tubular channel. In some cases, the plexus can partially persist favoring the formation of segmental duplication or fenestration. An example of duplication is presented in Fig. 3.24. An example of fenestration is presented in Fig. 3.25. The AcomA can maintain the primordial plexus configuration (Fig. 3.26).

The AcomA is rarely absent. Both ACA are directly connected or the connection is more distally located and so the peri-callosal artery arises at the level of the connection. This anomaly is rare in human and is reported by De La Torre-Netzky [24] to be frequent in some mammals, typically in dogs.

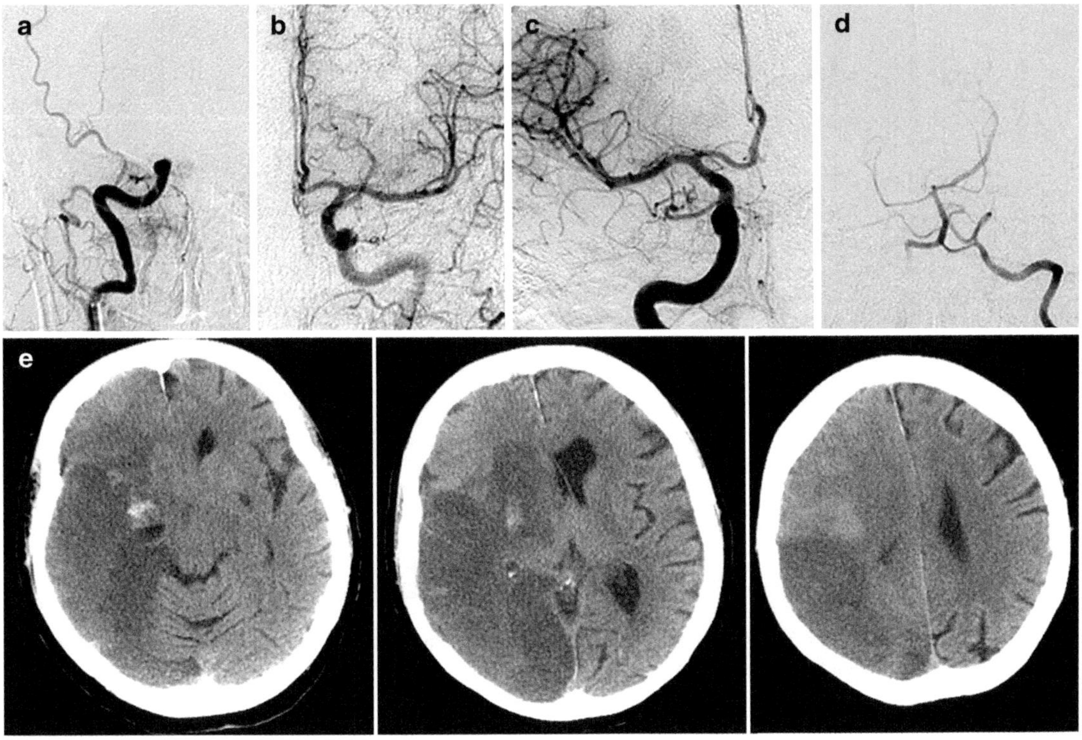

Fig. 3.23 (**a**) Distal occlusion of the right ICA. (**b**) There is no collateral circulation from the left ICA to the right. (**c**) Rapid re-canalization of the occluded right ICA. There is, however no flow through the AcomA, probably involved in the occlusion. Also the right PCA (fetal origin) remained occluded, as confirmed by the (**d**) vertebral angiogram. Extensive infarct on the (**e**) post-treatment CT

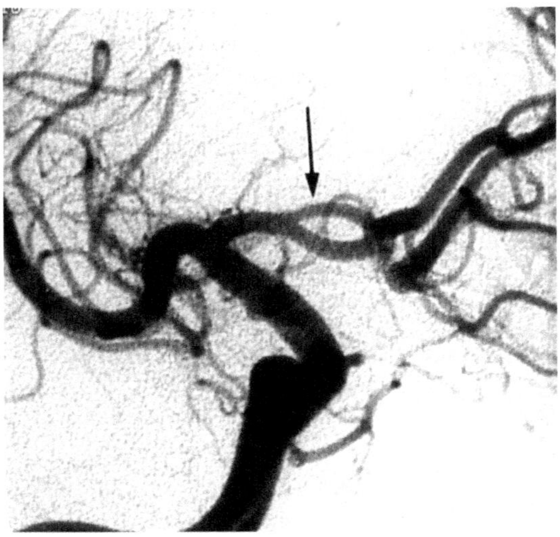

Fig. 3.24 Carotid right angiogram. Duplication of A1 (arrow). (Taken from Bradac [15])

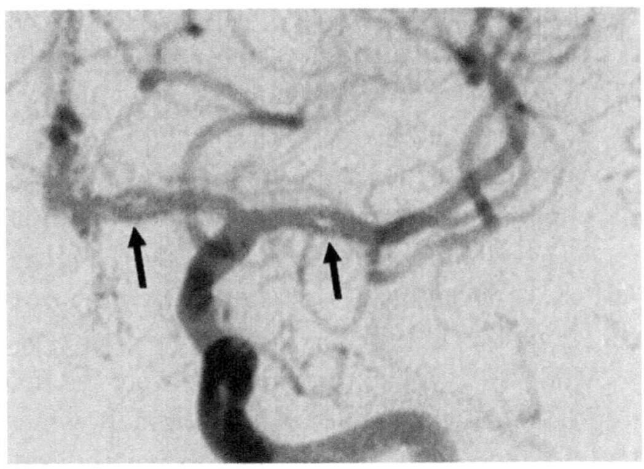

Fig. 3.25 Left Carotid angiogram. Fenestration of A1 (arrow), associated with fenestration of M1 (arrow)

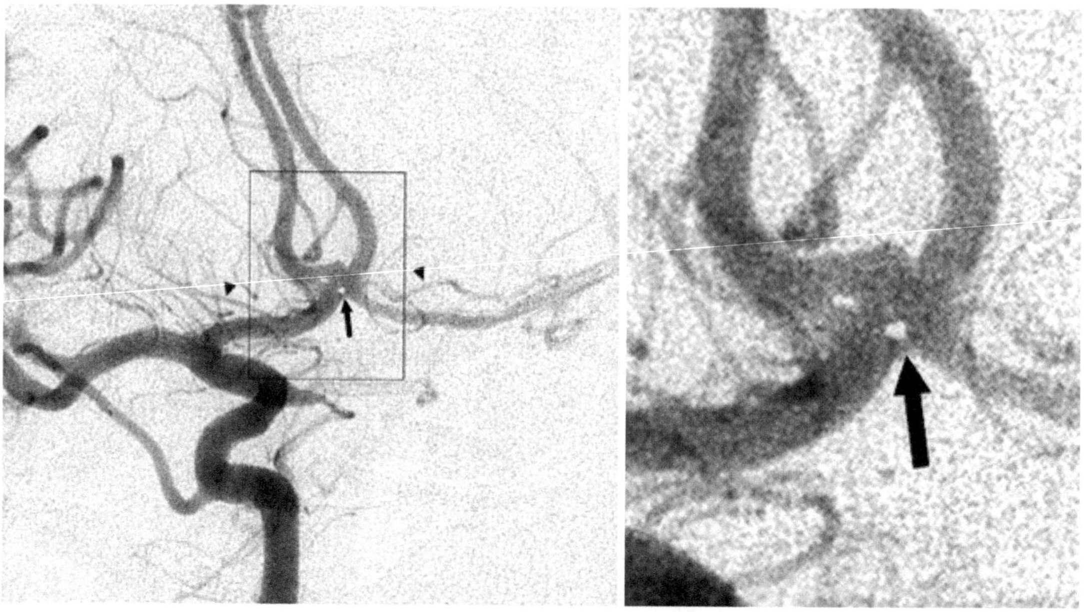

Fig. 3.26 Carotid angiogram. Persistence of the plexural structure of the AcomA (detail, arrow). Presence of Heubner Artery (arrowhead). (Taken from Bradac [15])

3.6 Infraoptic ACA

In this very rare variant, the artery arises from the cavernous portion of ICA, runs cranially passing inferiorly to the optic nerve, joining the A1-A2 segment. It can replace the normal course of the A1 segment or both the normal and anomalous branches can be present (Complete Duplication of ACA) (Fig. 3.27).

After the first description of Robinson [120], the anomaly has been reported by many authors [5, 11, 38, 48, 66, 83, 88, 96, 106, 107, 116, 159, 161]. It is frequently associated with other vessel anomalies [149].

Moffat [91, 92] and Bosma [13] were the first to propose an explanation of the anomaly which is now largely accepted. The authors have considered the early vascular structure of the optic vesicle (Chap. 6) supplied by the "periocular plexus" receiving branches from the Olfactory Artery, the Primary Maxillary Artery (PMA), and the Primary Dorsal Ophthalmic artery (PDO) all connected together. In the further evolution these connections disappear. In some cases, however, anastomoses between the olfactory artery and the PMA persist. The olfactory artery regresses, replaced by the Anterior Cerebral Artery which retains the connections with the PMA causing the anomaly. More recently other authors [42] considering that the Infra-optic ACA can sometimes arise from the supraclinoid ICA, have proposed that in these cases the anomaly is due to persistence of connections between the Olfactory artery and the Primary dorsal or Ventral ophthalmic artery.

3.6.1 Unique Peri-Callosal Artery (AZYGOS)

This rare anomaly is characterized by the presence of only one Peri-callosal artery [8, 48, 69, 70, 114, 136].

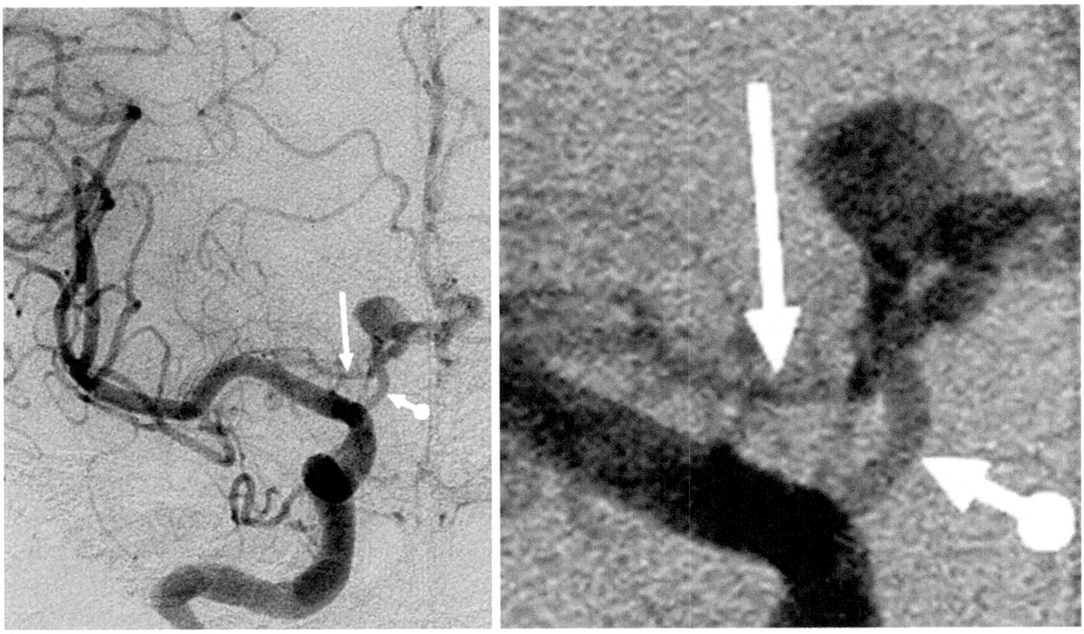

Fig. 3.27 Carotid angiogram. Example of infraoptic course of ACA. In this patient, the infraoptic segment (arrow with dot) was associated with a segment with a normal course (arrow). Aneurysm was present

The anomaly probably develops in the embryo phase of 18–20 mm in which both A1 and A2 connect together through the formation of the AcomA, giving off each the peri-callosal artery which fuse together in a unique vessel. An example is presented in Fig. 3.28.

A particular condition is that in which one well-developed peri-callosal artery divided distally gives off branches for both hemispheres. The contro-lateral peri-callosal is smaller, giving off only basal branches. This configuration, called by some authors [114] "*Bi-hemispheric Peri-callosal Artery*" has great similarity with that of Azygos. It is conceivable that it is a partial Azygos anomaly.

Further in this section the relationship of the Azygos with the sub-callosal artery is discussed. The anomaly is an incidental discovery without clinical consequences, provided that it is not associated with other vascular malformation.

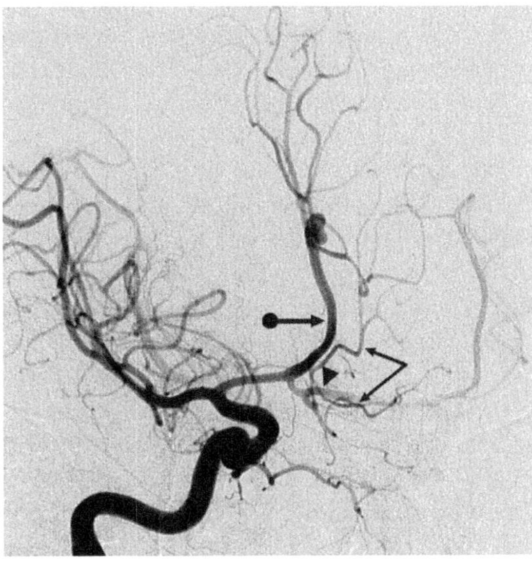

Fig. 3.28 Right carotid angiogram in patient studied for a ruptured aneurysm. The Peri-callosal Artery (arrow with dot) is unique (Azygos Artery). It divides distally in branches for both hemispheres. There is a small left A1 (arrow head) from which arise some basal branches for the right hemisphere (arrow with angle). (Taken from Bradac [15])

3.7 Median Artery of Corpus Callosum (Subcallosal Artery

The artery has been described first by De Vriese [25] (Chap. 2) as a branch arising from the AcomA at the embryo of 20–24 mm. The artery has been taken again into consideration in the study of Lazorthes [65]. The author described the artery which he called "*Artere du Corps Calleux*" appearing as a courte, moyenne, longue.

A few years later Baptista [8], similarly to the description of Lazorthes, described a short, small artery, and a long artery. He called this latter the "Accessory or Triplicate ACA."

A very important work appeared later by Marinkovicz et al. [83]. These authors in a micro-angiographic study described a small branch relatively short in 91% of the cases supplying the subcallosal area, the genu of corpus callosum, and anterior pillar of fornix. The authors called this vessel "the Subcallosal Artery." In the remaining 9% the vessel was large, extending along the corpus callosum supplying it. This artery was defined as the "Median Artery of corpus callosum" (Triplicated Peri-callosal artery).

Similar results have been reported later by Tao et al. [141] and Chenin et al. [18].

Interesting are also the results and considerations of another group of authors [127]. They reported the more frequent presence of a small branch they called the "Subcallosal Artery" and more rarely of a large branch called "Triplicate ACA." To these branches they added the Azygos artery. The authors concluded that all these vessels can be considered as a variation of the "Median artery of Corpus Callosum" described by De Vriese. These arteries can develop differently appearing with a pattern of one of the three branches described above.

The clinical importance and the consequences of the occlusion of the Subcallosal artery have been described by Meila et al. [84] on the basis of their experience and review of the literature. The occlusion can be due to a micro-angiopathy or to an inadvertently occlusion in treatment of AcomA aneurysms (endovascular or surgical). The patient presents with confusion and amnesia. These symptoms commonly regress, but can persist for a long time. On CT and MR, infarct involving the genu of corpus callosum and especially fornix are typically present. This explains clearly the clinical symptoms, considering that fornix is part of the circuit involved in the memory (Kandel) formed by connections from hippocampus, through fornix towards the mammillary bodies and further through the mammillo-thalamic tract to the cingulate gyrus and association areas.

Unfortunately, we can demonstrate the consequences of the occlusion of the Subcallosal artery, but we can rarely identify the artery on the angiogram.

In an internal study, involving 100 carotid angiograms performed in our department, aimed to identify the frequency of visible subcallosal artery, this was demonstrated in two cases (4%) (Fig. 3.29).

An example of triplicated peri-callosal artery is shown in Fig. 3.30.

We also experienced (Fig. 3.31), two cases of assumed occlusion of the subcallosal artery (SA) following treatment of AcomA aneurysm in patients who had the typical clinical symptoms with the corresponding ischemia on CT and MR. In one of these patients, the SA could not be identified with certainty. In the other, the SA was demonstrated before and after the treatment. It is conceivable that the occlusion was only temporary. In both patients there was a slow complete recovery.

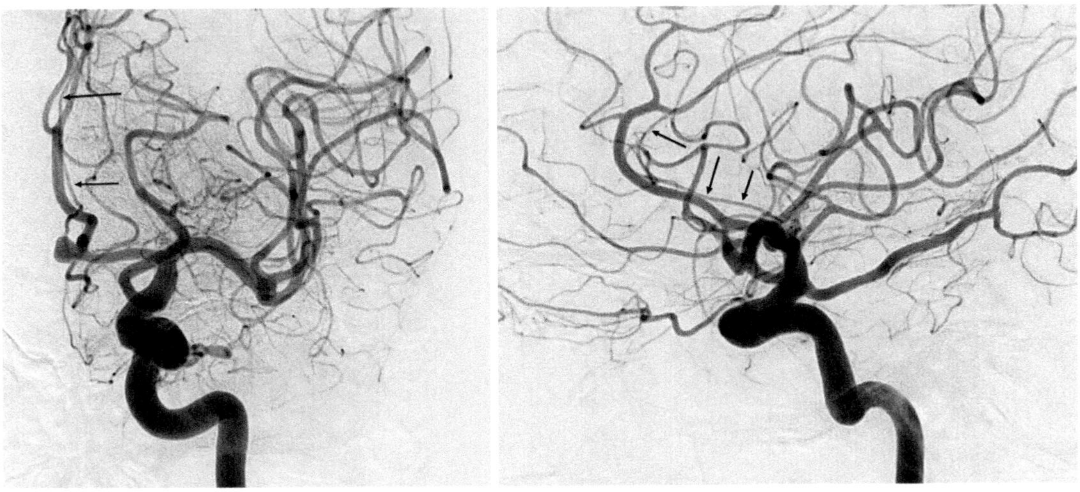

Fig. 3.29 Carotid angiogram (AP and Lateral views) showing an example of subcallosal artery (arrow)

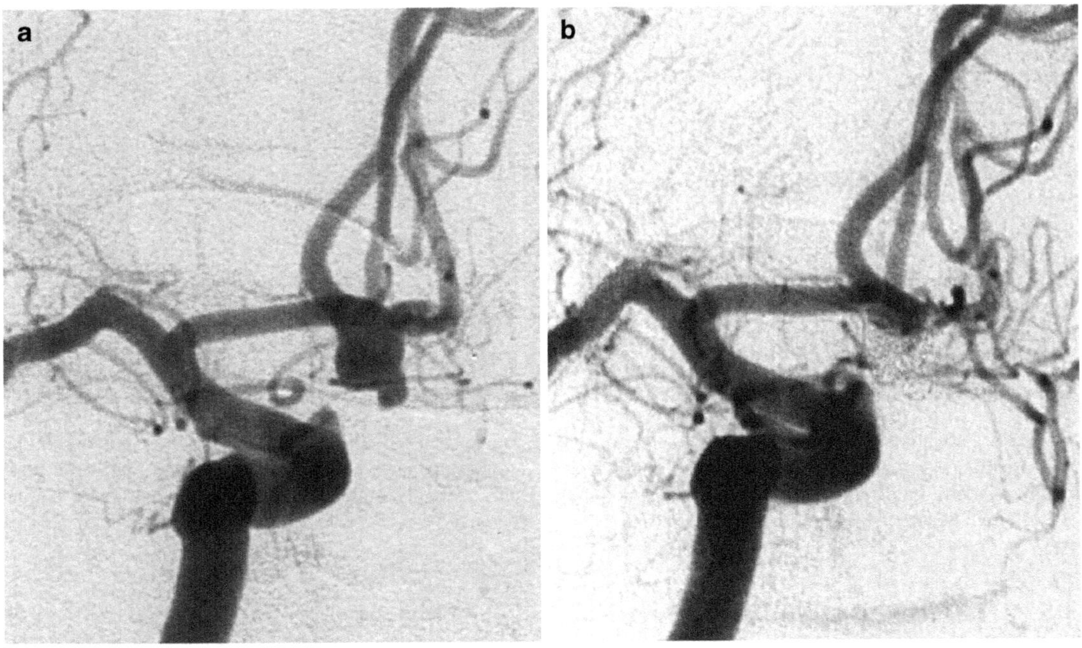

Fig. 3.30 (**a**) Carotid angiogram showing an example of Triplicated Peri-callosal Artery. (**b**) Angiogram post endovascular treatment. (Taken from Bradac [15])

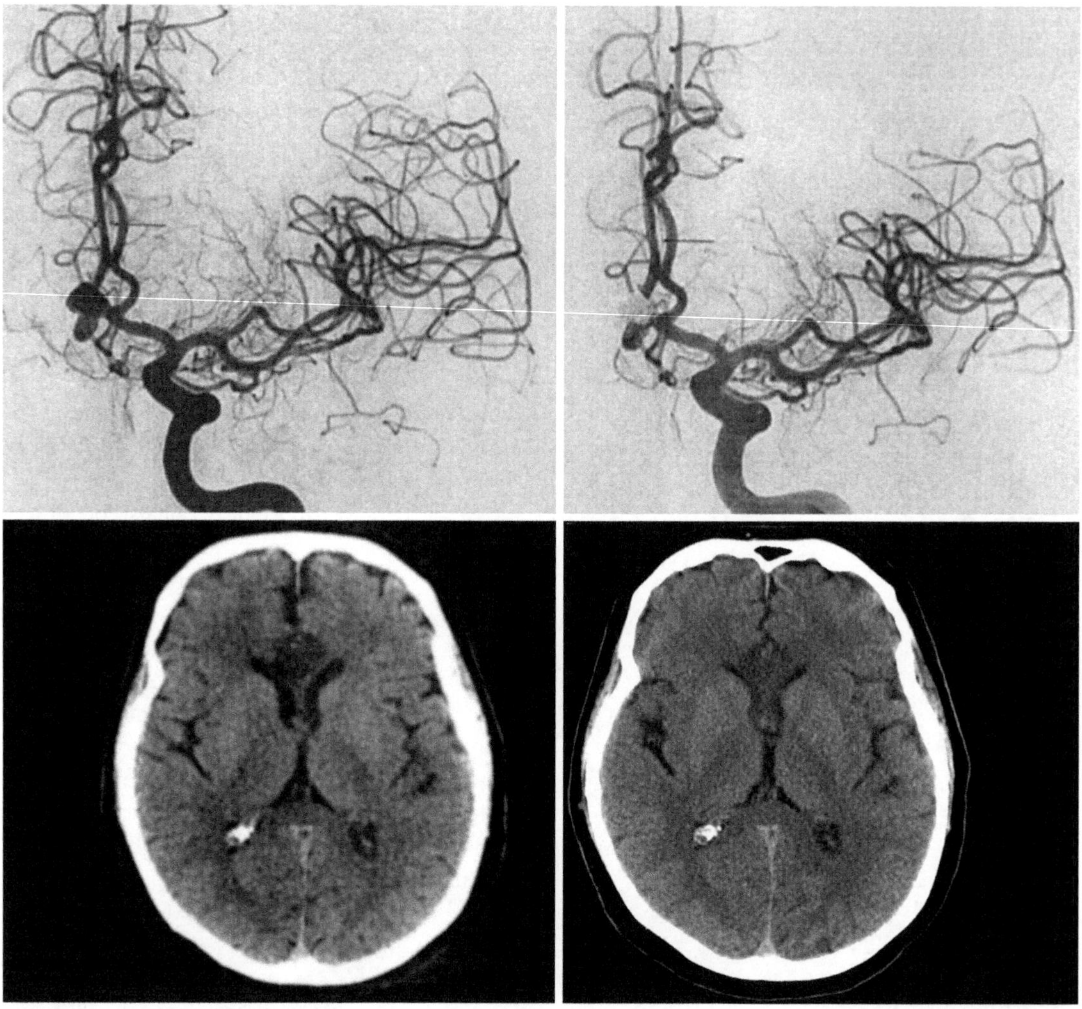

Fig. 3.31 Patient with AcomA aneurysm. The endovascular treatment was uneventful. However, the CT post-treatment showed an infarct involving Fornix and Genus of Corpus Callosum causing agitation and confusion. The comparison of the pre-treatment and post-treatment angiograms showed that the subcallosal artery was present, probably only temporary occluded. The patient recovered

3.8 Persistent Olfactory Artery

As described in Chap. 2, the olfactory artery is the first branch of the Cranial ICA division. The artery commonly regresses at the 12–18 mm embryo, replaced by the ACA arising from the same common trunk. Its persistence is extremely rare. It has been identified by Moffat [92] in an autoptic study performed on a 70-year-old man who died from a stomach carcinoma.

Sporadic cases of incidental discovery on angiographic study have been reported [106, 148]. In the reported cases, the artery had first a horizontal course along the frontal base. It made then a sharp curve continuing in the distal anterior cerebral artery. At the level of the curve an aneurysm was present.

On the diagram, the anomalous course of the ACA due to persistence of the olfactory artery is demonstrated (Fig. 3.32).

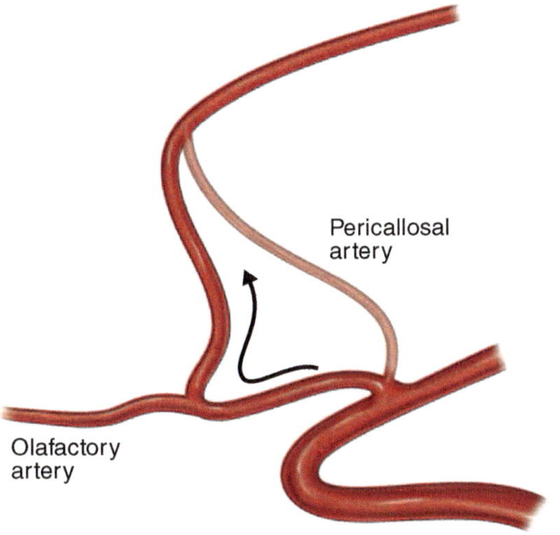

Fig. 3.32 Diagram showing the persistent Olfactory Artery, joining distally the Peri-callosal Artery

3.9 Middle Cerebral Artery (MCA)

At the end of the embryonic phase (embryo of 40–44 mm, 50–56 days of age), the configuration of the MCA with its essential components typical of the adult are developed. Following the continuous growth of the brain the MCA undergoes further changes.

At the beginning of the fetal phase, the trunk of the MCA (the future M1) has an oblique upwards course and the distal branches arising from it have a vertical, rectilinear course [54, 55, 118]. Following the growth of the temporal lobe especially of its anterior medial part, as well as the formation of Insula and progressive growth of the cerebral lobes and development of cortex with appearing of circumvolutions and sulci, the configuration of the MCA changes. The M1 becomes more horizontal, the distal branches run on the surface of the insula, and to reach the surface of the hemispheres are forced to make a double curve. On the cortex due to the presence of gyri and sulci the distal branches become more tortuous. The pattern becomes progressively that of the adult, even if some segment continues to show minimal changes still in young children.

Modifications involve also the perforators. The vessels have appeared at the embryo of 18–20 mm. Following the growth of the forebrain and the compression and displacement of the olfactory lobe, the perforators are forced to change their course [54, 55]. The more lateral which have first a vertical course, acquire progressively their typical adult configuration. The first segment is directed medially, then bends laterally continuing vertically passing through the APS to reach the ba. This evolution is shown in Fig. 3.33.

In Fig. 3.34, the adult configuration of the MCA which has been subdivided in a few segments has been demonstrated. The first segment is the so-called M1. It runs horizontally in the Sylvian fissure parallel 1 cm posterior to the sphenoid ridge. From the M1 arise the perforators as ascending branches which run through the APS to the basal ganglia (superior-lateral part of head of Nucleus Caudatus, sometimes to the entire head of Nucleus Caudatus, completely his body and entirely the superior part of the Internal Capsule, including the Supero-Lateral part of his anterior limb, most of the Putamen, part of Pallidum). Following the first description of Duret [31], many other authors have been involved in their study [28, 37, 68, 123, 132, 150, 154]. The arteries can develop as single branches or as a common trunk dividing in more branches distally. This latter configuration has been reported to occur up to 50% by Umansky et al. [150]. The role of the perforators arising from A1 has been described in the section of the Anterior cerebral artery. They can replace the medial perforator of M1 up to 26% [150].

As it will be described more in detail further in the section, the distribution of these branches is related to the length of M1.

At the anterior border of the insula, M1 divides in two-three branches (Bi-Trifurcation). These turn sharply running on the surface of the insula (M2 segment). The branches make then a double curve (M3 segment) to exit from the insular cistern, reaching the surface of the brain extending to the areas they supply (M4 segment).

The distal branches have been subdivided and named [87, 118] taking into consideration the vascular territory they supply (Fig. 3.35a, b).

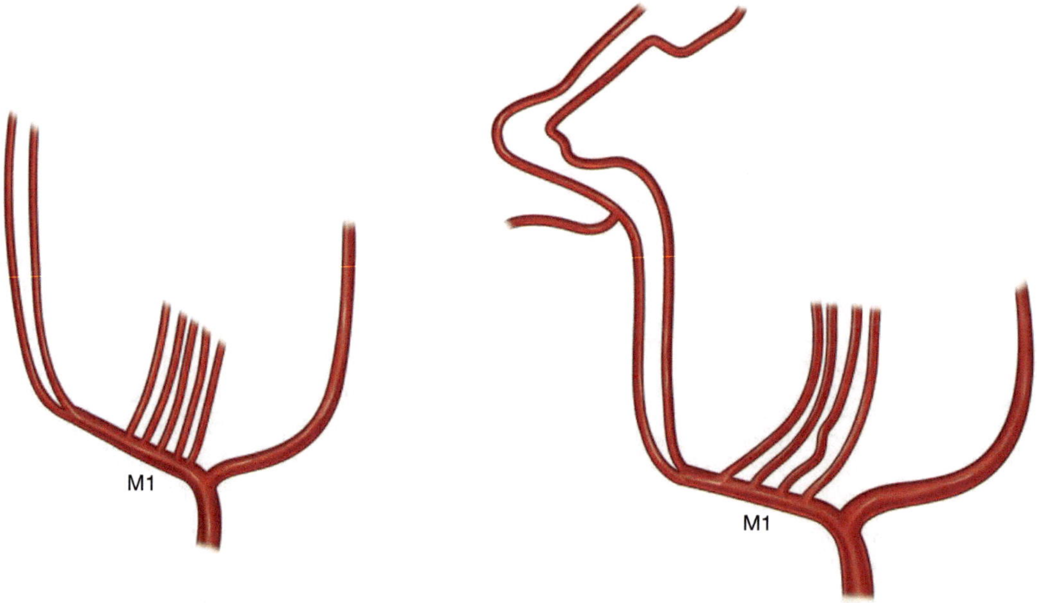

Fig. 3.33 Diagram showing the changes in course of the MCA during its evolution in the fetal phase involving the first segment (M1), the distal segments, and the perforators (see text)

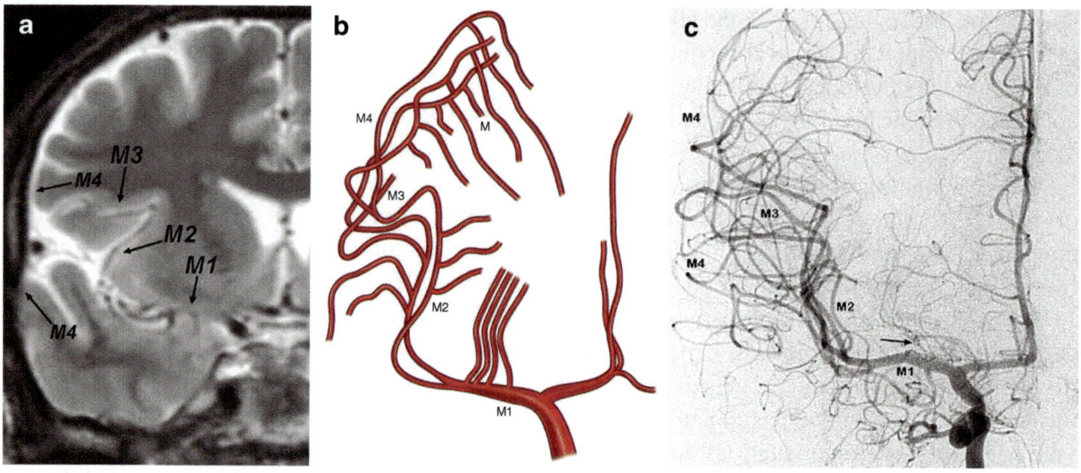

Fig. 3.34 Course and pattern of the adult MCA as shown on MR (**a**) on Diagram (**b**) and on angiogram (**c**). M1, M2, M3, M4 segments; perforators; Medullary branches (M). (Figs **a** and **c** taken from Bradac [15])

The orbitofrontal artery is the first branch to leave the Sylvian insular cistern. It can sometimes arise from the horizontal segment of M1. The artery which is in balance with the orbitofrontal branch of the ACA runs in the sulcus separating the *pars triangularis* from the pars orbitalis of the inferior frontal gyrus extending to the pars orbitalis. The operculo-frontal arteries leave the cistern at the level of the *pars triangularis* taking an ascending course. The artery can appear as a trunk dividing distally in two or three branches which can have also a separate origin.

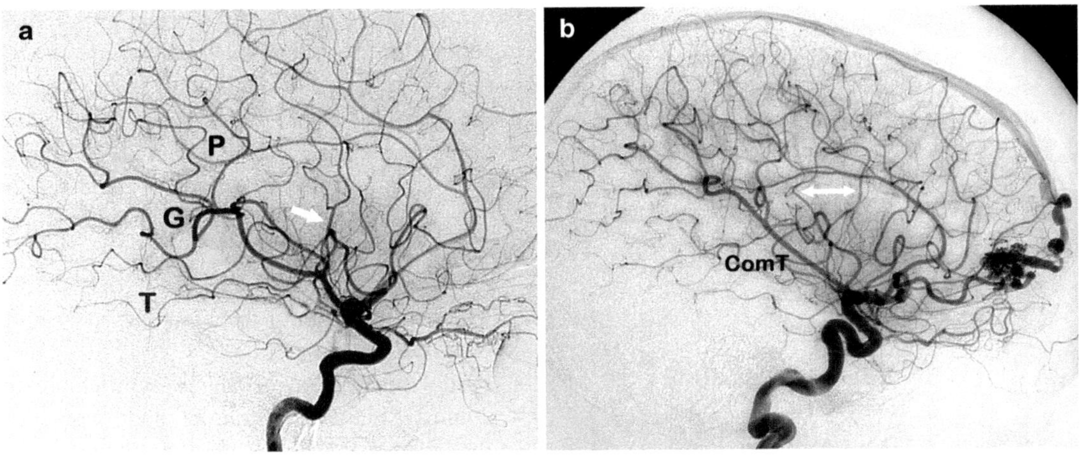

Fig. 3.35 Two examples of a lateral carotid angiogram. The Central Artery (white arrows). The Operculo-frontal arteries run anteriorly. On (**a**) the Parietal (P), the Temporal (T), and the Gyrur Angularis (G) arteries are shown. On (**b**) the posterior branches arise as a Common Trunk (ComT), there is a large Orbito-Frontal artery supplying a Fronto-Basal AVM

They supply the Broca area and the prefrontal-premotor areas. The central artery is the most posterior ascending frontal branch. It arises as a unique trunk dividing distally in two branches or as two branches arising separately It emerges from the Sylvian fissure at the level of the *pars opercularis* running cranially to the central fissure giving off branches supplying the precentral (primary premotor area) and the post-central (primary sensory area) gyrus.

The parietal arteries consist of two branches exiting from the posterior part of the Sylvian fissure, the anterior commonly is small and the posterior is well developed. They ran slightly posterior to the central artery. The parietal arteries supply the parietal and supra-marginal gyri.

The temporal branches emerge from the Sylvian fissure taking a descending course supplying the pole, the anterior, middle, and posterior part of the lateral temporal lobe. These branches have a variable extent and frequently the posterior is predominant.

The *Gyrus Angularis* Artery is considered the terminal branch of the MCA. It emerges from the distal part of the Sylvian fissure sometimes as a common trunk with the parietal or posterior temporal arteries, running towards the *gyrus supramarginalis* and *gyrus angularis*. It forms frequently an upward convex curve as it turns around the gyrus of Heschl leaving the Sylvian fissure. It is involved in the supply of the Wernicke area.

In a radioanatomical-angiographic study concerning the origin of the distal branches of the MCA from the M1 segment, some authors [87, 124] have identified two most frequent patterns of division: the bifurcation and trifurcation. Other configurations are extremely rare.

In the Bifurcation pattern, there are two groups of trunks, the antero-superior and the postero-inferior.

From the antero-superior arise the Orbitofrontal (O), the Operculo-Frontal (OF), and Central arteries (C).

From the postero-inferior arise the Parietal (P), the *Gyrus Angularis* (GA), and the Temporal Arteries (T).

In the Trifurcation pattern there are three groups, antero-superior, middle, and the postero-inferior.

From the antero-superior arise the orbitofrontal and the operculofrontal.

From the middle arise the central, the parietal, and the *Gyrus Angularis* arteries.

From the posterior-inferior arise the temporal arteries.

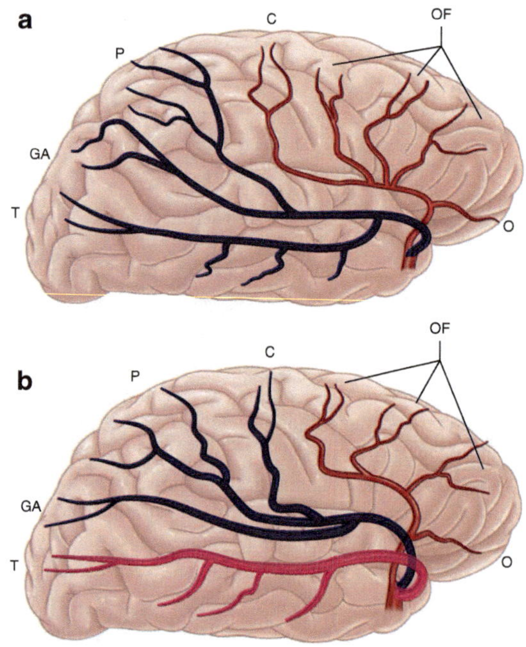

Fig. 3.36 Diagram showing the pattern of the distal branches of the MCA in the Bifurcation (**a**) and Trifurcation (**b**) division (modified from [87]). Orbito-frontal (O), Operculo-Frontal (OF) branches, Central artery (C), Parietal (P), Gyrus Angularis (GA), Temporal (T) branches

The above described configurations are useful in the study of the lateral carotid angiogram of the MCA (Fig. 3.36).

Basically it is relatively easy to recognize the specific groups of arteries. However, the frequent variations and overlapping can make the given case difficult to identify the single artery with certainty.

More about the distal branches are presented in Chap. 4.

3.10 Anomalous Evolution of the MCA

In this context, it is useful to remember that MCA develops at the embryo of 12 mm from many twigs arising from the distal ICA and partially from the trunk of the ACA. The twigs fuse together forming first a plexural structure changing in a tubular channel. It is conceivable that the twigs are not all equal. Some can be longer and extend more distally, others are short ending close to their origin, some others regress. The various evolution of the twigs can explain some variations of the M1.

- The configuration of the M1 can appear long or short.
- Partial persistence of the primordial plexus could explain fenestration and segmental duplication of M1.
- Two groups of twigs could have an independent evolution, each fusing separately, leading to the formation of a complete duplication of MCA.
- Some twigs of the ACA could develop independently resulting in the formation of an "Accessory MCA."

The different length of M1 can influence the origin of the perforators. In the short M1, the perforators are grouped in the short segment. The more distal arise commonly from the superior divisional distal branch (Fig. 3.37a, b). In the long M1, the perforators can be more generously distributed along the M1.

The different length of the M1, considered commonly as a normal variant, can have clinical consequences in pathological conditions, typically in presence of aneurysm, in which a short M1 with perforators located close to the aneurysm, can make the treatment more difficult and riskier (Figs. 3.38a, b and 3.39).

The MCA is the artery more frequently involved in stroke, typically at the level of M1. The site of occlusion, but also the configuration of M1 and its perforators, can play a role in the clinical consequences (Figs. 3.40 and 3.41).

In this context, a few considerations should be made: The rapid recanalization of the distal branches can avoid lesions in the cortical regions. Ischemia in the vascular territory of the perfora-

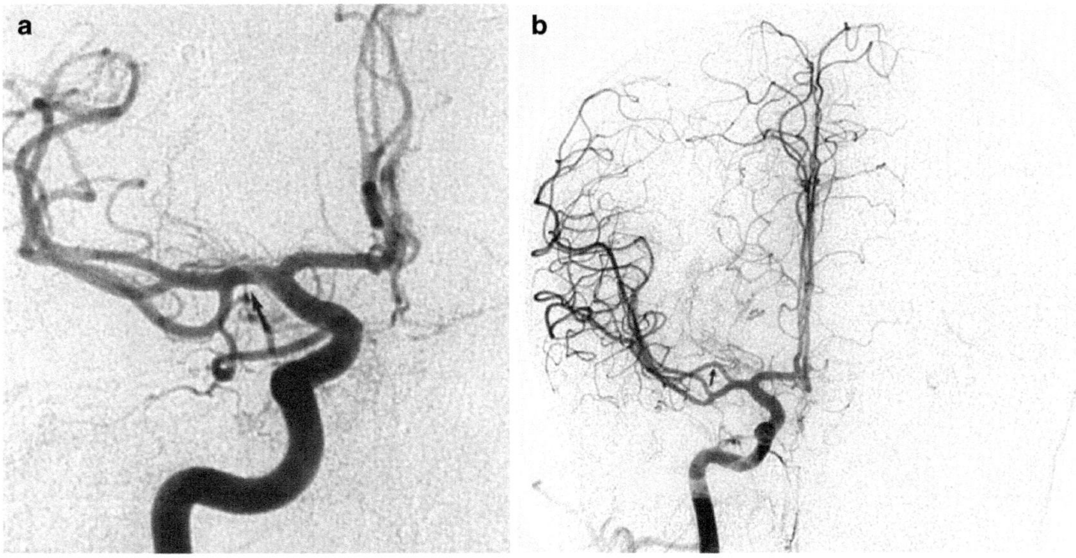

Fig. 3.37 Carotid angiogram in two different cases (**a**, **b**). Example of a short M1. In (**b**) the perforators arise from the superior branch (arrow). (Taken from Bradac [15])

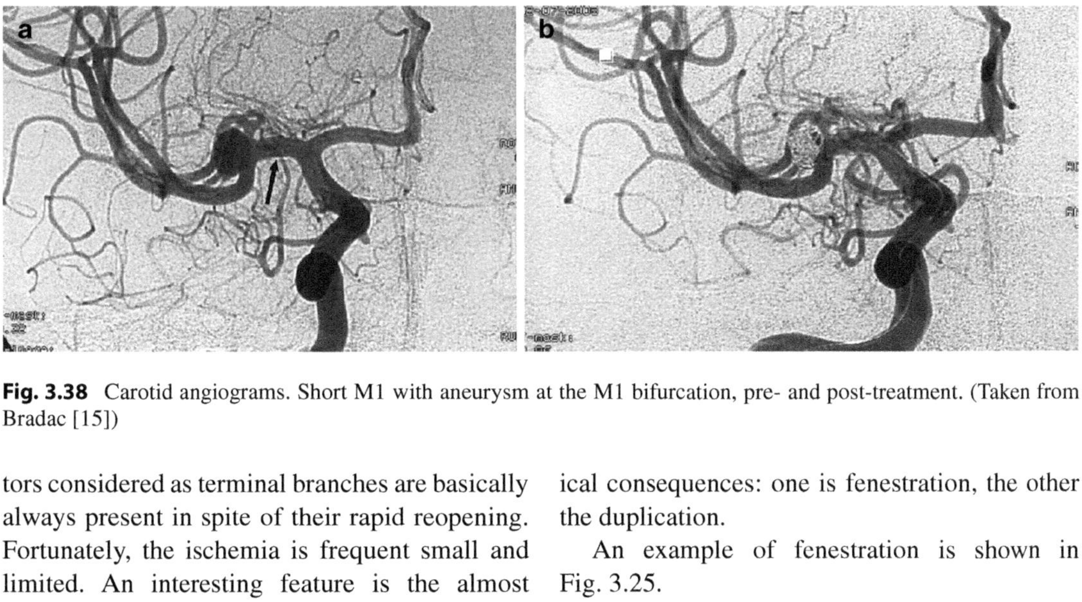

Fig. 3.38 Carotid angiograms. Short M1 with aneurysm at the M1 bifurcation, pre- and post-treatment. (Taken from Bradac [15])

tors considered as terminal branches are basically always present in spite of their rapid reopening. Fortunately, the ischemia is frequent small and limited. An interesting feature is the almost always sparing of the internal capsule. This is little surprising, considering that it is vascularized at least in the superior part by the perforators of M1. This will be discussed more in detail in Chap. 4.

There are other anomalies in which the pattern of M1 and origin of the perforators can have clinical consequences: one is fenestration, the other the duplication.

An example of fenestration is shown in Fig. 3.25.

As far as it concerns the duplication, in this condition, the MCA is formed by two separate branches arising from ICA or one from ACA. Crompton [19] who first described this anomaly introduced the term "Accessory MCA" including both configurations, the one with both branches arising from ICA and the other with one

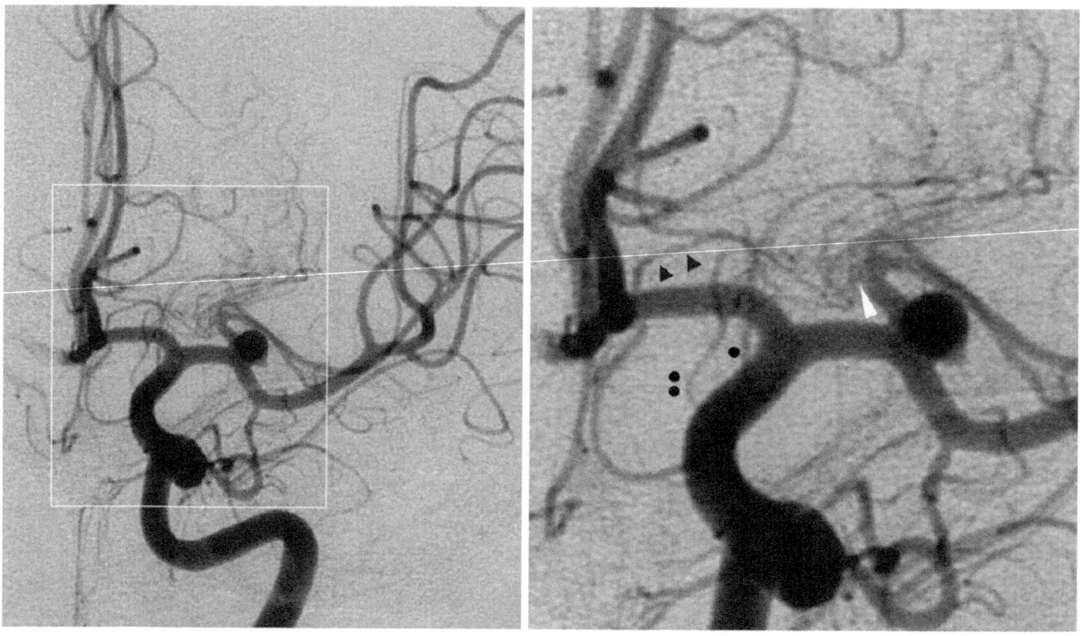

Fig. 3.39 Carotid angiogram. Short M1 with aneurysm at the bifurcation. The perforators arise from the Superior Trunk (white arrow head). A few perforators arise from A1. Heubner Artery (arrowheads). PcomA, AchA (small dots). (Taken from Bradac [15])

branch arising from ACA. Many reports followed [36, 137, 139].

Today it is preferring to distinguish the “Duplication” pattern in which both separate branches arise from ICA, from the condition called “Accessory MCA” in which the second branch arises from ACA. In this context, it is useful to report the position of other authors who have interpreted the accessory branch as a large recurrent artery of Heubner. However, this is not accepted by most authors, since the Heubner artery ends as perforators, while the accessory continues in cortical branches (Figs. 3.42, 3.43a, b, and 3.44a–c). As it has been described in previous parts of the chapter, both conditions can be considered as a “Complete Duplication” since both branches, the normal and the anomalous have a separate origin.

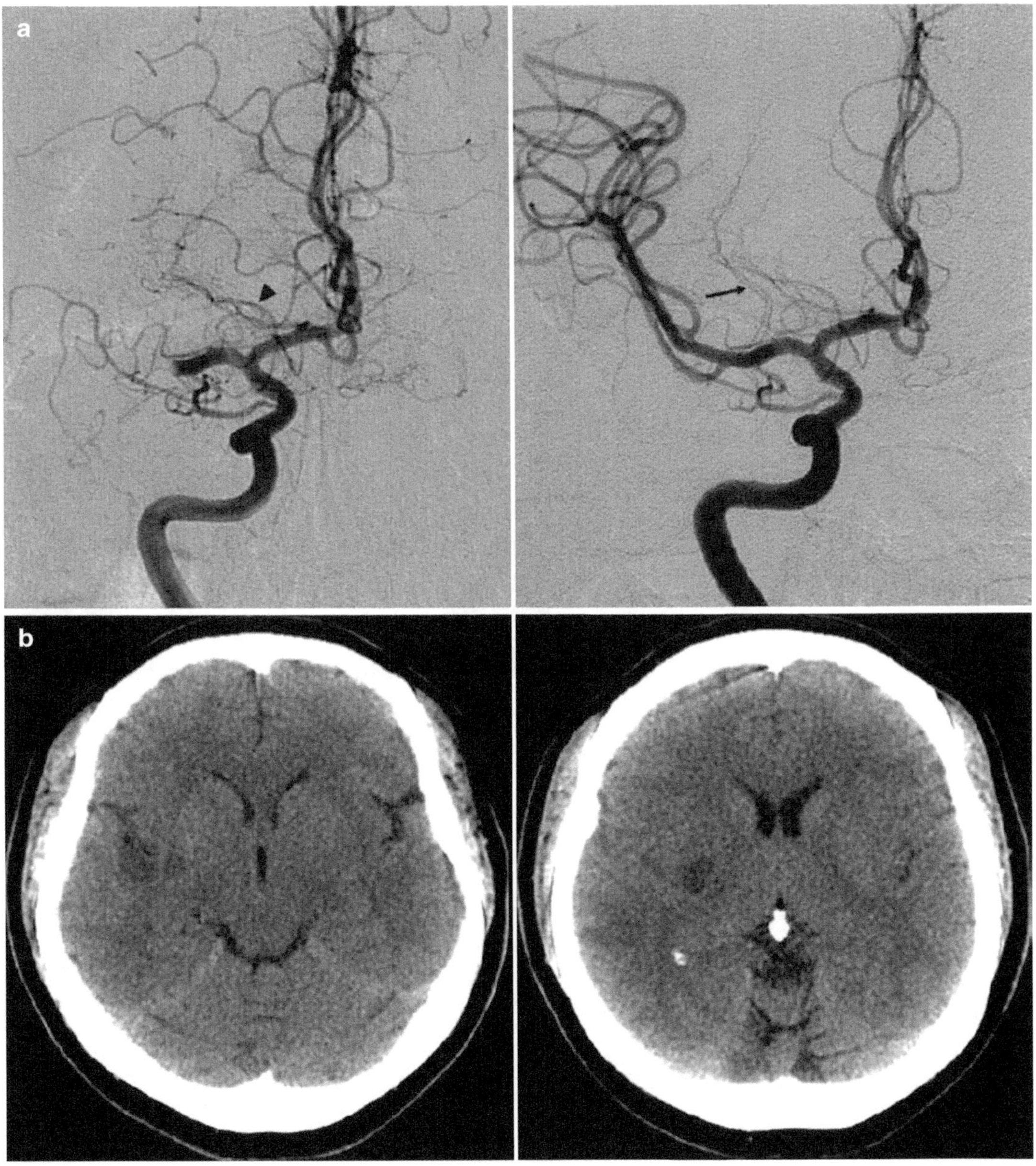

Fig. 3.40 (**a**) Carotid angiogram in patient with stroke due to occlusion of M1. Heubner artery (arrow head). On the right, rapid endovascular re-canalization. (**b**) On the post-treatment CT, there is a small infarct in the Insula region and Putamen. (Taken from Bradac [15])

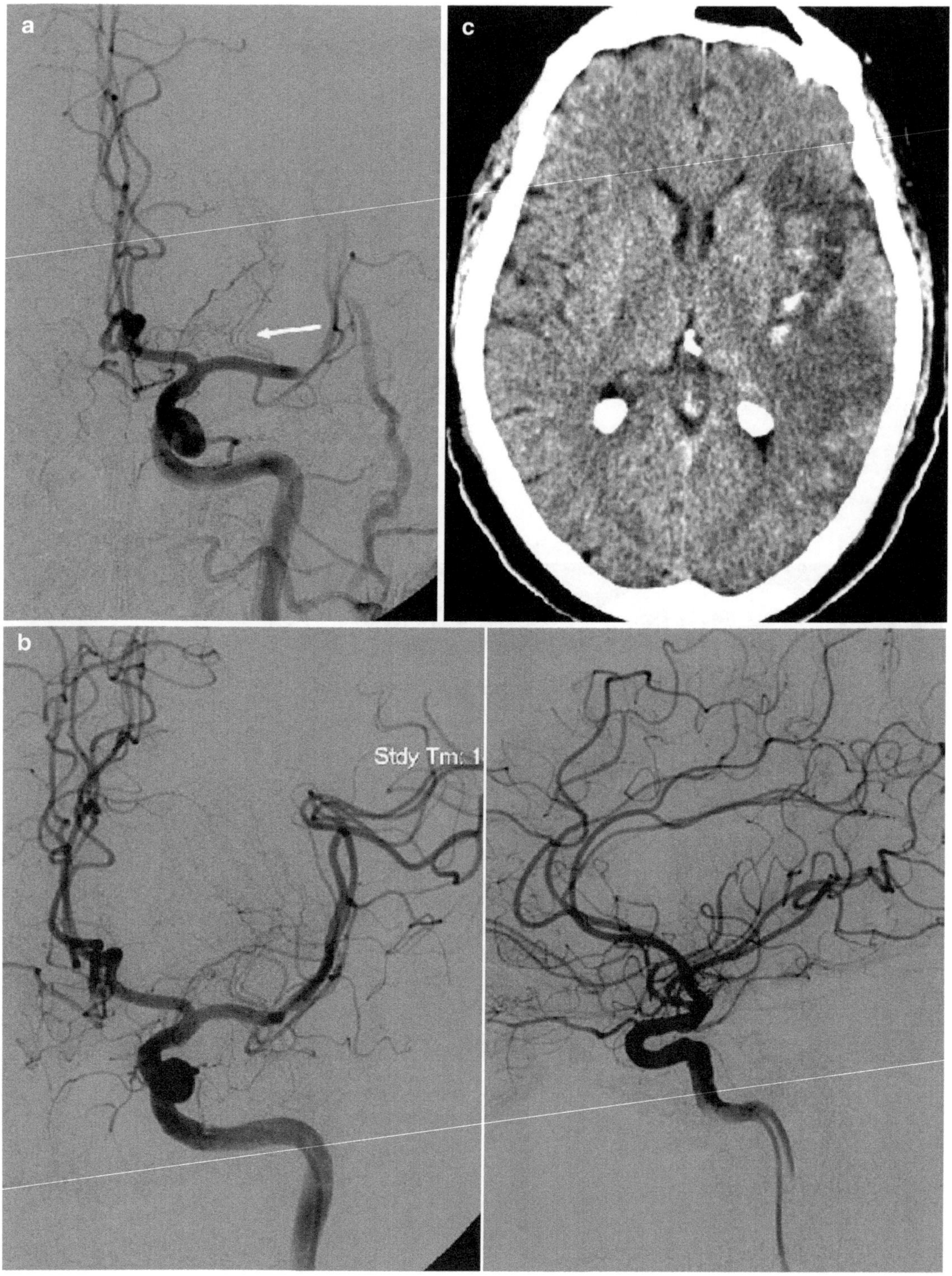

Fig. 3.41 (**a**) Carotid angiogram in patient with stroke due to occlusion of the distal long M1. The perforators (arrow) are not involved. (**b**) Partial re-canalization. (**c**) On the post-treatment CT, there is an infarct in the insula and temporal region. Basal ganglia are spared. (Taken from Bradac [15])

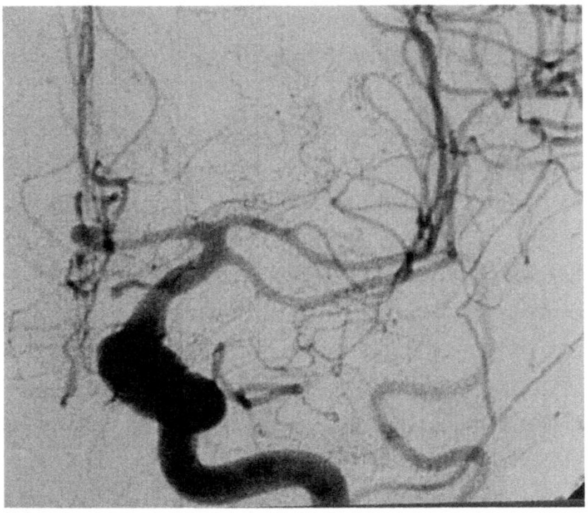

Fig. 3.42 Carotid angiogram. Duplication of M1. (Taken from Bradac [15])

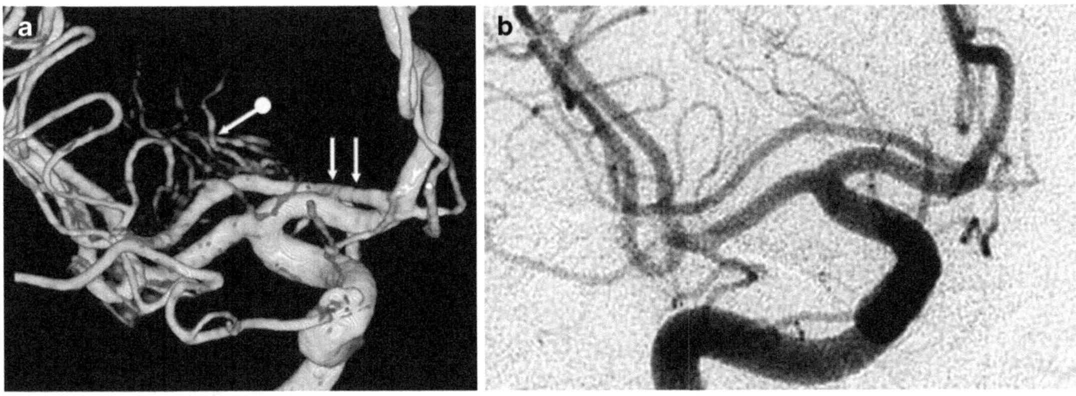

Fig. 3.43 Angio-CT (**a**) and Angiogram (**b**) in an accessory MCA (arrows). From the accessory branch arise a few perforators (arrow with dot). (Taken from Bradac [15])

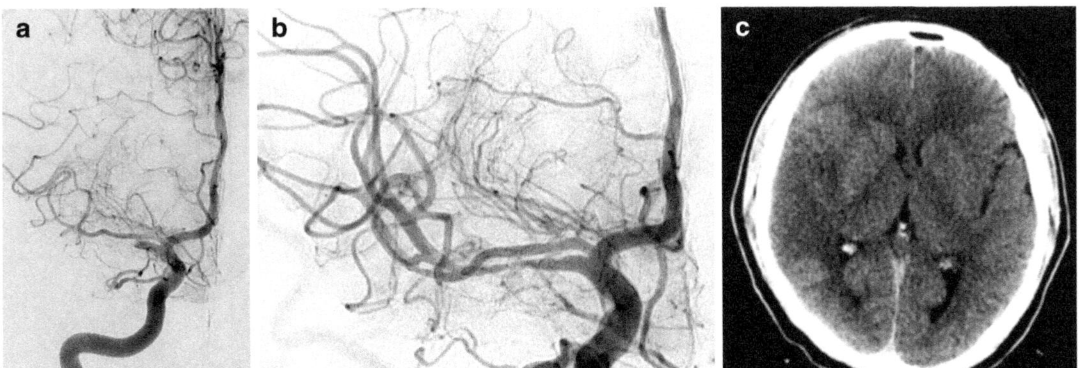

Fig. 3.44 (**a**) Carotid angiogram in patient with stroke. Duplicated M1. The occlusion involved the inferior branch. From the smaller superior branch arise the perforators, some arise from A1. (**b**) Recanalization with persistent small narrowing of the occluded branch. (**c**) On the post-treatment CT, infarct in the temporo-insular region

3.11 Anterior Choroidal Artery (AchA)

In the fetal phase, the AchA undergoes many changes, following the growth of the cerebral hemispheres, especially due to the formation of the occipital-temporal lobes with extension of ventricles and associated choroid plexus. The course of the artery is longer and complex and the supply of the choroid plexus becomes one of its important functions. *This latter as demonstrated in the comparative study* [25] *is a new acquirement which becomes progressively more important in mammals and typical in humans.*

The final adult configuration has been described by many authors in anatomic and angiographic examinations [1, 2, 17, 35, 40, 129, 144]. The most important points are summarized here. The artery has been subdivided in two different functional segments: the *Cisternal* and the *Plexal* (Figs. 3.45a–d and 3.46).

The cisternal arises from ICA 2–3 mm distal to the PcomA, crosses the optic tract from lateral to medial, continuing its course around the midbrain. The Basal vein lies above and the PCA below. The artery reaches the lateral geniculate body (LGB) to which it sends branches supplying its lateral part, while the medial part is supplied by branches of the posterior choroid artery arising from the PCA. There are anastomoses between the two vascular territories.

At the level of the LGB, from the cisternal segment, arises a branch which curves sharply laterally to enter the temporal horn at the choroid fissure. This is the plexal segment of the AchA which supplies the choroid plexus, the wall of the

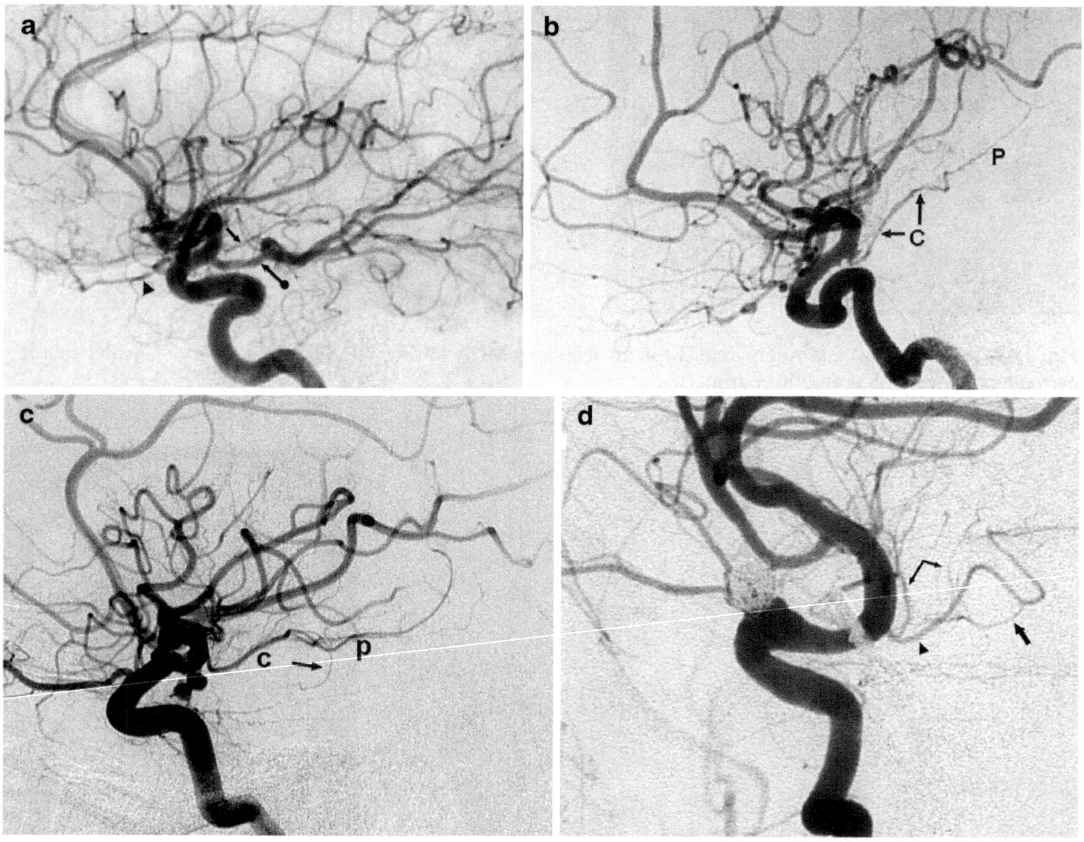

Fig. 3.45 Carotid angiograms showing the course of the AchA in four different patients. (**a**) Relation of the AchA (small arrow) with the PcomA (arrow with dot). (**b**) Cisternal (C) and Plexal (P) segments. (**c**, **d**) well-developed Uncal branch (arrow) and Perforators (arrow with angle). (Taken from Bradac [15])

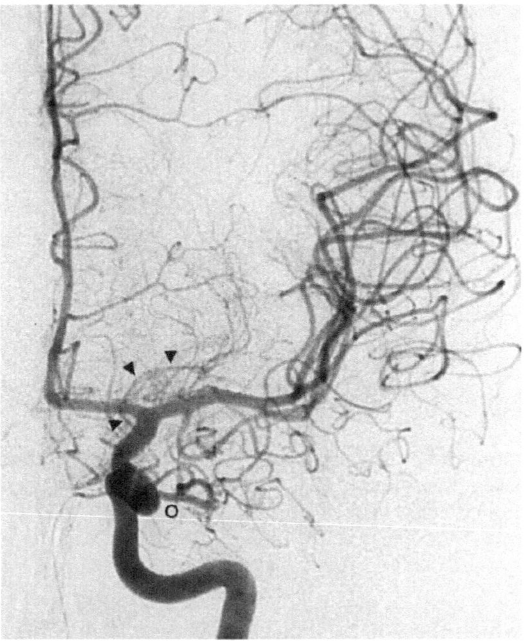

Fig. 3.46 Carotid angiogram. AP view. Course of the AchA (arrow head). (Taken from Bradac [15])

temporal horn and atrium and Hippocampus. It anastomoses with a branch of the lateral posterior choroidal artery (LPCA) of the PCA. A balance is present between the two groups, however, frequently the AchA is predominant taking over the supply of the LPCA at the atrium, and can sometimes also extend along the floor of the third ventricle anastomosing at the level of the foramen of Monro with the Medial Posterior Choroidal Artery of the PCA (MPCA).

In its long course, the artery gives off branches supplying the optic tract and midbrain anastomosing with branches of PcomA and PCA. From the cisternal segment arise many perforators which pass through the APS to supply the medial part of pallidum and the genu of internal capsule. These latter structures can be supplied by perforators arising directly from ICA. Other perforators are involved in the supply of the inferior part of the posterior limb of the internal capsule, its retro-lenticular and sub-lenticular part. Considering these anatomical conditions, it is clear that the clinical symptoms, following occlusion of the AchA selectively due to emboli or following occlusion of ICA are the consequence of involvement of the cisternal segment. In this context, it should be emphasized that the symptoms can be extremely various considering the connections with the PCA and the variations of the origin of the perforators.

3.12 Anomalies of the Anterior Choroidal Artery (AchA)

Considering the complex evolution of the artery, it is not surprising that anomalies develop. In this context, the phylogenetic study of Abbie [1, 2] is interesting about the evolution of the AchA from lower vertebrates to the humans. In his work, Abbie has shown some similarities in all groups, such as the tight relationship and connections between AchA and PCA and differences concerning the involvement of the AchA in the supply of the choroid plexus.

In the lower reptilian scale, the AchA appears as formed by two components with complete separate origin with distinctive vascular territories. One is a branch arising from the cranial division of ICA and the other arises from the already developed posterior cerebral artery.

Only in the higher reptilian scale (crocodile), the AchA appears as an entity, a vessel formed by the fusion of the above described components arising now from ICA. The artery which is mainly involved in the supply of the optic tract and lateral geniculate body presents many connections with the PCA in which it ends. Considering that the PCA in this group of animals is the essential vessels supplying the visual center (optic lobe), the above described connections are an important contribution to the visual function. The AchA is not involved in the supply of choroid plexus absent or very small in this group of animals.

In the higher evolution scale from mammal to the primates and humans, the AchA undergoes as described above great changes acquiring the human configuration maintaining many connections with the PCA but developing in the human the typical involvement of the choroid plexus.

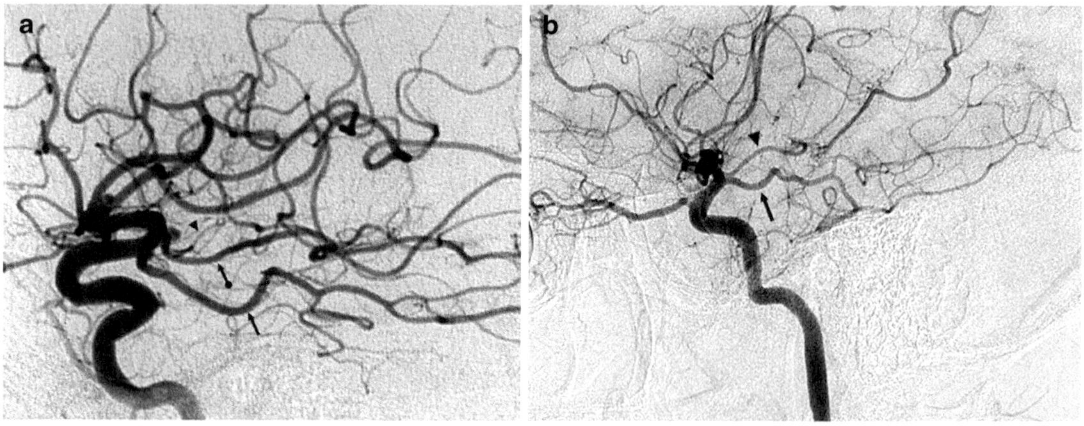

Fig. 3.47 Carotid angiogram. Anomalous pattern of the AchA in two different patients. (**a**) A well-developed AchA (arrow with dot) take over some branches of the PCA (arrow). Note the small perforator of the AchA (arrow head). (**b**) Same pattern. The AchA (arrow head) takes over some branches of the PCA (arrow). (Taken from Bradac [15])

3.12.1 Anomalies in the Human Adult

Some anomalies of the AchA appearing in the adult can be partially explained considering the above phylogenetic study. One is the so-called Hyper-plastic AchA. In this condition, the artery appears to take over partially or completely the vascular territories normally supplied by the PCA. This has been interpreted as an enlargement of the anastomoses between AchA and PCA, in cases of hypo-aplasia of segments of the PCA. The first case has been described on autoptic examination by Blackburn [12]. Later angiographic studies have been reported [40, 63, 138, 140, 161]. This anomaly occurs in about 1.8% and 2.7% in accordance to Takahashi M and Takahashi S respectively (Fig. 3.47a, b).

Cases of "Hypo-plasia," characterized by absence of the plexal segment, can occur, even if they are extremely rare. This configuration reproduces what normally occurs in the higher reptilian (crocodiles). As described above, the AchA is not involved in the supply of the plexus, absent or very small in this group of animals.

The AchA can take its origin proximal to the PcomA. This is an extremely rare variation for which there is no clear explanation. It has been reported in the study by Moyer et al. [98] and Nisho et al. [105].

A case of absence has been reported by Carpenter [17]. On the basis of the today experience, this could be explained by absence of the PcomA replaced by a large AchA.

3.13 Posterior Cerebral Artery

In the fetal phase, the primordial PCA undergoes further changes which have already begun at the end of the embryonic phase, mainly related to two processes. The one is the extent of the artery dorsally towards the occipital lobe contributing to the formation of the visual center, the second is the shift of its origin from ICA to the basilar artery to compensate the increased distance.

At birth, the artery has reached its final "adult" configuration which later on the basis of radio-anatomical and angiographic studies has been divided in a few segments [82, 124, 153, 161].

The first segment arising from the BA is called the P1. It runs in the interpeduncular fossa surrounding the cerebral pedoncules. It gives off perforators-branches described by Foix and

Hillemand [34] as "Thalamo-perforating branches" and later by Percheron [112, 113] as "Para-median Thalamic Arteries" (Fig. 3.48a, b).

They can appear as a group of arteries in which each branch has a separate course supplying its specific territory or as a common trunk dividing distally in their specific branches. The branches are subdivided in anterior supplying the anterior part of Thalamus and Mesencephalon and Posterior for the Middle-Posterior part of Thalamus and Mesencephalon [37, 132, 155]. The different origin of the PCAS will influence the origin of the perforators. The branches can arise prevalently from PcomA or P1, or can be distributed on both PcomA an P1 if both are present. Furthermore, the perforators can arise prevalently or completely from one P1 or PcomA [32, 66] (Fig. 3.49a–c).

Other arteries arising from P1 are the Mesencephalic branches, running around the midbrain, supplying it. They extend dorsally to the quadrigeminal area anastomosing with branches of the superior cerebellar artery. One of these branches, sometimes larger has been called the Collicular or Quadrigeminal artery [37, 132].

One particular artery arising from P1 is a meningeal branch. It runs along the inferior margin of the tentorium towards the falco-tentorial area. It has been described by Wollschlaeger and Wollschlaeger [156], who called it the *"Davidoff-Schechter"* artery, in homage to their supporters. The very small branch is frequently present. It is, however, recognizable on the angiogram only in pathological conditions (Fig. 3.50).

The second segment is called P2. This runs around the midbrain lying below the AchA and Basal Vein and above the superior cerebellar artery. It gives off the thalamo-geniculate artery,

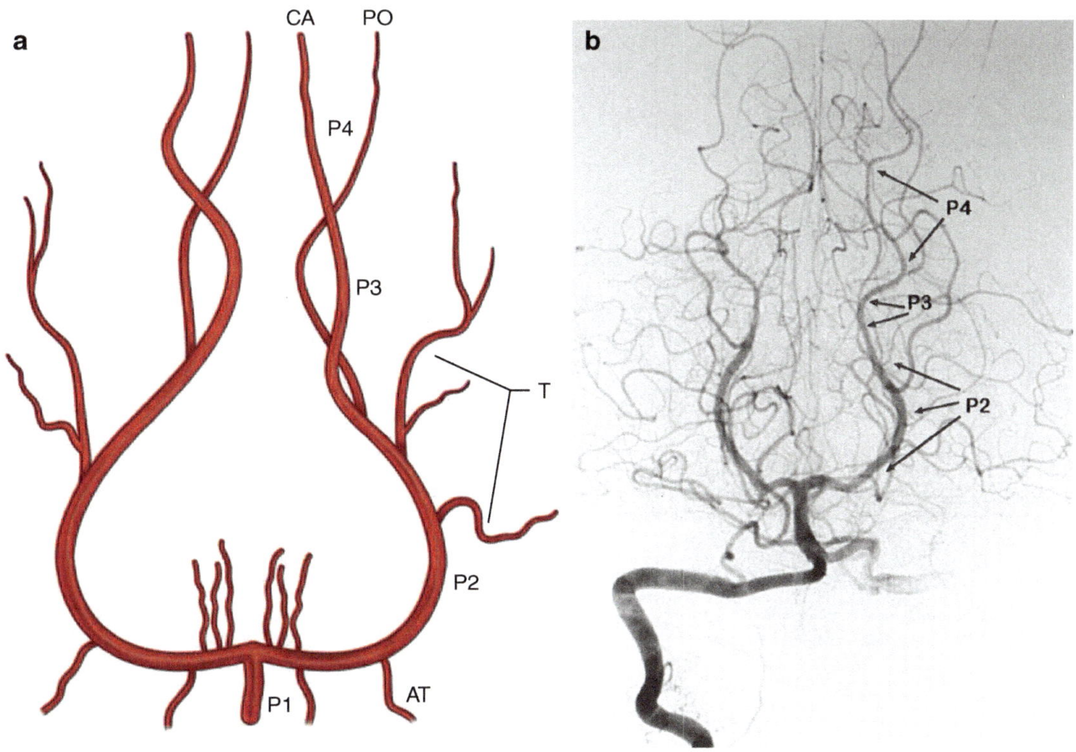

Fig. 3.48 (**a**) Diagram showing the course of the PCA with its segments (P1–P4). Anterior temporal branch (AT). Temporal branches (T). Calcarine Artery (CA). Parieto-Occipital (PO). (**b**) Vertebral angiogram, same indications. (Fig b taken from Bradac [15])

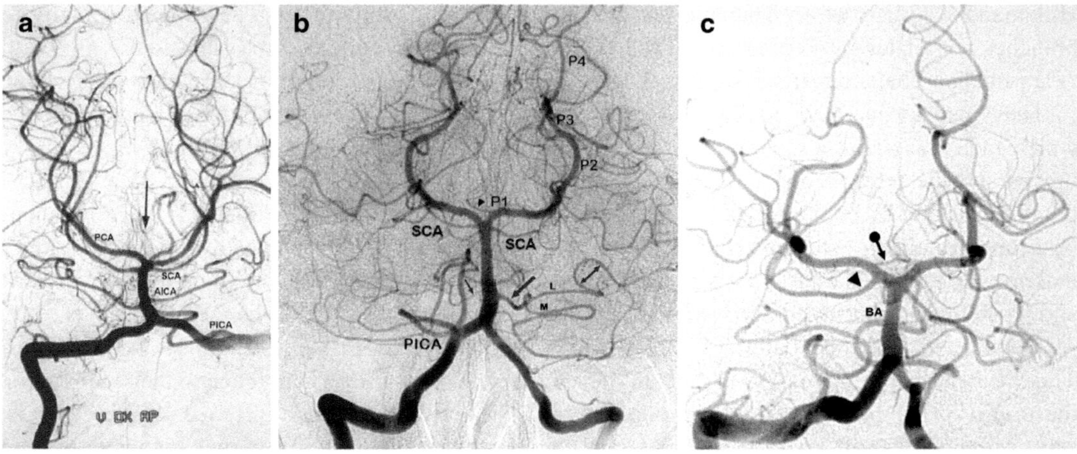

Fig. 3.49 Vertebral angiograms. (**a**) Origin of the Thalamo-Perforate branches (arrow) from both P1. Superior Cerebellar Artery (SCA), Anterior Inferior Cerebellar Artery (AICA), Posterior Cerebellar Artery (PICA). (**b**) The Thalamo-Perforate branches (arrow head) seem to arise predominantly from the left P1. SCA, Lateral (L) and Medial (M) branches of the AICA. Typical curve of its lateral branch at the level of the VII, VIII nerves (arrow). Right well-developed PICA. (**c**) Another example of unilateral origin of the Thalamo-Perforate branches (arrow with dot). SCA on the right arises from the P1 (arrowhead). (Figs a and b taken from Bradac [15])

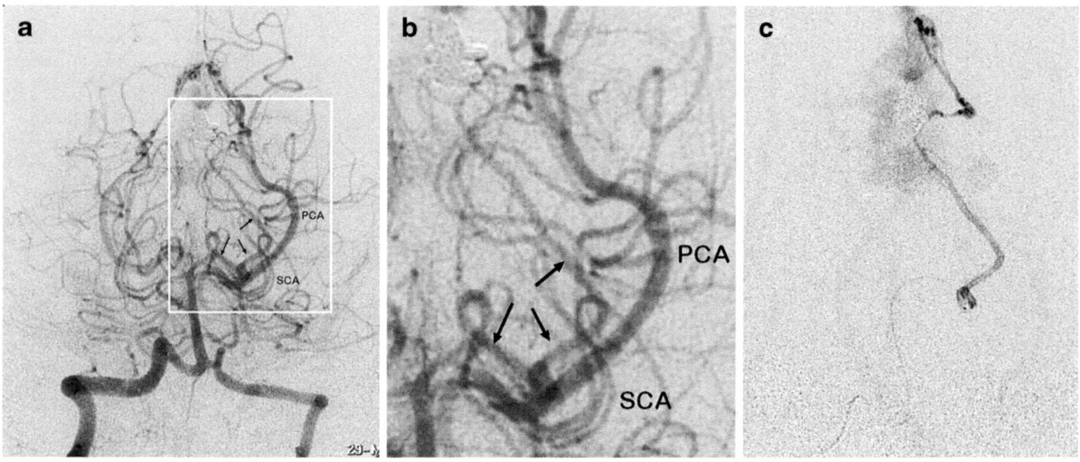

Fig. 3.50 (**a**) Angiogram showing an example of the "Davidoff–Schechter Artery" in DAVF (arrows). Posterior Cerebral Artery (PCA), Superior Cerebellar Artery (SCA). (**b**) Magnification. (**c**) Selective study

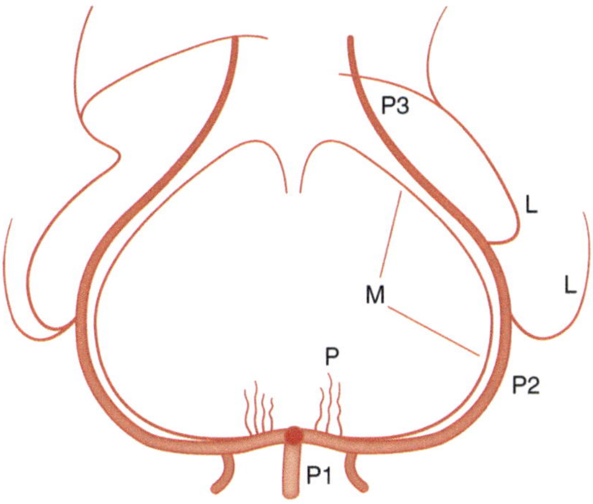

Fig. 3.51 Diagram showing the course of the Posterior Medial (M) and Lateral (L) choroidal branches. P1, P2, and P3 segments of the PCA. Thalamo-perforated branches (P). (Taken from Bradac [15])

supplying the lateral thalamus and the choroidal branches.

The choroidal branches deserve a special description. These branches similar to the AchA have a first part (cisternal) involved in the supply of parenchyma and a second "Plexal" devoted to the choroid plexus [35]. The posterior middle choroid artery arises from P1, runs along the midbrain reaching the posterior thalamus supplying it. It turns then anteriorly, enters the roof of the third ventricle, coursing towards the foramen of Monro where it can be sometimes anastomoses with branches of the AchA. The posterior lateral choroid artery arises from P2, runs around the midbrain reaching the posterior thalamus supplying these structures. At the level of the lateral geniculate body, it sends a branch to supply its medial part anastomosing with branches of the AchA devoted to its lateral part. Another branch enters the choroid fissure contributing to the supply of the posterior part of the plexus of the temporal horn and extending to the atrium. There are anastomoses with the AchA. In the diagram in Fig. 3.51, the course of the medial and lateral choroidal arteries is shown.

The P2 segments end at the quadrigeminal cistern, where the segments of both side run close to each other forming the so-called P3 segment.

From the P3 arise the distal branches forming the P4 segment. These are the Parieto-occipital (PO), the Calcarine (CA), and the Splenial (S) Arteries. These branches arise frequently from P3 or sometimes from P2 as a common trunk dividing distally or as separate branches. Independently from their origin, they run to the vascular territory for which they are programmed. The PO runs towards the parietal area supplying the cuneus and partially the precuneus anastomosing with the parietal branches of the ACA and inferiorly with the CA. The CA runs inferiorly to the PO towards the calcarine fissure. Not rarely, the CA divides in a superior and inferior trunk, from which arise branches directed to the calcarine fissure [130].

As far as it concerns the splenial artery, it can have a different origin. It runs around the splenium anastomosing with the corresponding branch of the ACA.

Other cortical branches, arising from the P2 segment, are devoted to the inferior medial surface of the temporal lobe including the supply of the hippocampus and partially the inferior part of the occipital lobe. They anastomose laterally with the branches of the MCA and at the level of the uncus with the AchA. The most posterior branches, sometimes very large (temporo-occipital artery) can contribute to the supply the visual cortex. The course of the distal branches is shown in Fig. 3.52.

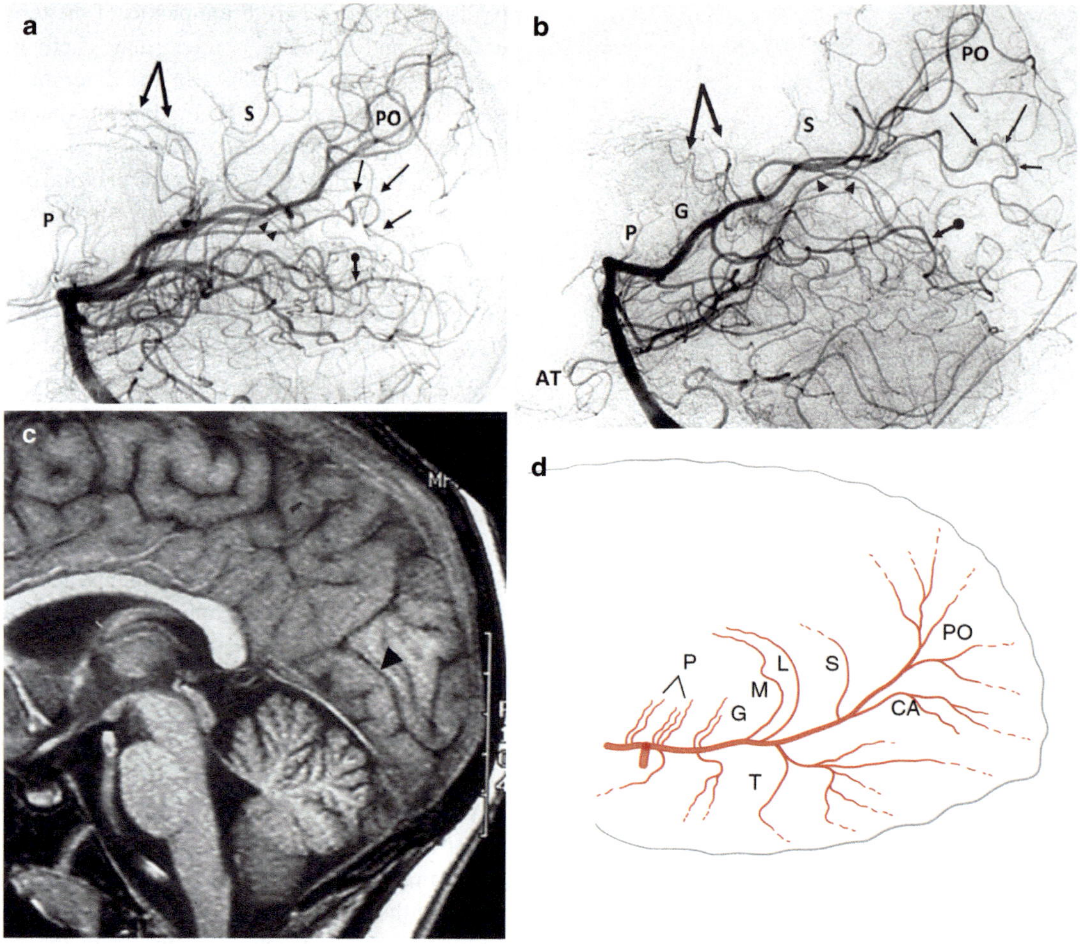

Fig. 3.52 (**a**) Lateral vertebral angiogram, Perforating branches (P), Posterior Choroidal branches (arrow with angle), Splenial Artery (S), Calcarine (arrow), Posterior-Occipital (PO), Temporal (arrow with dot) arteries. (**b**) Same indications. There is a better demonstration of the cerebellar branches of the SCA (arrowhead) and of the Thalamo-Geniculate (arrow with angle) and of the Anterior Temporal branches (AT). (**c**) MR showing the Calcarine fissure (arrow head). (**d**) Diagram with the same indications. (Taken from Bradac [15])

3.14 Anomalies of the PCA

A discussed in Chap. 2, the PCA changes: in the fetal phase its origin shifting from the PcomA to the basilar artery. In the adult, its origin from the BA is in 70%, from the PcomA in 30%. In 20% the artery can have a double origin. An example is shown in Fig. 3.53.

This different configuration can influence the distribution of the perforators which can furthermore as already described above have a predominant origin from one side. Other variations are:

- Cases of segmental duplication have been reported [157].

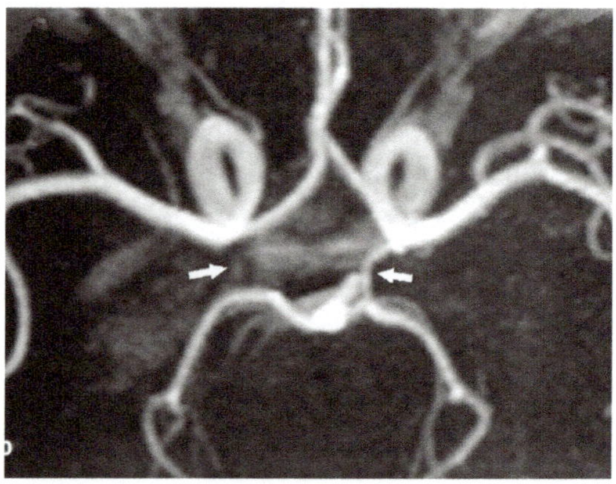

Fig. 3.53 MR angiogram showing the well-developed P1 (arrow) on one side, and aplasia (arrow) on the other side. (Taken from Bradac [15])

- Anomalies due to connections with the AchA have been described in the chapter (AchA).
- Anomalies, developing through persistence of the primary trigeminal artery or other pre-segmental branches are discussed in Chap. 4.

3.15 Further Evolution of the Vertebrobasilar System

As described in Chap. 2, the Vertebro-basilar system (VB) has developed by the junction of its two main components: the basilar artery appearing at the 9–10 mm embryo and the subclavian-vertebral arteries at the 12 mm embryo as described in Chap. 2. In the further evolution, the VB, at the end of the embryonic phase, reaches the configuration similar to that of the adult.

In the fetal phase, the system undergoes further changes involving especially the posterior cerebral artery, as already described above in this chapter. Other changes involve the vascularization of brainstem and little later of cerebellum, as well as that of the cervical spinal cord, through the spinal arteries.

In the diagram (Fig. 3.54) the typical adult course of the extra-intracranial VA joining the BA is shown.

From its origin from the subclavian artery now branches on the left of the aortic arch and on the right of the innominate trunk, each VA takes a dorsal course to reach the transverse foramen of the sixth cervical vertebra. The artery runs further cranially through the foramina of the transverse processes from C6 to C2 surrounded by the vertebral venous plexus. Between C2–C1, the arteries curve laterally and exiting from C1 the VAs take a horizontal dorsal course on the sulcus of the posterior arch of C1. Then each VA forms a second curve directed anteriorly to enter the foramen magnum. It perforates the dura, then runs in the subarachnoid space lateral to the medulla then anteriorly to it, joining commonly at the level of the ponto-medullary sulcus the contralateral continuing in the basilar artery.

As far as it concerns the BA, the artery courses upwards behind the *clivus* in the pre-pontine cistern, close to the surface of the pons on the midline showing sometimes lateral deviation. At the level of the interpeduncular cistern, between the cerebral peduncles, the Ba ends dividing in the P1 segments continuing in the PCAs.

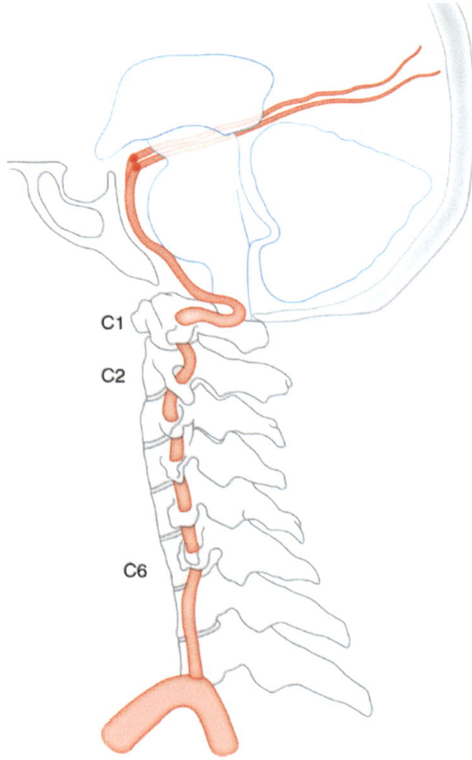

Fig. 3.54 Diagram showing the course of the extra cranial Vertebral Artery (VA). The artery runs from the sixth cervical vertebra, cranially through the foramina of the transverse processes towards the skull basis. At the Foramen magnum the VA enters the cranial cavity, perforates the Dura running in the Subarachnoid Space. It joins the contro-lateral VA continuing in the Basilar artery (BA). As far as it concerns the BA, it runs behind the clivus in the pre-pontine cistern continuing at the level of the Interpeduncular cistern in the P1 and further in the PCA. (Taken from Bradac [15])

3.16 Extracranial Branches of the Vertebral Artery

On his cervical course, the vertebral artery gives off several branches. These are the radiculo-medullary arteries, commonly arising at C4–C5 level, sometimes also more caudally located, in descending and ascending branches. These latter anastomose with the developed anterior spinal artery, arisen from the intracranial VA (Fig. 3.55). The origin and course of the ASA and as well as of the posterior spinal artery from VA are described separately further in this section.

Other branches arising from the extracranial VAs are the musculo-cutaneous branches. These can have potential anastomoses with branches of ECA. The most frequent and well developed are the connections at the level of C1–C2 with the occipital artery and at C3–C4 with the ascending pharyngeal artery. Anastomoses can develop also with the cervical arteries (ascending and deep cervical arteries) [63, 96]. These connections can be an important collateral circulation between these vascular territories and should be taken into consideration by endovascular treatment performed in these regions (Figs. 3.56 and 3.57).

Short before its entry in the cranial cavity, at the level of the foramen magnum, from the VA arises frequently a meningeal branch. More about the meningeal branches is in Chap. 8.

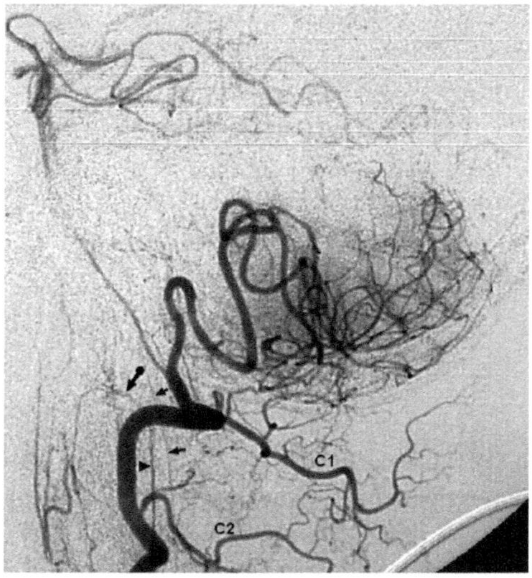

Fig. 3.56 Angiogram. Hypoplastic VA ending in the PICA There are large musculocutaneous branches at the C1–C2 level, potential anastomoses with the Occipital artery. Anastomosis between the Hypoglossal branch of the AphA (arrow with dot) and the Meningo-meningeal branch of the VA (arrow head). Anterior spinal artery (arrow). (Taken from Bradac [15])

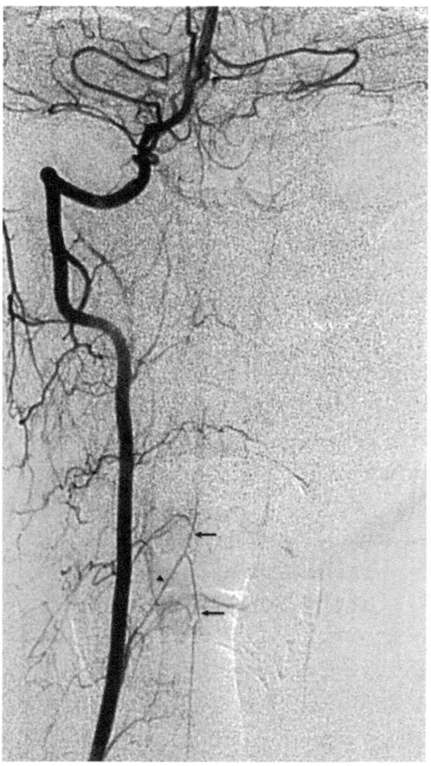

Fig. 3.55 Vertebral angiogram. Radiculo-Meningeal branch dividing in descending and ascending branches (arrow). (Taken from Bradac [15])

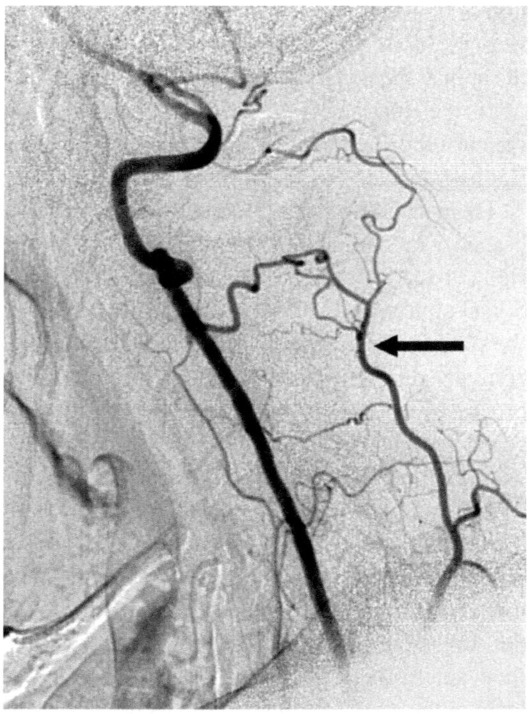

Fig. 3.57 Angiogram of the Subclavian Artery. There is a small Vertebral Artery. Well-developed Deep Cervical Artery (arrow) supplying also the territory of the hypo plastic ascending Cervical Artery. Anastomoses of both Cervical Arteries with the VA. (Taken from Bradac [15])

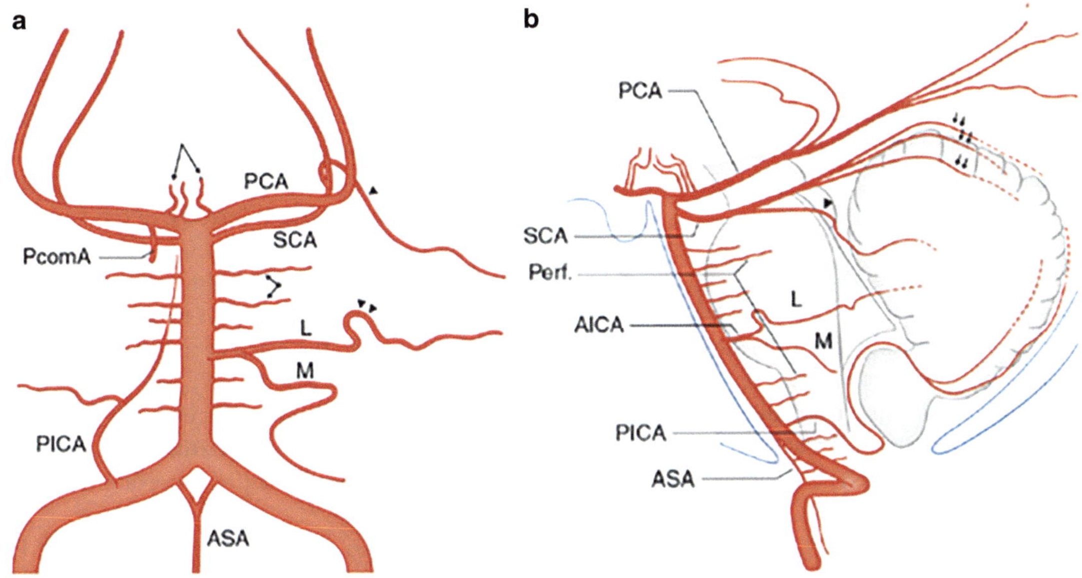

Fig. 3.58 Diagram showing the course of the VA and BA and their branches in the intracranial sector. (**a**) AP view. The VA unite forming the BA, continuing in the PCAs. Bilateral symmetric origin of the Thalamo-Perforate branches (arrow with angle). Right well-developed PICA, absent on the left. Well-developed left AICA. Lateral branch, Medial branch (M) taking over the territory of PICA. Branches of the BA (arrow). Anterior Spinal artery (ASA). Typical course of the SCA. (**b**) Lateral view. Same indications as in (**a**). Cerebellar branches of the SCA (arrows). Marginal branch (M). Note the different segments of PICA: Anterior-Lateral Medullary, Retro Medullary, Supra-tonsillar, Vermian Hemispheric branches (H). Anterior spinal artery (ASA). (Taken from Bradac [15])

Intra-cranially, from the vertebro-basilar sector, arise many branches involved in the supply of brainstem and cerebellum. These are shown in the diagram (Fig. 3.58).

3.17 Intracranial Branches

In the vascularization of pons and medulla, many vessels are involved, arising from BA and VA. As far as it concerns the mesencephalon, a contribution comes also from the PCA and AchA. These arteries have been subdivided in anterior (antero-medial, antero-lateral), lateral and posterior, considering the point where these vessels penetrate the parenchyma [32, 37, 65, 143].

These arteries can perforate in short after their origin from the main trunk, others run first on the surface of the parenchyma before entering it. There are many anastomoses between the superficial branches, while the perforators are end-arteries, without possibility of collateral circulation similarly as it has been described in other sectors.

3.17.1 Arteries of the Medulla

The antero-medial arise from the anterior spinal and vertebral arteries. They enter the medulla at the anterior-medial sulcus. Some other runs first on the surface of medulla before entering it (antero-lateral).

The lateral arises from the VA and PICA. The contribution of the PICA depends on the extent of its medullary course, which can sometimes be very limited.

The posterior arise from PICA and posterior spinal arteries.

3.17.2 Arteries of the Pons

The antero-medial arise from the BA, entering the parenchyma and the basilar sulcus. Others (antero-lateral group) enter the parenchyma more lateral after a short superficial course.

The laterals arise from BA and for the Middle Cerebellar Peduncles from AICA.

The posterior are branches of the Superior Cerebellar Artery.

3.17.3 Mesencephalon

The anterior-medial are branches of the thalamo—perforating branches (P1).

The laterals arise from the SCA, PCA, and AchA, anastomosing to each other before entering the parenchyma. The posterior is mainly the collicular branch of the PCA, which, at the level of the superior colliculus forms a reach anastomoses with the inferior collicular artery, branch of the SCA.

3.17.4 Cerebellar Arteries

Considering the particular evolution of the Cerebellar Arteries, these are described separately.

As described in Chap. 2, the *Superior Cerebellar Artery* (SCA) appears early at the embryo of 9–10 mm following the development of the basilar artery. The pattern of the SCA is relatively constant. It arises from the distal BA, it runs antero-laterally on the surface of the pons, being inferior to the oculomotor nerve which separates the artery from the PCA. It runs further around the midbrain (midbrain segment) inferiorly to the edge of the tentorium to which it can have a contact. The trunk or one of its branches can make a loop caudally coming in contact with the trigeminal nerve [43]. At the level of the quadrigeminal plate both SCA approach to each other, then each artery continues in a vermis branch which is considered the terminal branch of the SCA. In its pontine, midbrain and quadrigeminal course the SCA giving off branches anastomosing with branches of PCA, then penetrate the superior part of pons and midbrain supplying them. Other branches are devoted to the vascularization of cerebellum. The first of these is the marginal branch running latero-caudally, its extent is in balance with the lateral branch of the AICA. Other branches extend dorsally to supply the superior vermis and the superior cerebellar hemispheres. These branches arise from the midbrain portion of the SCA which lies inferiorly to the superior surface of the cerebellum. To reach it, the branches are forced to run first upwards towards the cerebellar convexity, then curve downwards extending along the surface of the cerebellar hemispheres (Fig. 3.59d).

The course of the artery is relatively constant, the changes of its configuration are rare and basically they modify little the pattern of the artery.

Among these, there is its origin from the P1 and the possible duplication or triplication [81].

As far as it concerns the AICA and PICA, as described in Chap. 2 their development is slower, reaching the final typical configuration in the advanced fetal phase, around the embryo aged of 180–190 days. This evolution is connected to the late appearing of the cerebellar hemispheres, of which AICA and PICA are the essential contributor vessels. The cerebellar hemispheres begin to appear at the embryo of 90 days, and this development becomes faster at the embryo of 150 days [61, 62, 111, 122]. This growth is also associated with that of the Pons, with development of the cortico-pons cerebellar fibers.

In the phylogenetic scale, the growth of cerebellum appears first in animal with complex body movement as in the birds and swimming reptiles. The growth is greater in the primates, reaching his maximum development in human.

In the adult configuration, the typical anterior inferior cerebellar artery (AICA) arises from the middle segment of the BA, it runs laterally on the inferior surface of the pons and the middle cerebellar peduncles, dividing them in lateral and medial branches [101].

The lateral branch (L) extents to the *flocculus*, where it forms frequently a complex loop around the seventh-eighth nerves, extending sometimes into the *meatus acusticus*. At this level the artery gives off three important branches: the one is the auditory—labyrinth artery. This branch can arise

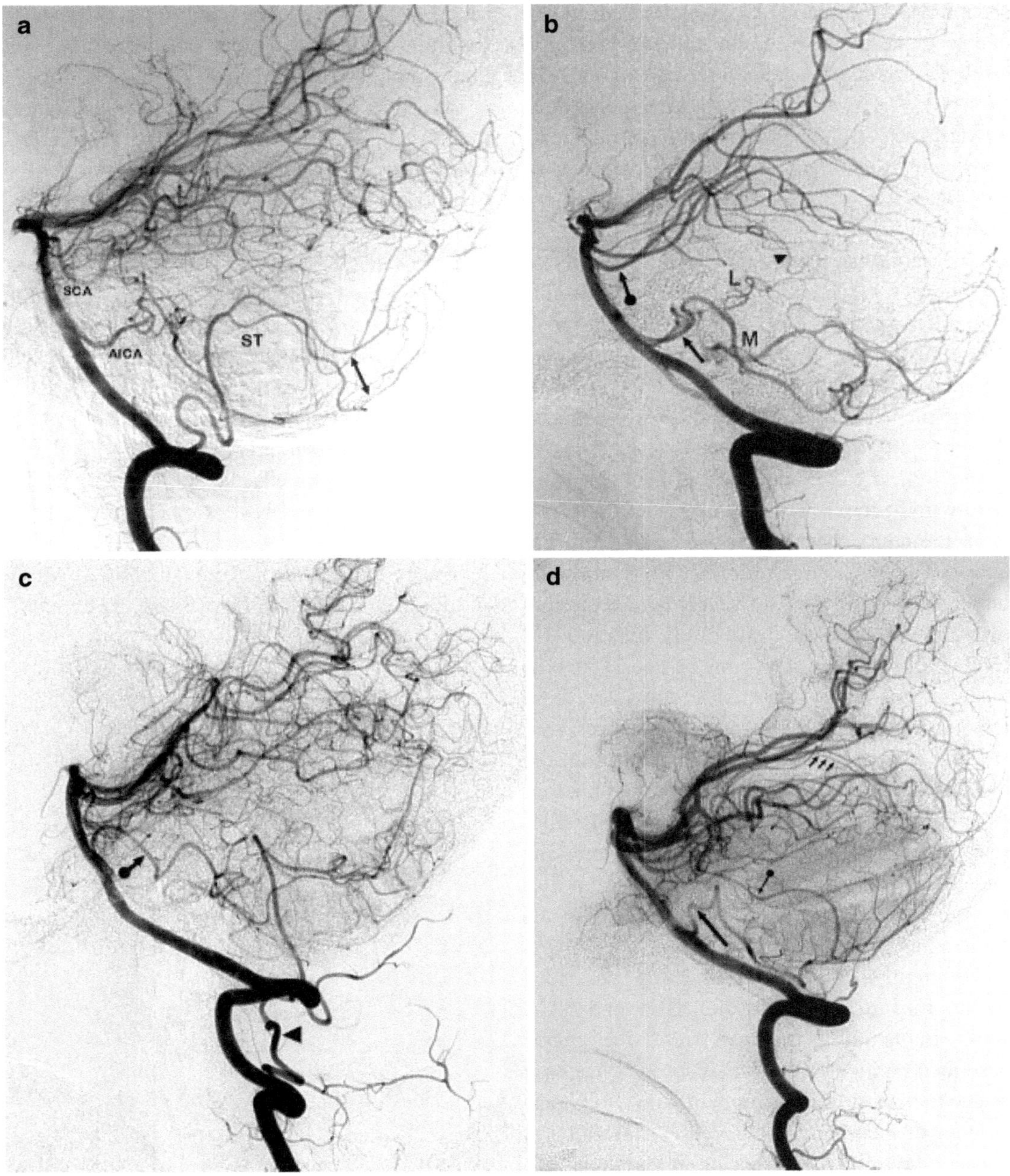

Fig. 3.59 (**a**) Typical course of SCA. AICA with a well-developed Medial branch. PICA with a well-developed Supra-tonsillar segment (ST). Distal cerebellar branches (arrow). (**b**) SCA (arrow with dot). Marginal branch (arrow head). PICA is absent. Well-developed AICA (arrow). Its Medial branch (M) takes over the territory of PICA. (**c**) Origin of PICA from C2 (arrow). The trunk of AICA is not recognizable. There is a branch, probably its superior accessory component (arrow wit dot), which contributes to the vascularization of PICA. (**d**) PICA is absent, its territory is taken over by the AICA (arrow) and by the Marginal branch of SCA (arrow with dot). Hemispheric cerebellar branches of SCA (arrows). (Taken from Bradac [15])

separately from the BA, as described in the embryogenic phase by Padget. It has been precisely described in the adult by some authors [53, 54, 100]. The second is the dural vessels which anastomoses on the surface of the petrous bone, with petro-squamous branches of the middle meningeal artery. The third is a recurrent branch to the Pons.

The lateral branch extents further laterally on the anterior surface of cerebellum, connecting with the marginal branch of the SCA. It gives off also some branches for the lateral part of the choroid plexus of the fourth ventricle.

The medial branch (M) is frequently smaller, it runs on the anterior-medial surface of cerebellum, it can enlarge when involved in the supply in the hypo-plastic or a-plastic PICA.

In the adult, the posterior inferior cerebellar artery (PICA) arises from the VA commonly intra-cranially. It can, however, take its origin extra-cranially at the C1 and rarely at the C1–C2 level [82]. It runs first antero-lateral to the medulla (medullary segment), having a close relationship with 9th, 10th, and 11th nerves.

It takes then an upwards course between the surface of medulla and antero-surface of the tonsilla. It makes then a typical curve (supratonsillar segment) where branches arise, supplying the choroid plexus, descending then along the posterior surface of the tonsillar, dividing in its Vermian and Hemisphere branches.

Differently from the SCA, as already described by Stopford in 1916 [135], the AICA and PICA show frequently variations from the above described configuration. This can be considered as due to their slow development with a long persistence of their plexural structures, described in Chap. 2, favoring the appearing of variations.

AICA and PICA appear with their typical configuration in about 50% of the cases. In 40%, both or one AICA is dominant, replacing partially or completely the PICA. In 10% PICA is dominant. It can also occur that the SCA, especially with its marginal branch, takes over the vascular territories of the hypo-plastic AICA and PICA.

Another variation involving the AICA is the presence, in association with the main trunk, of one or two accessories branches [101]. The one is running superiorly to the main trunk, close to the trigeminal nerve, the other one inferiorly. This latter can replace the medial branch of AICA.

As far as it concerns the PICA, an extremely rare anomaly is its duplication [64, 72, 73, 110, 160]. In this condition, the PICA is formed by two branches which have a separate origin and unite in the distal trunk. More about this variation is described in the section "Posterior Spinal Artery."

Another extremely rare anomaly is its origin from the posterior meningeal artery as reported by some author [108].

Anomalies associated with trigeminal artery and the hypoglossal artery, as well as is relation with the hypoglossal and jugular branch of ascending pharyngeal artery are described in Chap. 5.

The normal and variant course of SCA, AICA, and PICA are shown in Figs. 3.49b, 3.58, 3.59a–d, 3.60, and 3.61.

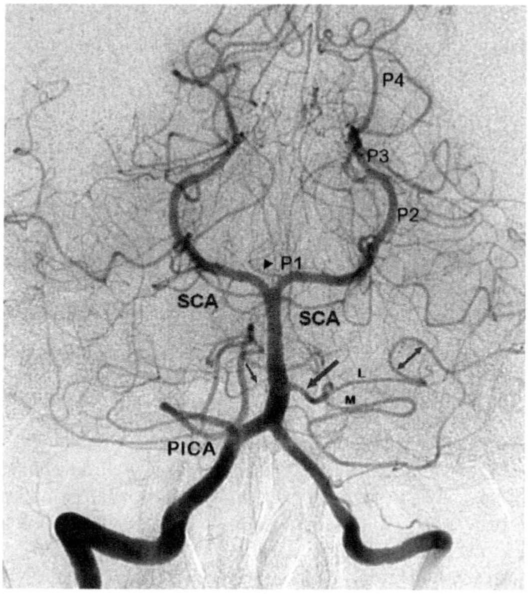

Fig. 3.60 Vertebral Angiogram, AP view. PICA well-developed on the right. Absent on the left. Its territory is taken over by a great AICA. Lateral (L) and Middle (M) branches. Typical curve surrounding the VII and VIII nerves. Normal SCA. Asymmetric origin of the Thalamo-Perforate Arteries (arrow head). (Taken from Bradac [15])

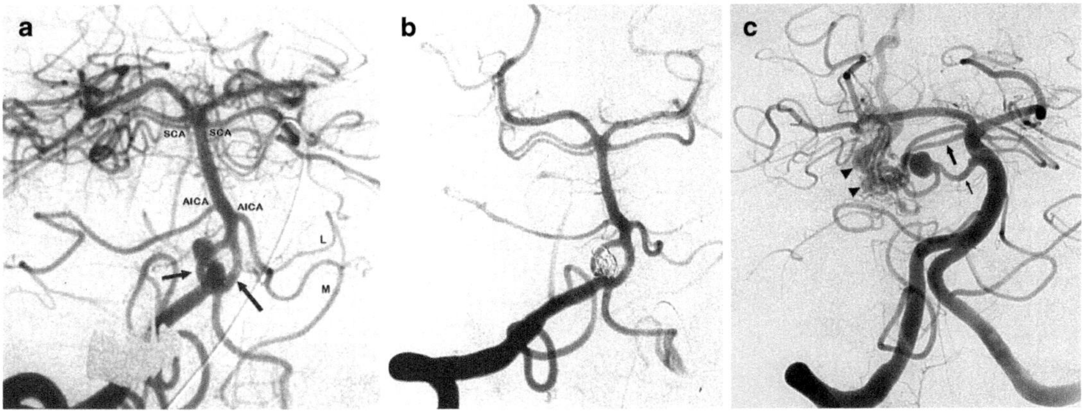

Fig. 3.61 (**a**) Duplication of the proximal BA (arrow), developed at the junction of the two VAs with the BA. The anomaly was associated with an aneurysm, presenting with hemorrhage. (**b**) The same angiogram post-treatment. The duplication is better visible. The duplication of the right SCA is also better recognizable. (**c**) Vertebral angiogram in patient with AVM supplied by a duplicated right SCA (arrow). Another feeding artery arises from the BA (small arrow). This could be also a superior accessory AICA. There is a Stress-aneurysm. Venous drainage (arrow head). (Taken from Bradac [15])

3.18 Other Anomalies of Vertebro-Basilar Sector

Duplication (Complete and Segmental) and Fenestration of the Vertebro-Basilar Sector.

These anomalies, as described also in the previous sections, can involve all cerebral vessels, but are more frequent in the vertebro-basilar sector. The definition of fenestration and duplication, reported in the literature, is not unanimous. This is due to the fact that the same findings are interpreted differently by the various authors.

Basically, fenestration on anatomical studies, is defined when the vessels present with two separate lumens, each lined with the typical endothelium. In the duplication, the vessels have two separate origins, which can, but not always, converge distally.

The angiographic configuration can be variable. In this work, for convenience, the ***fenestration*** *is described as a short division of the lumen of the vessels. In the case in which the division extends for a few segments, the term* ***segmental duplication*** *is used. Furthermore, in this condition both segments arise from a common trunk which distally fuse again together. In the* ***complete duplication****, the vessels have a separate origin.*

These anomalies can involve the extra-cranial and intra-cranial vertebro-basilar system.

Complete Duplication, Fenestration, and Segmental Duplication of the Extra-cranial Vertebral Artery.

As described in the section about variations of the aortic arch, the VA can take its origin from the aortic arch between the left common carotid and the left subclavian arteries or more rarely from the distal left subclavian artery. The anomalous VA can be associated with a normal VA, resulting in duplicated VA (Fig. 3.62, 3.63, and 3.64). Another possible duplication can develop distally more frequently at the C1–C2 level where the VA with the normal course is associated with an anomalous VA having taken its origin from the first intersegmental artery (Fig. 3.64).

As far as it concerns the fenestration and the segmental duplication of the VA, it should be considered that the primordial vertebral artery, developed from longitudinal anastomosis, between the cervical segmental arteries, appears first with an irregular pattern, characterized by dilatation and narrowing. Anomalous evolution from this primordial pattern can explain the configuration presenting with segmental duplication or fenestration. An example of fenestration is shown in Fig. 3.65a.

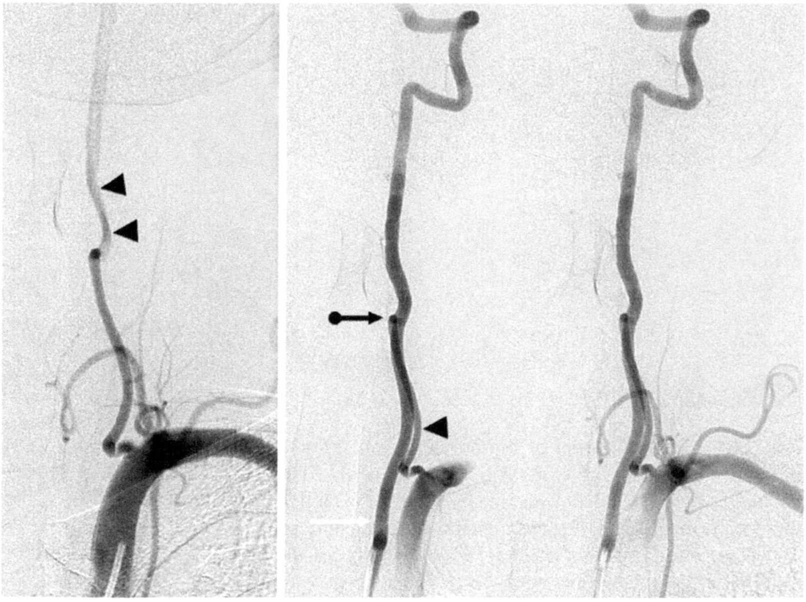

Fig. 3.62 Duplication of Vertebral artery. The normal branch (arrow head) has a typical origin from the subclavian artery. The anomalous branch (arrow with dot) arise from aortic arch. Both branches join together at the fifth transverse foramen. (Taken from Bradac [15])

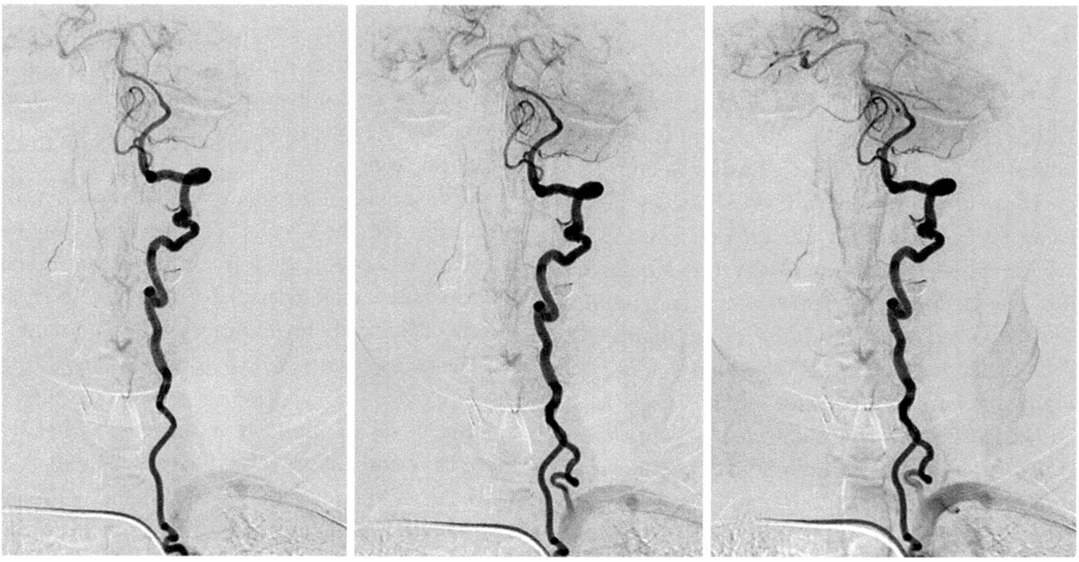

Fig. 3.63 Duplication of VA. One branch arises from the proximal subclavian artery. The second anomalous branch from the distal subclavian artery. Both branches join together at the seventh Foramen

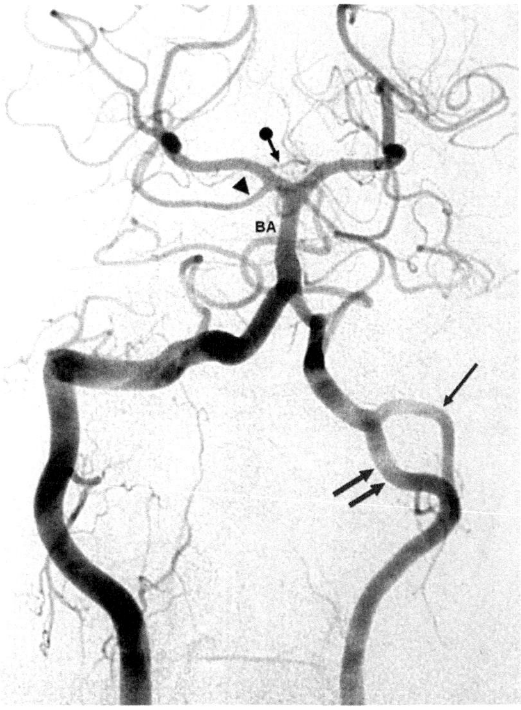

Fig. 3.64 Another example of duplicated VA at the C1–C2 level. Normal (arrow) and anomalous (arrows) branches. Note the anomalous origin of the SCA from the P1 (arrowhead) and the asymmetric origin of the thalamo-perforated branches (arrow with dot)

After having considered the above presented anomalies, it seems useful to make a short consideration about the DISSECTION. This is not an anomaly developed as a deviation from the normal evolution, instead is a real pathological condition. The origin and course of this pathological process has been already described in the section concerning the dissection in the carotid sector which are the same in the dissection of the vessels in the vertebro-basilar sector. On the angiogram, the lumen of the involved artery can present with a narrowing of different lengths, frequently associated with dilatation forming pseudo-aneurysm. It can also show the presence of double lumen or the artery is occluded (Fig. 3.65b). All these changes differ greatly from the segmental duplication or segmentation, where the lumen appear regular as in the normal case. Furthermore, the dissection presents acutely with symptoms depending on the site and type of vessel involved, whereas the anomalies are commonly incidental discovery, provided that are not associated with other pathologies.

3.18.1 Fenestration and Segmental Duplication Involving Intracranial Vertebral and Basilar Artery

These anomalies could be interpreted as a failure of the BLC and of the more cranially primordial irregular structure of the VA to evolve in the typical tubular vessel. Examples involving the BA are presented in Figs. 3.61, 3.67, and 3.68. Segmental duplication of VA is presented in Fig. 3.66.

3.18.2 Segmental and Complete Aplasia of the BA

These are very rare anomalies, for which there is not a clear explanation. In the segmental form, one segment of the BA does not develop. All segments can be involved; the anomaly is more frequent at the level of the middle segment (Fig. 3.69).

An extremely rare aplasia involves the complete BA. In this condition, each VA continues separately in two trunks which replace the Aplastic BA. One could also think that the BA does not develop as a unique trunk, from the fusion of the VAs, but two BAs with separate origin develop.

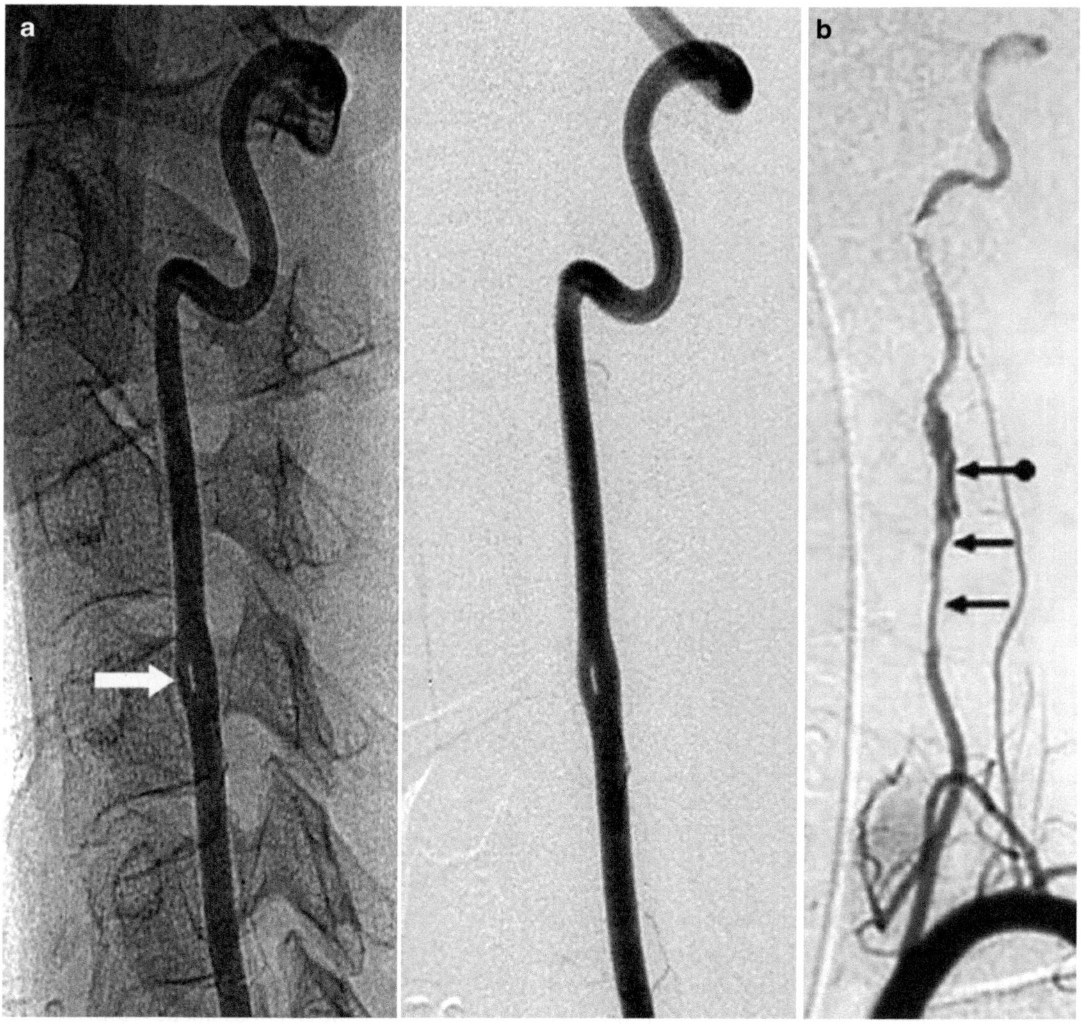

Fig. 3.65 (**a**) Fenestration of the cervical VA (arrow). (**b**) Vertebral angiogram in a case of dissection. Young patient presenting with symptoms of brainstem involvement. Irregularity of the VA, with narrowing (arrows) dilatation (arrow with dot), where also double lumen is recognizable. (Taken from Bradac [15])

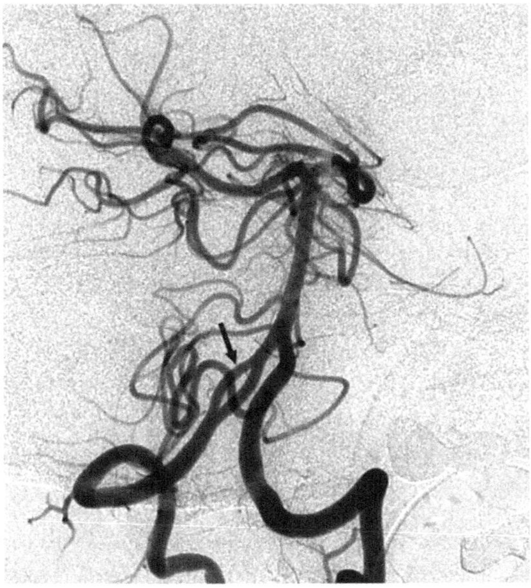

Fig. 3.66 Segmental Duplication of the VA (arrow) shortly before its junction with the BA. (Taken from Bradac [15])

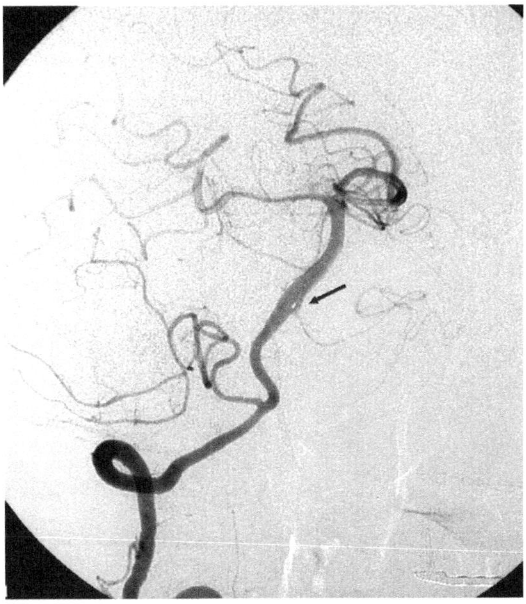

Fig. 3.67 Fenestration of the BA at its middle segment, at the origin of the AICA (arrow). (Taken from Bradac [15])

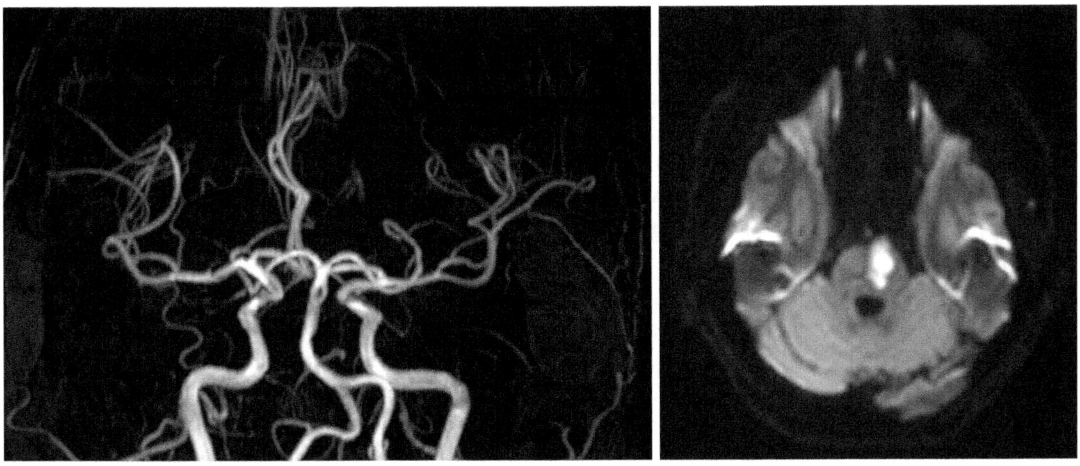

Fig. 3.68 Fenestration of the distal BA in patient with stroke involving the Anterior-Medial perforators arising only from one segment of the fenestrated BA

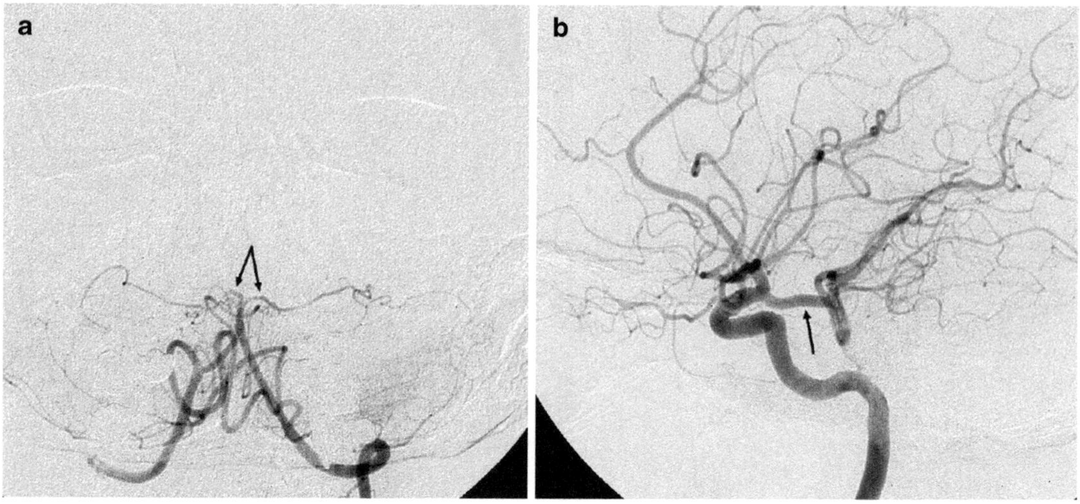

Fig. 3.69 (**a**) Example of a segmental aplasia of the proximal BA at the level of the AICAs (arrow with angle). (**b**) The distal BA is filled through the PcomA (arrow). (Taken from Bradac [15])

3.19 Spinal Arteries

3.19.1 Anterior Spinal (ASA)

The Anterior Spinal Artery (ASA) arises from the developed VA, identified by Padget on the embryo at 14–18 mm. Further detailed anatomo-angiographic studies in the adult [27, 63, 65, 145] have shown that the artery is formed by the fusion of two branches arising each from the VA, intracranially a little more distal to the origin of the future PICA.

The ASA runs first on the anterior surface of the medulla, then on the anterior median sulcus of the cervical spinal cord, connecting with the ascending branch of the cervical ASA, formed by a radiculo-medullary artery, commonly at the level of C4–C6.

The two branches of the ASA are frequently asymmetric, one being larger. The formed ASA can be duplicated, one branch having only a short course ending caudally in the sulcal artery. In 10% of the cases, the artery can have a unilateral origin, and it can also occur that the unique branch arises from the hypoplastic VA.

The artery is involved in the supply of the medulla, through its anterior medial branches, and of the cervical spinal cord through its sulcal branches entering the medial sulcus supplying the anterior horns, partially the posterior horns and the great part of the white matter.

From the sulcal arteries arise superficial branches, running on the lateral surface of the spinal cord, anastomosing with the corresponding superficial branches of the PSA.

3.19.2 Posterior Spinal (PSA)

As far as it concerns the PSA, it has been recognized by Padget at the embryo of 40 mm. Further micro-angiographic studies [63, 121, 145] have shown that the PSA is formed by two branches arising from the intracranial or extracranial VA or from the PICA, running separately on the dorso-lateral surface of the medulla, continuing caudally on the dorso-lateral surface of the spinal cord. The artery supplies the posterior part of the medulla and part of the posterior horn and part of the white matter of the cervical spinal cord.

Other studies have shown the presence of an additional trunk [46, 64, 80, 86, 145] running on the latero-dorsal surface of the cord, ventral to the dorsal nerve, differently from the trunk of the PSA, which are dorsal to the dorsal nerve. This new described system, called Lateral Spinal Artery (LSA), arises from PICA or frequently from VA at the level of C1–C2. Through the LSA, anastomosis develops between the PCA cranially and the VA caudally. The artery is continuing then caudally at the C3–C4 level in the classical postero-lateral trunk of the PSA.

In some cases, these anastomoses can enlarge, explaining in accordance to some authors [64] the presence of some anomalies of the PICA, already described in the section "Cerebellar arteries." The one is the origin of the PICA from extracranial VA (Fig. 3.59c). The other is the duplication (complete) of the PICA (Fig. 3.70). In this case, the artery is formed by two branches having a separate origin. The superior branch corresponds to the normal origin of PICA, the inferior branch is the anastomotic branch of the LSA. Another very rare anomaly related to the presence of the enlarged anastomosis of the LSA and is the condition in which the ascending branch arises from the extracranial VA continuing directly in the VA, which runs vertically without forming a typical course on the other [64].

The ASA is frequently visible on the angiogram (Figs. 3.71, 3.72, and 3.73). Differently the PSA is more rarely identified on the angiogram, unless it is involved in pathological conditions (Fig. 3.74). In other cases, its involvement can be indirectly suspected on the base of angiographic and MR findings (Fig. 3.75).

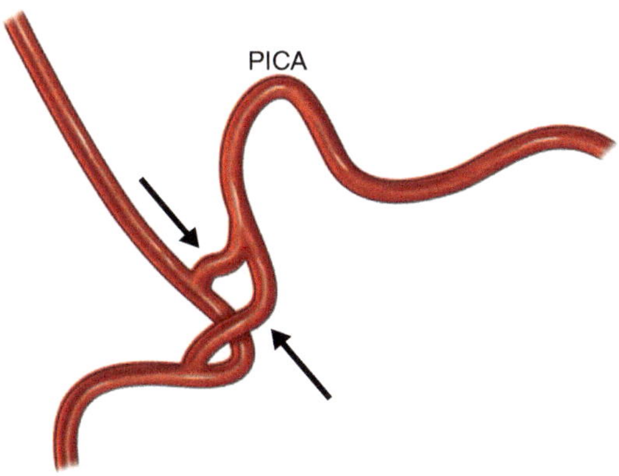

Fig. 3.70 Diagram showing the anomaly of the PICA with its duplicated origin (see also text of PSA). One superior branch arises from the intracranial VA (arrow), the inferior from the VA at the C1 level

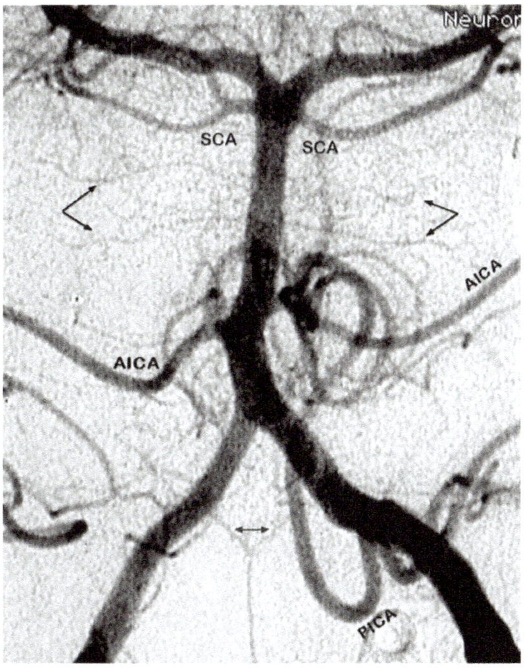

Fig. 3.71 AP vertebral angiogram showing the typical pattern of the ASA (arrow). The PICA, AICA. and SCA are also indicated. Basal branches (arrow with angle). (Taken from Bradac [15])

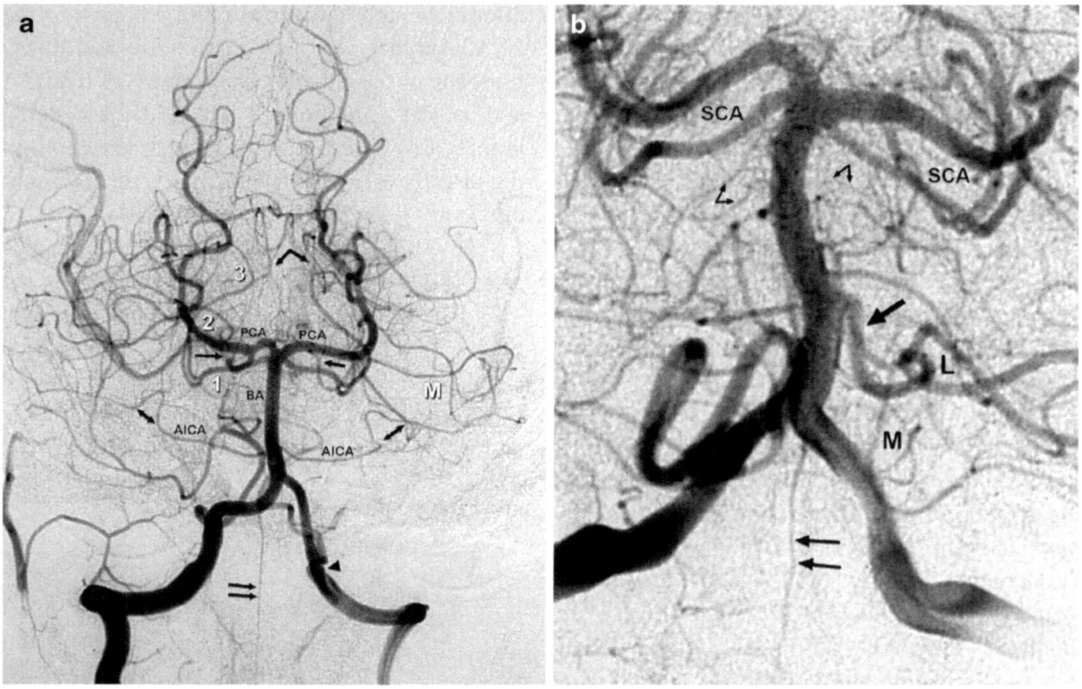

Fig. 3.72 Unilateral origin of the ASA (arrows) from the right VA (**a**) and from the left VA (**b**). The course of the SCA, AICA, and PICA as well as of the branches of the BSA is also indicated. (Taken from Bradac [15])

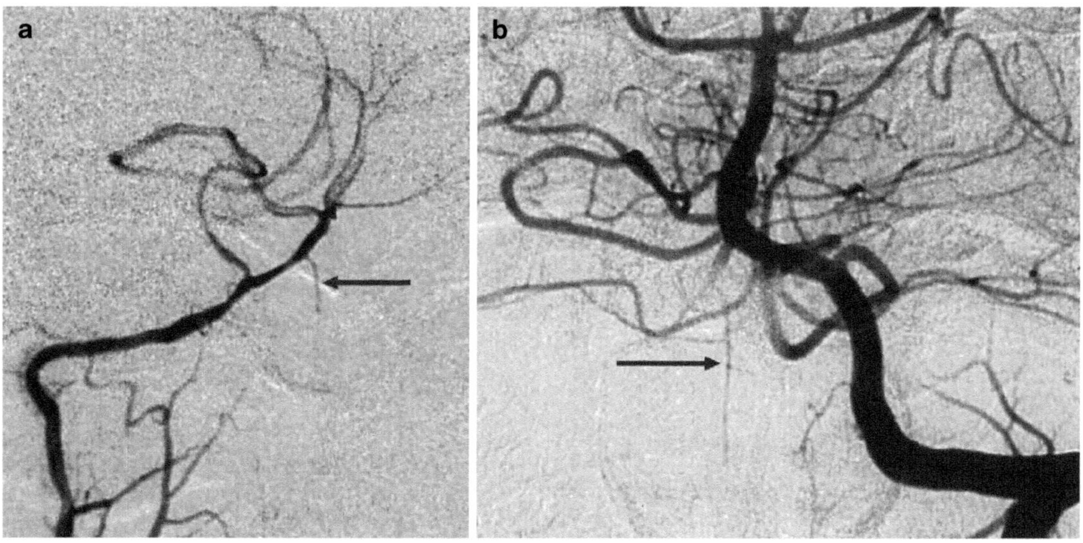

Fig. 3.73 Right hypoplastic VA and left well-developed VA. Unilateral origin of the ASA (arrow) from the right hypoplastic VA. (Taken from Bradac [15])

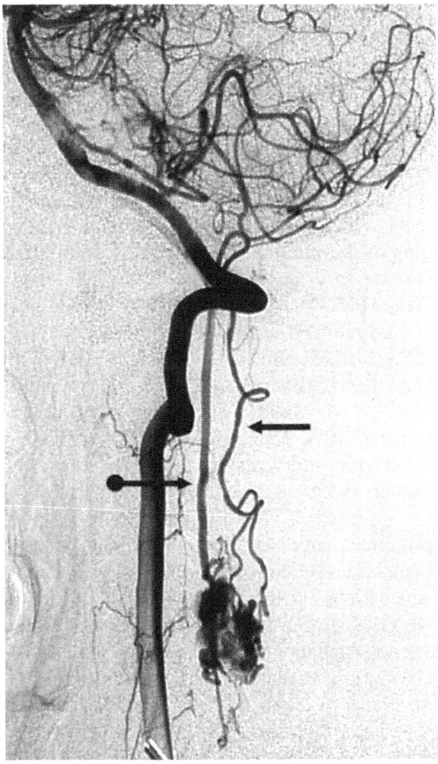

Fig. 3.74 Vertebral angiogram in patient with AVM of cervical spinal cord supplied by a dilated ASA (arrow with dot) and enlarged and tortuous PSA (arrow). (Taken from Bradac [15])

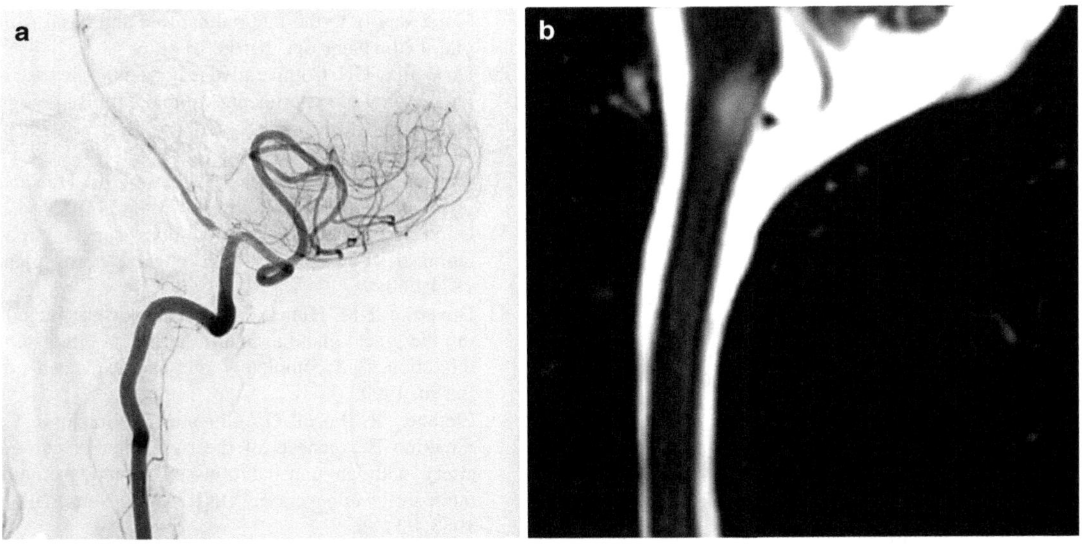

Fig. 3.75 Patient with stroke indicating involvement of Medulla. On the vertebral angiogram, there is a severe narrowing of the proximal VA. The PICA is normal. On CT with contrast there is an infarct in the dorsal medulla indicating involvement of PSA

References

1. Abbie AA. The blood supply of the lateral geniculate body, with a note on the morphology of the choroidal arteries. J Anat. 1933a;67(Pt 4):491.
2. Abbie AA. The clinical significance of the anterior choroidal artery. Brain. 1933b;56(3):233–46.
3. Adachi B, Kihara T. Das Arteriensystem der Japaner, Verlag der Kaiserlich-Japanischen Universitat, zu Kyoto. Kommission bei Maruzen Co. 1928:26–46.
4. Adams WE. The extracanial carotid rete and carotid fork in Nycticebus Coucang. Acad Zool. 1957;2:21–38.
5. Al-Qahtani S, Tampieri D, Brassard R, Sirhan D, Mellanson D. Coil embolization of an aneurysm associated with an infraoptic anterior cerebral artery in a child. Am J Neuroradiol. 2003;24(5):990–1.
6. Andersen CA, Collins GJ Jr, Rich NM, Mcdonald PT. Spontaneous dissection of the internal carotid artery associated with fibromuscular dysplasia. Am Surg. 1980;46:263–6.
7. Apley J. Congenital anomalies of the aortic arch and its branches. Proc R Soc Med. 1949;42(11):918–22.
8. Baptista AG. Studies on the arteries of the brain: II. The anterior cerebral artery: some anatomic features and their clinical implications. Neurology. 1963;13(10):825.
9. Barry A. The aortic arch derivatives in the human adult, vol. 111; 1951. p. 221.
10. Bayford D. An account of a singular case of obstructed deglutition. Mem Med Soc Lond. 1789:275–86.
11. Bernini FP, Cioffi FA, Muras I, Rinaldi F. Carotid syphon-pericallosal arterial anastomosis: case report. Acta Neurochir. 1982;66:61–9.
12. Blackburn IW. Anomalies of the encephalic arteries among the insane. A study of the arteries at the base of the encephallon in two hundred and twenty consecutive cases of mental disease, with special reference to anomalies of the circle of Willis. J Comp Neurol Psychol. 1907;17(6):493–517.
13. Bosma NJ. Infra-optic course of anterior cerebral artery and low bifurcation of the internal carotid artery. Acta Neurochir. 1977;38(3–4):305–12.
14. Bosniak MA. An analysis of some anatomic-roentgenologic aspects of the brachiocephalic vessels. Am J Roentgenol Radium Therapy, Nucl Med. 1964;91:1222–31.
15. Bradac GB. Applied cerebral angiography. Normal anatomy and vascular pathology. Cham: Springer; 2017. https://doi.org/10.1007/978-3-319-57228-4. 497 pages, ISBN 978-3-319-57227-7.
16. Bradač GB, Kaernbach A, Bolk-Weischedel D, Finck GA. Spontaneous dissecting aneurysm of cervical cerebral arteries. Neuroradiology. 1981;21(3):149–54.
17. Carpenter M, Noback C, Moss M. The anterior choroidal artery; its origins course, distribution, and variations. AMA Arch Neurol Psychiatry. 1954;71(6):714–22.
18. Chenin L, Kaoudi A, Foulon P, Havet E, Peltier J. Microsurgical anatomy of the subcallosal artery. Surg Radiol Anat. 2019;41:1037–44.
19. Crompton MR. The pathology of ruptured middle cerebral aneurysms with special reference to the difference between the sexes. Lancet. 1962;2:421–5.
20. Dahn MS, Kaurich JD, Brown FR. Independent origins of the internal and external carotid arteries: a case report. Angiology. 1999;50(9):755–60.
21. Daniel PM, Dawes JDK, Prichard MM. Studies of the carotid rete and its associated arteries. Philos Trans R Soc Lond Ser B Biol Sci. 1953;237(645):173–208.
22. Danziger J. Bilateral rete carotidis in man-a case report. S Afr Med J. 1972;46(40):1487–8.
23. Daseler EHE, Anson B. Surgical anatomy of the subclavian artery and its branches. Surg Gynecol Obstet. 1959;108(2):149–74.
24. De La Torre E, Netsky MG. Study of persistent primitive maxillary artery in human fetus: some homologies of cranial arteries in man and dog. Am J Anat. 1960;106:185.
25. De Vriese B. Sur la signification morphologique des artères. Arch biol (Liege). 1905;21:357.
26. Del Zotto E, Ritelli M, Pezzini A, Drera B, Gamba M, Giossi A, et al. Clinical, neuroradiological and molecular features of a patient affected by pseudoxhantoma elasticum associated to carotid rete mirabile: case report. Clin Neurol Neurosurg. 2012;114(6):758–61.
27. Djindjian R. L'angiographie de la moelle épinière. Angiography of the spinal cord. Paris: Masson et Cie; 1970.
28. Djulejić V, Marinković S, Georgievski B, Stijak L, Aksić M, Puškaš L, et al. Clinical significance of blood supply to the internal capsule and basal ganglia. J Clin Neurosci. 2016;25:19–26.
29. Du Boulay GH. Comparative neuroradiologic vascular anatomy of experimental animals. In: Radiology of the skull and brain. St. Louis: Mosby; 1974. p. 2763–86.
30. du Boulay GH, El Gammal T, Trickey SE. True and false carotid retia. Br J Radiol. 1973;46(543):205–12.
31. Duret H. Recherches anatomiques sur la circulation de l'encéphale. Arch physiol norm path. 1874;I:60–91.
32. Duvernoy HM. Human brain stem vessels: including the pineal gland and information on brain stem infarction. 2nd completely rev. and expanded ed. Berlin; 1999.
33. Elefante R, Fucci G, Granata F, Graziussi G, Smaltino F. Agenesis of the right internal carotid artery with an unusual transsellar intracavernous intercarotid connection. AJNR Am J Neuroradiol. 1983;4(1):88.
34. Foix C. Les artères de l'axe encéphalique jusqu'au diencéphale inclusivement. Rev Neurol. 1925;2:160–79.

35. Fujii K, Lenkey C, Rhoton AL. Microsurgical anatomy of the choroidal arteries: lateral and third ventricles. J Neurosurg. 1980;52(2):165–88.
36. Gibo H, Carver CC, Rhoton AL, et al. Microsurgical anatomy of the middle cerebral artery. J Neurosurg. 1981;54(2):151–69.
37. Gillilan LA. The arterial and venous blood supplies to the forebrain (including the internal capsule) of primates. Neurology. 1968;18(7):653–70.
38. Given CA, Morris PP. Recognition and importance of an infraoptic anterior cerebral artery: case report. Am J Neuroradiol 2002;23(3):452–454.
39. Given CA II, Huang-Hellinger F, Baker MD, Chepuri NB, Morris PP. Congenital absence of the internal carotid artery: case reports and review of the collateral circulation. Am J Neuroradiol. 2001;22(10):1953–9.
40. Goldberg HL. The anterior choroidal artery. In: Newton TH, Potts, editors. Angiography. Radiology of skull and brain. St Louis: Mosby; 1974.
41. Gozzoli L, Crasto S, Leombruni S, Bradac GB. Magnetic resonance angiography in a case of agenesis of the left carotid artery associated with transellar intercarotid anastomosis. Rivista Neuroradiol. 1998;11(6):883–6.
42. Gregg L, San Millán D, Tamargo RJ, Gailloud P. Ventral and dorsal persistent primitive ophthalmic arteries. Oper Neurosurg. 2016;12(2):141–52.
43. Hardy DG, Rhoton AL. Microsurgical relationships of the superior cerebellar artery and the trigeminal nerve. J Neurosurg. 1978;49(5):669–78.
44. Harnsberger HR. Handbook of head and neck imaging. St. Louis: Mosby; 1995.
45. Haughton VM, Rosenbaum EE. The normal and anomalous aortic arch and brachiocephalic arteries. In: Radiology of the skull and brain, vol. 2; 1974. p. 1145–63.
46. Hiramatsu M, Sugiu K, Yasuhara T, Hishikawa T, Haruma J, Nishi K, et al. Angioarchitecture of the normal lateral spinal artery and craniocervical junction arteriovenous fistula using contrast-enhanced cone-beam CT. Clin Neuroradiol. 2022;33:375.
47. Hong JM, Lee JH, Yong SW. Asymtomatic rete mirabile in carotid and vertebral circulation systems. J Neurol Neurosurg Psychiatry. 2010;81(9):1022–3.
48. Huber P. Zerebrale Angiographie fuer klinik und praxis. (No Title). 1979.
49. Jentzer A. Dissecting aneurysm of the left internal carotid artery. Angiology. 1954;5(3):232–4.
50. Kakou M, Destrieux C, Velut S. Microanatomy of the pericallosal arterial complex. J Neurosurg. 2000;93(4):667–75.
51. Kantor H. Tiefe Teilung der Arteria carotis communis. Anat Anz. 1905;26:492–6.
52. Kemmetmüller H. Über eine seltene Varietät der Art. Vertebralis Anatomische Hefte. 1911a;44:305–60.
53. Kemmetmüller H. Ueber eine seltene Varietät der Art. vertebralis. Anatomische Hefte. 1911b;44:305–60.
54. Kier EL. Fetal cerebral arteries: a phylogenetic and ontogenetic study. In: Radiology of the skull and brain. Vol. II, Book 1. St. Louis: Mosby; 1974a. p. 1089–130.
55. Kier EL. Development of cerebral vessels. In: Radiology of the skull and brain. St. Louis: Mosby; 1974b. p. 1089–130.
56. Killien FC, Wyler AR, Cromwell LD. Duplication of the internal carotid artery. Neuroradiology. 1980;19:101–2.
57. Kishore PR, Kaufman AB, Melichar FA. Intrasellar carotid anastomosis simulating pituitary microadenoma. Radiology. 1979;132(2):381–3.
58. Klinkhamer AC. Esophagography in anomalies of the aortic arch system. Excerpta Medica Foundation. 1969:1–62.
59. Kommerell B. Verlagerung des Oesophagus durcheine abnorm verlaufende Arteria subclavia dextra (Arteria Lusoria). Fortschr Geb Roentgenstr. 1936;54:590–5.
60. Kung DK, Liu W, Smoker WR, Hasan DM. Duplication of the internal carotid artery presenting with severe atherosclerotic stenosis. J Clin Neurosci. 2011;18(7):982–3.
61. Kuntz A. A textbook of neuroanatomy. Acad Med. 1950;25(2):158.
62. Larsell O. The development of the cerebellum in man in relation to its comparative anatomy. J Comp Neurol. 1947;87(2):85–129.
63. Lasjaunias P, Berenstrein A. Surgical nueroangiography. Berlin: Springer; 1990.
64. Lasjaunias P, Vallee B, Person H, Ter Brugge K, Chiu M. The lateral spinal artery of the upper cervical spinal cord: anatomy, normal variations, and angiographic aspects. J Neurosurg. 1985;63(2):235–41.
65. Lazorthes G. Vascularisation et circulation cérébrales: par G. Lazorthes, avec la collaboration de F. Amaral-Gomes, G. Bastide, L. Campan, J. Espagno ... [etc.]. [Internet]. Masson et Cie (Villeneuve-Saint-Georges, l'Union typographique); 1961. Disponibile su: https://books.google.it/books?id=IbK_oQEACAAJ.
66. Lazzaro NA, Wright B, Castillo M, Fischbein NJ, Glastonbury CM, Pg H, et al. Artery of percheron infarction: imaging patterns and clinical spectrum. Am J Neuroradiol. 2010;31(7):1283–9.
67. Lee JH, Oh CW, Lee SH, Han DH. Aplasia of the internal carotid artery. Acta Neurochir. 2003;145:117–25.
68. Leeds NF. The striate arteries and the artery of Heubner. In: Newton, Potts, editors. Angiography. Radiology of the skull and brain. St Louis: Mosby; 1974.
69. Lehmann G, Vincentelli F, Ebagosti A. Rare abnormalities of the circle of Willis: infra-optic pathway of the anterior cerebral arteries (author's transl). Neuro-Chirurgie. 1980;26(3):243–6.
70. Lemay M, Gooding CA. The clinical significance of the azygos anterior cerebral artery. Am J Roentgenol. 1966;98:602.
71. Lemke AJ, Benndorf G, Liebig T, Felix R. Anomalous origin of the right vertebral artery:

review of the literature and case report of right vertebral artery origin distal to the left subclavian artery. Am J Neuroradiol. 1999;20(7):1318–21.
72. Lesley WS, Dalsania HJ. Double origin of the posterior inferior cerebellar artery. Am J Neuroradiol. 2004;25(3):425–7.
73. Lesley WS, Rajab MH, Case RS. Double origin of the posterior inferior cerebellar artery: association with intracranial aneurysm on catheter angiography. Am J Roentgenol. 2007;189(4):893–7.
74. Lie TA, Foundation EM. Congenital anomalies of the carotid arteries: including the carotid-basilar and carotid-vertebral anastomoses. An angiographic study and a review of the literature [Internet]. Excerpta Medica. 1968; Disponibile su: https://books.google.it/books?id=17tqAAAAMAAJ.
75. Liechty JD, Shields TW, Anson BJ. Variations pertaining to the aortic arches and their branches; with comments on surgically important types. Q Bull Northwest Univ Med Sch. 1957;31(2):136.
76. Lin J, Kircheff I, Newton TH, Potts DG. Normal anterior cerebral artery complex. In: Radiology of the skull and brain: angiography, vol. 2. St. Louis: Mosby; 1974. p. 1319–410.
77. Lippert H, Pabst R. Arterial variations in man: classification and frequency [Internet]. Munchen: J.F. Bergmann Verlag; 1985. Disponibile su: https://books.google.it/books?id=nZhLAQAAIAAJ.
78. Lo WW, Solti-Bohman LG, McElveen JT Jr. Aberrant carotid artery: radiologic diagnosis with emphasis on high-resolution computed tomography. Radiographics. 1985;5(6):985–93.
79. Mahadevan J, Batista L, Alvarez H, et al. Bilateral segmental regression of the carotid and vertebral arteries with rete compensation in a Western patient. Neuroradiology. 2004;46:444–9.
80. Maillot C, Koritké JG. Origins of the posterior spinal artery trunk in man. C R Assoc Anat. 1970;149:837–47.
81. Mani RL, Newton TH, Glickman MG. The superior cerebellar artery: an anatomic-roentgenographic correlation. Radiology. 1968;91(6):1102–8.
82. Margolis MT, Newton TH. Posterior cerebral artery. In: Newton, Potts, editors. Angiography. Radiology of skull ad brain. St Louis: Mosby; 1974.
83. Marinković S, Milisavljević M, Marinkovis Z. Branches of the anterior communicating artery. Acta Neurochir. 1990;106(1):78–85.
84. Meila D, Saliou G, Krings T. Subcallosal artery stroke: infarction of the fornix and the genu of the corpus callosum. The importance of the anterior communicating artery complex. Case series and review of the literature. Neuroradiology. 2015;57:41–7.
85. Mellado JM, Merino X, Ramos A. Agenesis of the internal carotid artery with a trans-sellar anastomosis: CT and MRI findings in late-onset congenital hypopituitarism. Neuroradiology. 2001;43:237–41.
86. Mercier PH, Brassier G, Fournier HD, Picquet J, Papon X, Lasjaunias P. Vascular microanatomy of the pontomedullary junction, posterior inferior cerebellar arteries, and the lateral spinal arteries. Interv Neuroradiol. 2008;14(1):49–58.
87. Michotey P, Grisoli F, Raybaud C, Salamon G. Anatomical and radiologic study of the middle cerebral artery. Technics of reference marles. Ann Radiol. 1974;17:721–41.
88. Milenković Z. Anastomosis between internal carotid artery and anterior cerebral artery with other anomalies of the circle of Willis in a fetal brain. J Neurosurg. 1981;55(5):701–3.
89. Minagi H, Newton TH. Carotid rete mirabile in man: a case report. Radiology. 1966;86(1):100–2.
90. Mizutani T, Kojima H, Asamoto S, Miki Y. Pathological mechanism and three-dimensional structure of cerebral dissecting aneurysms. J Neurosurg. 2001;94(5):712–7.
91. Moffat DB. Developmental changes in the aortic arch system of the rat. Am J Anat. 1959;105:1–35.
92. Moffat DB. The embryology of the arteries of the brain: Arris and Gale Lecture delivered at the Royal College of Surgeons of England on 27th February 1962. Ann R Coll Surg Engl. 1962;30(6):368.
93. Mokri B, Sundt TM, Houser OW. Spontaneous internal carotid dissection, hemicrania, and Horner's syndrome. Arch Neurol. 1979;36(11):677–80.
94. Morgagni G. De sedibus, et causis morborum per anatomen indagatis libri quinque: Dissectiones, et animadversiones, nunc primum editas complectuntur propemodum innumeras, medicis, chirurgis, anatomicis profuturas. Multiplex praefixus est index... Vol. 2. Ex typographia Remondiniana; 1761.
95. Morimoto T, Nitta K, Kazekawa K, Hashizume K. The anomaly of a non-bifurcating cervical carotid artery: case report. J Neurosurg. 1990;72(1):130–2.
96. Morris P. Practical neuroangiography. Philadelphia: Lippincott Williams & Wilkins; 2007.
97. Moscow N. Anatomy of the cortical branches of the anterior cerebral artery. In: Radiology of the skull and brain, vol. 3. St. Louis: Mosby; 1974. p. 1411–20.
98. Moyer DJ, Flamm ES. Anomalous arrangement of the origins of the anterior choroidal and posterior communicating arteries: case report. J Neurosurg. 1992;76(6):1017–8.
99. Müller M, Schmitz BL, Pauls S, Schick M, Röhrer S, Kapapa T, et al. Variations of the aortic arch—a study on the most common branching patterns. Acta Radiol. 2011;52(7):738–42.
100. Nadgir RN, Loevner LA, Ahmed T, Moonis G, Chalela J, Slawek K, et al. Simultaneous bilateral internal carotid and vertebral artery dissection following chiropractic manipulation: case report and review of the literature. Neuroradiology. 2003;45:311–4.
101. Naidich TP, Kricheff II, George AE, Lin JP. The normal anterior inferior cerebellar artery: anatomic-radiographic correlation with emphasis on the lateral projection. Radiology. 1976;119(2):355–73.
102. Nakai K, Kaji T, Uchino A, Kawauchi T, Tamura C, Otani N, et al. Congenital external carotid–internal carotid artery anastomosis associated with con-

tralateral non-bifurcating cervical carotid artery. Neuroradiology. 2012;54:521–3.

103. Natsis KI, Tsitouridis IA, Didagelos MV, Fillipidis AA, Vlasis KG, Tsikaras PD. Anatomical variations in the branches of the human aortic arch in 633 angiographies: clinical significance and literature review. Surg Radiol Anat. 2009;31(5):319–23.
104. Newton TH. The vertebral artery. St. Louis: Mosby; 1974.
105. Nishio A, Yoshimura M, Yamauchi S, Masamura S, Kawakami T, Goto T, et al. Anomalous origin of the anterior choroidal artery. Interv Neuroradiol. 2009;15(1):73–6.
106. Nozaki K, Taki W, Kawakami O, Hashimoto N. Cerebral aneurysm associated with persistent primitive olfactory artery aneurysm. Acta Neurochir. 1998;140:397–402.
107. Nutik S, Dilenge D. Carotid anterior cerebral artery anastomosis. Case report. J Neurosurg. 1976;44:378.
108. Ogawa T, Fujita H, Inugami A, Shishido F, Higano S, Uemura K. Anomalous origin of the posterior inferior cerebellar artery from the posterior meningeal artery. AJNR Am J Neuroradiol. 1991;12(1):186.
109. Padget DH. The development of the cranial arteries in the human embryo. Contribution to embryology. Carnegie Institution of Washington DC; 1948.
110. Pasco A, Thouveny F, Papon X, Tanguy JY, Mercier P, Caron-Poitreau C, et al. Ruptured aneurysm on a double origin of the posterior inferior cerebellar artery: a pathological entity in an anatomical variation. Report of two cases and review of the literature. J Neurosurg. 2002;96(1):127–31.
111. Patten BM. Human Embryology. New York: McGraw Hill Book Co. Inc; 1953. p. 523.
112. Percheron G. Les arteres du thalamus humain. I. Artere et territoire thalamique polaires de l'artere communicante posterieure. 1976a.
113. Percheron G. Les artères du thalamus humain. II. Artères et territoires thalamiques paramédians de l'artère basilaire communicante. 1976b.
114. Perlmutter D, Rhoton AL. Microsurgical anatomy of the anterior cerebral-anterior communicating-recurrent artery complex. J Neurosurg. 1976;45(3):259–72.
115. Perlmutter D, Rhoton AL. Microsurgical anatomy of the distal anterior cerebral artery. J Neurosurg. 1978;49(2):204–28.
116. Quain R. The anatomy of the arteries of the human body: and its applications to pathology and operative surgery with a series of lithographic drawings. London: Taylor and Walton; 1844.
117. Redekop GJ. Extracranial carotid and vertebral artery dissection: a review. Can J Neurol Sci. 2008;35(2):146–52.
118. Ring BA. The middle cerebral artery. In: Radiology of the skull and brain: angiography. St Louis: Mosby; 1974. p. 1442–78.
119. Roberts LK, Gerald B. Absence of both common carotid arteries. Am J Roentgenol. 1978;130(5):981–2.
120. Robinson LR. An unusual human anterior cerebral artery. J Anat. 1959;93(Pt 1):131.
121. Rojas S, Ortega M, RodríGuez-Baeza A. Variable anatomic configuration of the posterior spinal arteries in humans. Clin Anat. 2018;31(8):1137–43.
122. Romer AS, Parsons TS. The vertebrate body. 5th ed. Philadelphia, PA: Saunders College; 1977.
123. Rossner SS, Rhoton AL, Ono M, et al. Microsurgical anatomy of the anterior perforating arteries. J Neurosurg. 1974;61:468.
124. Salamon G, Huang YP. Radiologic anatomy of the brain. Berlin: Springer; 1976.
125. Schievink WI. Spontaneous dissection of the carotid and vertebral arteries. N Engl J Med. 2001;344(12):898–906.
126. Schievink WI, Mokri B, Piepgras DG. Spontaneous dissections of cervicocephalic arteries in childhood and adolescence. Neurology. 1994;44:1607.
127. Serizawa T, Saeki N, Yamaura A. Microsurgical anatomy and clinical significance of the anterior communicating artery and its perforating branches. Neurosurgery. 1997;40(6):1211–8.
128. Shellshear JL. The arterial supply of the cerebral cortex in the chimpanzee (Anthropopithecus troglodytes). J Anat. 1930;65(Pt 1):45.
129. Sjogren SE. The anterior choroidal artery. Acta Radiol. 1956;46(1–2):143–57.
130. Smith CG, Richardson WF. The course and distribution of the arteries supplying the visual (striate) cortex. Am J Ophthalmol. 1966;61(6):1391–6.
131. Staples GS. Transsellar intracavernous intercarotid collateral artery associated with agenesis of the internal carotid artery: case report. J Neurosurg. 1979;50(3):393–4.
132. Stephens RB, Stilwell DL. Arteries and veins of the human brain. (No Title). 1969.
133. Stewart JR, Kincaid OW, Titus JL. Right aortic arch: plain film diagnosis and significance. Am J Roentgenol. 1966;97(2):377–89.
134. Stoesslein F, Porstmann W, Schueler F, Schoepke W. Aberrant vertebral artery originating from the descending aorta. Eur J Radiol (Germany, Federal Republic of). 1982;2(2):157–9.
135. Stopford JSB. The arteries of the pons and medulla oblongata. J Anat Physiol. 1916;50(Pt 2):131.
136. Szdzuy D, Lehmann R, Nickel B. Common trunk of the anterior cerebral arteries. Neuroradiology. 1972;4(1):51–6.
137. Tacconi L, Johnston FG, Symon L. Accessory middle cerebral artery: case report. J Neurosurg. 1995;83(5):916–8.
138. Takahashi M, Arii H, Tamakawa Y. Anomalous arterial supply of temporal and occipital lobes by anterior choroidal artery: angiographic study. Am J Neuroradiol. 1980;1(6):537–40.
139. Takahashi S, Hoshino F, Uemura K, et al. Accessory middle cerebral artery: is it a variant form of the recurrent artery of Heubner? Am J Neuroradiol. 1989;10(3):563–8.

140. Takahashi S, Suga T, Kawata Y, et al. Anterior choroidal artery: angiographic analysis of variations and anomalies. Am J Neuroradiol. 1990;11(4):719–29.
141. Tao X, Yu XJ, Bhattarai B, Li TH, Jin H, Wei GW, et al. Microsurgical anatomy of the anterior communicating artery complex in adult Chinese heads. Surg Neurol. 2006;65(2):155–61.
142. Taptas JN. The so-called cavernous sinus: a review of the controversy and its implications for neurosurgeons. Neurosurgery. 1982;11(5):712–7.
143. Tatu L, Moulin T, Bougosslavsky J. Arterial vascular territory of human brain. 2001.
144. Theron J, Newton TH. Anterior choroidal artery. I. Anatomic and radiographic study. J Neuroradiol. 1976;3(1):5–30.
145. Thron AK. Vascular anatomy of the spinal cord: neuroradiological investigations and clinical syndromes. Vienna: Springer; 1988.
146. Tiedemann F. Abbildungen der Pulsadern des menschlichen Körpers, vol. 1. CF Müller; 1822.
147. Tode JC. Sundhed og underholdning. 1787.
148. Tsuji T, Abe M, Tabuchi K. Aneurysm of a persistent primitive olfactory artery: case report. J Neurosurg. 1995;83(1):138–40.
149. Uchino A, Saito N, Takahashi M, et al. Variations of the origin of the vertebral artery and its level of entry into the transverse foramen diagnosed by CT angiography. Neuroradiology. 2013;55:585.
150. Umansky F, Gomes FB, Dujovny M, Diaz FG, Ausman JI, Mirchandani HG, et al. The perforating branches of the middle cerebral artery: a microanatomical study. J Neurosurg. 1985;62(2):261–8.
151. Verbiest MH. [Intradural arteriovenous aneurysm]. Rev Neurol. 1951;85(3):189–99. PMID: 14921378.
152. Vitek JJ, Reaves P. Thoracic bifurcation of the common carotid artery. Neuroradiology. 1973;5(3):133–9.
153. Wackenheim A, Braun JP. Angiography of the mesencephalon: normal and pathological findings. Berlin: Springer; 1970.
154. Westberg G. Recurrent artery of Heubner and the arteries of the cerebral ganglia. Acta Radiol. 1963;1:949.
155. Westberg G. Arteries of the basal ganglia. Acta Radiol Diagn. 1966;5(P1):581–96.
156. Wollschlaeger PB, Wollschlaeger G. Eine infratentorielle, meningeal Arterie [An infratentorial meningeal artery]. Radiologe. 1965;5(11):451–2. German. PMID: 5888134.
157. Wollschlaeger PB, Wollschlaeger G. The circle of Willis. In: Newton, Potts, editors. Angiography. Radiology of skull and brain. St Louis: Mosby; 1974.
158. Wolpert S. Vascular studies of congenital anomalies. In: Radiology of the skull and brain. St. Louis: Mosby; 1974.
159. Wong ST, Yuen SC, Fok KF, Yam KY, Fong D. Infraoptic anterior cerebral artery: review, report of two cases and an anatomical classification. Acta Neurochir. 2008;150:1087–96.
160. Wong K, Udani SD, Makalanda HLD, Bhogal P. Posterior inferior cerebellar artery aneurysm: spontaneous subarachnoid hemorrhage secondary to a dissecting aneurysm of a double origin PICA. In: The aneurysm casebook: a guide to treatment selection and technique; 2020. p. 1463–8.
161. Zeal AA, Rhoton AL. Microsurgical anatomy of the posterior cerebral artery. J Neurosurg. 1978;48(4):534–59.

4 Distal Superficial Branches and Branches for the Deep Structures

As shown in the previous sections, the growing of the brain with the formation of cerebral lobes and deep nuclei, request the development of specific vessels.

Considering the pattern of the arteries developing on the surface of the cerebral hemispheres, it is amazing how great is their variety. At the same time, it is remarkable as pointed out already by Duret [11] *and later by Shellhear* [24, 25] *how great is the constancy of the branches in reaching their specific terminal areas, independently, from their various origin. It is further emphasized that this variety is of secondary importance. This depends on the various external factors, especially hemodynamic, influencing the branches in choosing the most convenient course. Taking this into consideration, it is appropriate as proposed earlier by some authors* [2, 9] *to name these branches according to the territory they supply. This particular aspect has been confirmed later through detailed radio-anatomic and angiographic studies.*

4.1 Morphology and Function of the Distal Cortical Branches

As it has been described in Chaps. 1 and 2, the surface of the brain in the first phases of the evolution is "Smooth" (Fig. 4.1). This configuration, known as "Lissencephaly," is typical in lower vertebrates. In the humans, in normal evolution, it is temporarily changing in the advanced fetal phase, with the formation of cortex with circumvolutions and sulci.

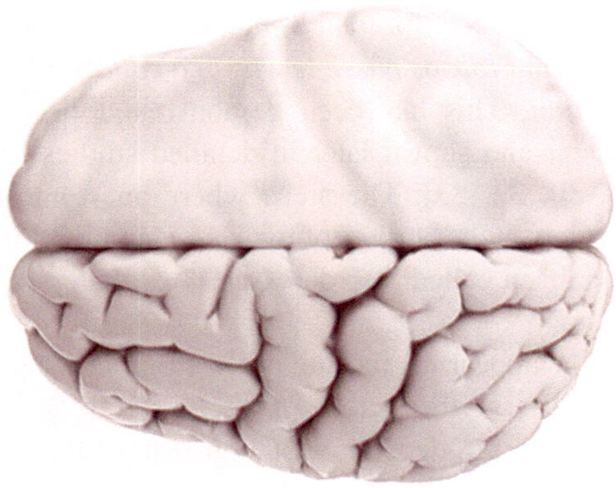

Fig. 4.1 Diagram of cerebrum comparing one half with a smooth surface (Lissencephaly) with a normal developed cortex where circumvolution and sulci are present

The evolution is linked to the neuronal migration towards the surface of the brain, beginning in the human at the 90–100 days of age, being complete at the fetus of 200 days [20, 26]. The distal vessels running on the smooth surface have a simple, rectilinear course. Following the appearing of gyri and sulci, the course becomes more tortuous with curves and angles. Disorders involving the process of migration lead to various forms of heterotopia and cortical dysplasia. In these cases, the arterial vessels maintain the primordial above described configuration associated

G. B. Bradac, *Origin and Development of Cerebral Vessels*,
https://doi.org/10.1007/978-3-031-78436-1_4

with various anomalies of the venous channels. These latter appear frequently greatly enlarged in the area of anomalous parenchyma [3]. This can lead to a misleading interpretation of a vascular malformation.

Where the distal branches of different sectors meet, connections develop, which have been already demonstrated in the early phase of the embryo by Beevor [4]. In the phase of smooth surface, due to their rectilinear course, the vessels develop a simple end-to-end anastomoses. Later, due to their tortuous course, the anastomoses acquire a more complex configuration.

Considering this evolution, it has become progressively clear that the cortical branches not only supply the parenchyma, but can play an important role as possible way of a collateral circulation. This has been demonstrated first by Beevor and shown later in detailed studies [21, 23, 30, 32, 33]. The areas where anastomoses develop, at the borders of two vascular territories, have been called "Border Zones" or Watersheds areas."

The appearing and site of the "Border Zones" depends on the extent of the distal branches which in turn depends on the growth of the specific parenchymal areas. The first developing is that between the ACA and MCA in the fronto-parietal regions. Anastomoses between PCA and ACA and MCA appeared later following the growth of the occipital and temporal areas.

In this context, however, further studies [28] have demonstrated that branches supplying a specific vascular territory can have an individual variable extent and so, branches of one vascular territory can extend to the adjacent territory and take over partially its vascularization. The consequence is that the "Border Zones" are not constant but can show great variability.

In the adult, in normal condition, the pressure of blood flow on both sides of the anastomoses is basically the same, and so no flow through the anastomoses is present. This situation can change due to different causes, responsible of minimal or complete absence of flow in one territory resulting in immediately activation of a collateral circulation at the level of the anastomotic connections.

Detailed angiographic studies, and especially the endovascular treatment in patients with stroke, as well as the possibility to examine directly on CT-MR the involved parenchyma, have confirmed the importance of the collateral circulation at the Border Zones as well as its variability giving further information:

1. The efficiency of the collateral circulation is temporary. The normal flow should be restored as quick as possible.
2. The efficiency is great near the origin of the collateral, but dwindles progressively increasing the distance from it.
3. Variations of circle of Willis as well as which segment of it is involved can be important.
4. The location of the Border Zones can have individual variation. The richness of anastomoses in one specific sector can be variable. One vascular territory can predominantly extend to the adjacent territory.
5. Further information has come from microanatomic and labor studies which have shown that the efficacy of collateral can be impaired due to changes of the microvasculature in the ischemic area such as swelling of endothelial and glial cells [1]. Other studies have shown that changes of white blood cells and platelets can favor thrombosis [18] and other authors [29] have emphasized the role of hyperglycemia.

4.2 Border Zones Involving Deep Structures

Another important "Border Zones" which should be considered, is that in the deep structures, developed between the so-called Deep and Superficial Perforators. The deep arise from A1-M1, having an ascending course supplying the basal ganglia and the adjacent white matter. The superficial arise from the superficial branches, penetrate the parenchyma extending with a descending perpendicular course towards the white matter in the periventricular area, towards the ascending perforators branches.

In accordance to the studies of some authors [10, 21] the superficial perforators (Medullary Branches) can be subdivided in branches with a short course supplying mainly the cortex and branches with a longer course, extending to the superficial white matter and further in the deep region towards the periventricular area.

All perforators are surrounded by a thin space, called *perivascular space*, identified in anatomical studies by Virchow [31], a German pathologist, and since then known as Virchow—Robin spaces. The space can enlarge with age, becoming well visible on CT and MR, being an incidental discovery or presenting with clinical symptoms consequences of the atrophy.

As far as it concerns the space surrounding the superficial and deep perforators, an interesting observation has been made by Hutchings and Weller [16], made on studies of electromicroscopy. The author demonstrated that the pia matter forms a continuous sheet separating the superficial subarachnoid space, from the sub-pial and perivascular space. The pia matter is an effective barrier impeding the passage of blood in the perivascular spaces, in case of acute subarachnoid bleeding.

Between the superficial (medullary) and deep perforators, in the area where they meet, there are basically no connections. Both group are end-arteries: Impaired blood flow in these branches results in ischemia.

It is not the aim of this work to describe the pathology of these branches, which has been described already in details in previous work [5–8, 15, 22].

It will be only shortly mentioned here that the perforators can be occluded by emboli arisen from ICA or its branches or cardiac in origin. Impairment of flow can be due to a long lasting hypotension in case of stenosis of ICA or his branches. Narrowing can be also due to a specific particular form of atherosclerosis called *lipohyalinosis.* It can be also associated to a rupture of the vessels resulting in hemorrhage. The ischemia due to occlusion of a single perforator is commonly small, called *lacunar infarct* (from Latin *lacuna,* small cavity). Its peculiar aspect and clinical relevance have been described and comprehensively discussed by Fischer [12, 13] who introduced the term *lacunar syndrome*. The number of the vessels involved can be variable, resulting in pathological process called *small vessels disease*. Involving of more than one perforator in adjacent areas can lead to formation of great lacunes, called by Fischer [13] *giant lacunes,* located in the basal ganglia (*Striato-capsular infarcts*) or in the white matter.

The same angio-architecture described in the cerebral hemispheres is present at the level of the cerebellar hemispheres [10], which develops later, following the slowly appearing of the cerebellum. On the surface of the cerebellar cortex, connections develop between the cerebellar arteries (SCA, AICA, PICA) where the branches meet at the level of border zones. From the superficial arteries arise with a perpendicular course branches extending towards the cerebellar white matter and further to the deep nuclei. These branches are end-arteries without possibility of collateral circulation.

As far as it concerns the vessels of brainstem (pons, medulla, mesencephalon) and Diencephalon, the vascularization is characterized by branches (see also Chap. 3) arised from the main trunk (BA, VA, AchA, and PCA) which run on the surface of the parenchyma, having numerous connections. From these branches arise branches penetrating the parenchyma, which are end-arteries, with no possibility of collateral circulation: their occlusion results in infarct.

Considering the above described configuration, it seems to be clear that in the brain there are two different well defined vascular structures. The one developed on the surface where the vessels present connections allowing in critical situation the developing of a collateral circulation, the other involving the perforators arising from the same above described vessels, being, however, end-arteries.

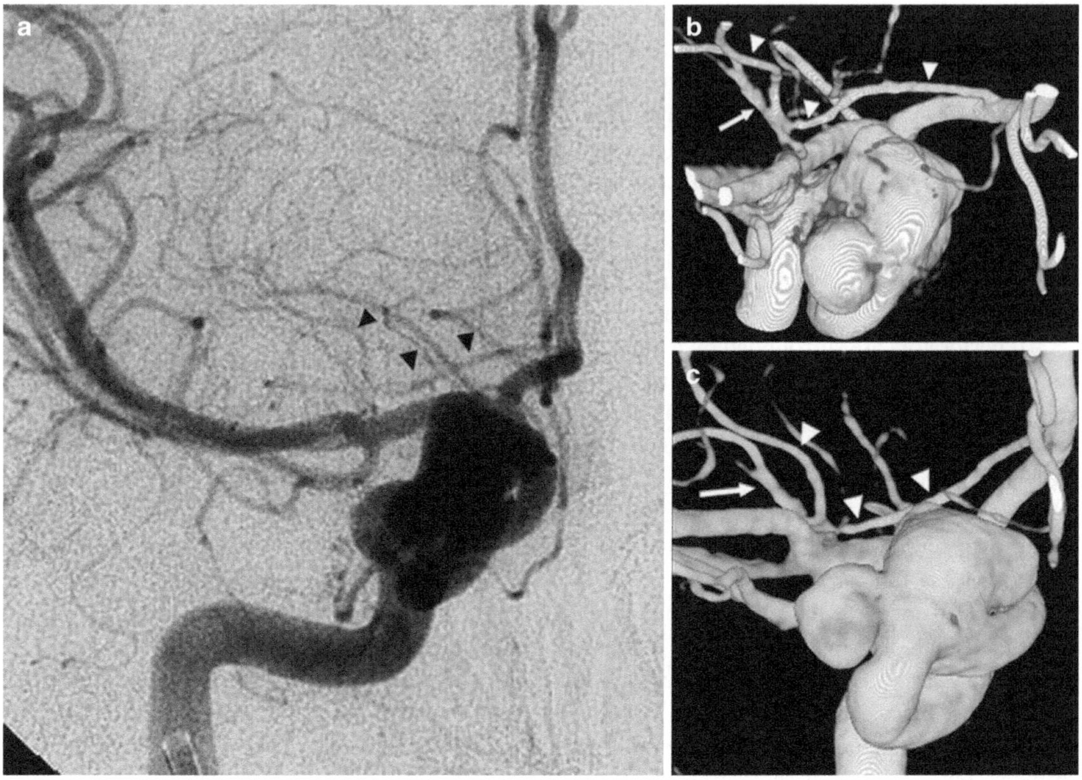

Fig. 4.2 Carotid angiogram and CT-angiography. Demonstration of connections between Heubner Artery (arrowhead) and a perforator branch (arrow) of M1. (Taken from Bradac [8])

Why in the evolution of the cerebral vessels this occurs, at the present time is not clear. In this context, however, concerning the vascular sector of the perforators, some observations should be made.

Already Kaplan and Ford [17] have suggested the possibility of anastomoses between the perforators. Hillal et al. [14] have identified anastomoses between the Heubner Artery and M1 perforators in children.

An interesting micro-angiographic study came later performed by Kodama and Suzuki [19] on fetuses, children, and adults. In all these cases, arterial anastomoses between the single deep perforators arising from A1 and M1 and between these and the medullary branches were demonstrated. The authors also observed a diminution of the numbers of deep perforators and medullary branches in the aged. They explained it with a *"diminishing demand for cerebral blood with aging."*

Other micro-angiographic studies [27] have demonstrated anastomoses between the Heubner Artery and perforators of M1 in 9% of the cases.

These latter can be occasionally demonstrated on routine angiogram (Fig. 4.2).

Taking all this into consideration, it is not completely unrealistic to think that in critical conditions such as the stroke, some "sleeping anastomoses" become temporary active. This could explain some limited ischemic lesions at the level of the basal ganglia and internal capsule as discussed in the previous chapters.

Variability of the supplied vascular territories related to the different extent of the perforators, could also in the single case play a role.

References

1. Ames A 3rd, Wright RL, Kowada M, Thurston JM, Majno G. Cerebral ischemia. II. The no-reflow phenomenon. Am J Pathol. 1968;52(2):437.
2. Baptista AG. Studies on the arteries of the brain: II. The anterior cerebral artery: some anatomic features and their clinical implications. Neurology. 1963;13(10):825–35.
3. Barkovich, AJ. Abnormal vascular drainage in anomalies of neuronal migration. Am J Neuroradiol. 1988;9(5):939–942.
4. Beevor CE. On the distribution of the different arteries supplying the human brain. Philo Trans R Soc Lond Ser B Biol Sci. 1909;200(262–273):1–55.
5. Bogousslavsky J, Van Melle G, Regli F. The Lausanne Stroke Registry: analysis of 1,000 consecutive patients with first stroke. Stroke. 1988;19(9):1083–92.
6. Boiten J, Lodder J, Lacunar infarcts. Pathogenesis and validity of the clinical syndromes. Stroke. 1991;22(11):1374–8.
7. Bradač GB, Daniele D, Bergui M, Cerrato P, Ferrio MF, Stura G, et al. Lacunes and other holes: diagnosis, pathogenesis, therapy. Neuroradiol J. 2008;21(1):35–52.
8. Bradac GB. Applied cerebral angiography: normal anatomy and vascular pathology. Cham: Springer; 2017. https://doi.org/10.1007/978-3-319-57228-4. 497 pages, ISBN 978-3-319-57227-7.
9. Critchley M. The anterior cerebral artery, and its syndromes. Brain. 1930;53(2):120–65.
10. De Reuck J. The cortico-subcortical arterial angio-architecture in the human brain. Acta Neurol Belg. 1972;72(5):323–9.
11. Duret H. Recherches anatomiques sur la circulation de l'encéphale. Arch Physiol Norm Path. 1874;I:60–91.
12. Fisher CM. The arterial lesions underlying lacunes. Acta Neuropathol. 1969;12(1).
13. Fisher CM. Lacunes: small, deep cerebral infarcts. Neurology. 1965;13(30).
14. Hilal SK, Solomon G, Gold AP, Carter S. Primary cerebral arterial occlusive disease in children: part I: acute acquired hemiplegia. Radiology. 1971;99(1):71–86.
15. Horowitz DR, Tuhrim S. Stroke mechanisms and clinical presentation in large subcortical infarctions. Neurology. 1997;49(6):1538–41.
16. Hutchings M, Weller RO. Anatomical relationships of the pia mater to cerebral blood vessels in man. J Neurosurg. 1986;65(3):316–25.
17. Kaplan HA, Ford DH. The brain vascular system [Internet]. London: Elsevier; 1966. Disponibile su: https://books.google.it/books?id=vJNZirNgVBkC.
18. Kleinschnitz C, De Meyer SF, Schwarz T, Austinat M, Vanhoorelbeke K, Nieswandt B, et al. Deficiency of von Willebrand factor protects mice from ischemic stroke. Blood J Am Soc Hematol. 2009;113(15):3600–3.
19. Kodama N, Suzuki J. Cerebrovascular Moyamoya disease. IIIrd report—the study on the aging of the perforating branches and the possibility of collateral pathway. Neurol Med Chir (Tokyo). 1974;14 pt 1:55–67.
20. Kuntz A. A textbook of neuroanatomy. Acad Med. 1950;25(2):158.
21. Lazorthes G. Vascularisation et circulation cérébrales: par G. Lazorthes, avec la collaboration de F. Amaral-Gomes, G. Bastide, L. Campan, J. Espagno ... [etc.]. [Internet]. Masson et Cie (Villeneuve-Saint-Georges, l'Union typographique); 1961. Disponibile su: https://books.google.it/books?id=IbK_oQEACAAJ.
22. Levine RL, Lagreze HL, Dobkin JA, Turski PA. Large subcortical hemispheric infarctions: presentation and prognosis. Arch Neurol. 1988;45(10):1074–7.
23. Meyer JS, Denny-Brown D. The cerebral collateral circulation. I. Factors influencing collateral blood flow. Neurology. 1957;7(7):447–58.
24. Shellshear JL. The basal arteries of the forebrain and their functional significance. J Anat. 1920;55(Pt 1):27–35.
25. Shellshear JL. The arteries of the brain of the Orang-utan. J Anat. 1927;61(Pt 2):167–97.
26. Truex RC. Human neuroanatomy. Acad Med. 1959;34(9):955.
27. Umansky F, Gomes FB, Dujovny M, Diaz FG, Ausman JI, Mirchandani HG, et al. The perforating branches of the middle cerebral artery: a microanatomical study. J Neurosurg. 1985;62(2):261–8.
28. van der Zwan A, Hillen B, Tulleken CA, Dujovny M, Dragovic L. Variability of the territories of the major cerebral arteries. J Neurosurg. 1992;77(6):927–40.
29. van Seeters T, Biessels GJ, Kappelle LJ, van der Graaf Y, Velthuis BK, Investigators DASS (DUST). Determinants of leptomeningeal collateral flow in stroke patients with a middle cerebral artery occlusion. Neuroradiology. 2016;58:969–77.
30. Vander Eecken HM, Adams RD. The anatomy and functional significance of the meningeal arterial anastomoses of the human brain. J Neuropathol Exp Neurol. 1953;12(2):132–57.
31. Virchow R. Die krankhaften Geschwülste: dreissig Vorlesungen gehalten während des Wintersemesters 1862–1863 an der Universität zu Berlin. Vol. 4. A. Hirschwald; 1867.
32. Zülch KJ. Über die entstehung und lokalisation der hirninfarkte. Zentralbl Neurochir. 1961;21:158–78.
33. Zülch KJ. Some basic patterns of the collateral circulation of the cerebral arteries. In: Cerebral circulation and stroke. Berlin/Heidelberg/New York: Springer; 1971. p. 106–22.

5 Considerations About Temporary Arteries

5.1 Trigeminal Artery

It appears early in the embryogenesis at the embryo of 4–5 mm [25, 30]. It arises from distal ICA joining the dorsally located BLC becoming its most important supply. Following the development of the vetebro-basilar system at the embryo of 9–12 mm and the development of the PcomA, the artery loses its function and progressively dwindles and regresses. In accordance to Padget, its regression could also be to an unfavorable direction of flow due to origin of the artery from ICA forming a downwards directed angle while the flow in the developed PcomA is more directed.

The artery can persist in the adult where its pattern has been progressively described in detailed anatomic-angiographic studies [3, 16, 20, 36, 41, 43]. Its frequency has been evaluated to be between 0.1% and 0.6% [16, 17].

The artery arises from the cavernous portion of ICA near the MHT giving off, sometimes branches for territories, normally supplied by the MHT [26]. It runs dorsally passing through or over the *Dorsum Sellae*, taking, sometimes a medial intrasellar course, which should be considered in case of trans-sphenoidal surgery [27]. It can run more laterally giving off branches for pons and *Ganglion Gasseri* [24, 28, 35].

Two types of Persistent Trigeminal Artery (PTR) have been described [29]. In one, the PTR supplies the distal BA from which arise the SCA and PCA. The PcomA is hypo-aplastic. The BA proximal to the insertion of the SCA can be normal joined by the VA. It can be hypoplastic with the VA supplying PICA and AICA. In the other one the PTR is connected with the BA from which arises the SCA. The PCA arises from ICA. There is a normal connection with the VA.

Another rarer form of PTR is the so-called Trigeminal Variant, in which the cerebellar arteries, more frequently the AICA arise from ICA at the level of the Trigeminal artery without interposition of the BA. This variant has been interpreted as a partial remnant of the regressed Trigeminal artery [15, 20, 22, 32–34, 39, 41].

The various configurations of the PTR are shown in Figs. 5.1, 5.2, and 5.3.

The trigeminal artery can play an important role as collateral circulation between BA and ICA. It can, however, be the cause of symptoms due to steal syndrome in one of these vascular sectors and be the way of emboli arising from ICA or from vertebra-basilar sector taking an opposite direction (Fig. 5.4).

G. B. Bradac, *Origin and Development of Cerebral Vessels*,
https://doi.org/10.1007/978-3-031-78436-1_5

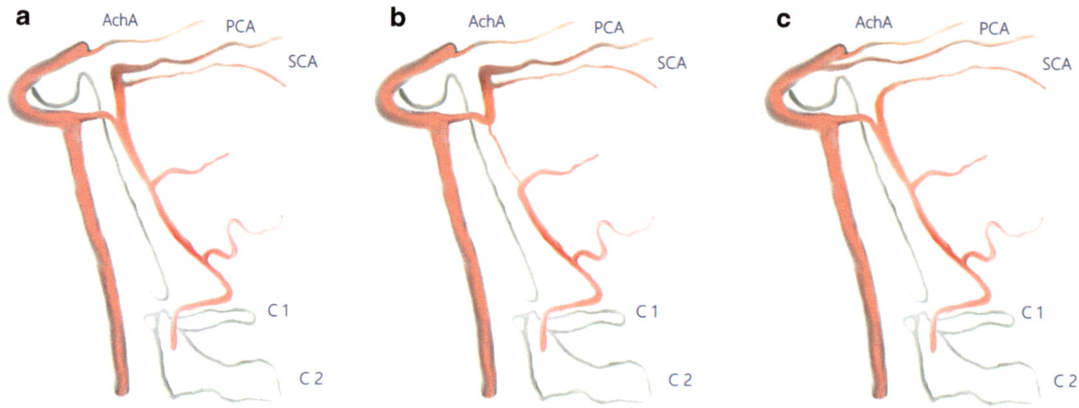

Fig. 5.1 (**a**) Trigeminal artery (PTR) is connected with the distal basilar artery, supplying the SCA and the Posterior Cerebral artery (PCA). The PcomA is aplastic. Anterior Choroidal artery (AchA). The Vertebral Artery (VA) is normal joining distally the BA. (**b**) Same indications. The VA is hypo-aplastic in its distal segment. (**c**) The PTR joins the distal BA supplying the SCA. The PCA arises from ICA

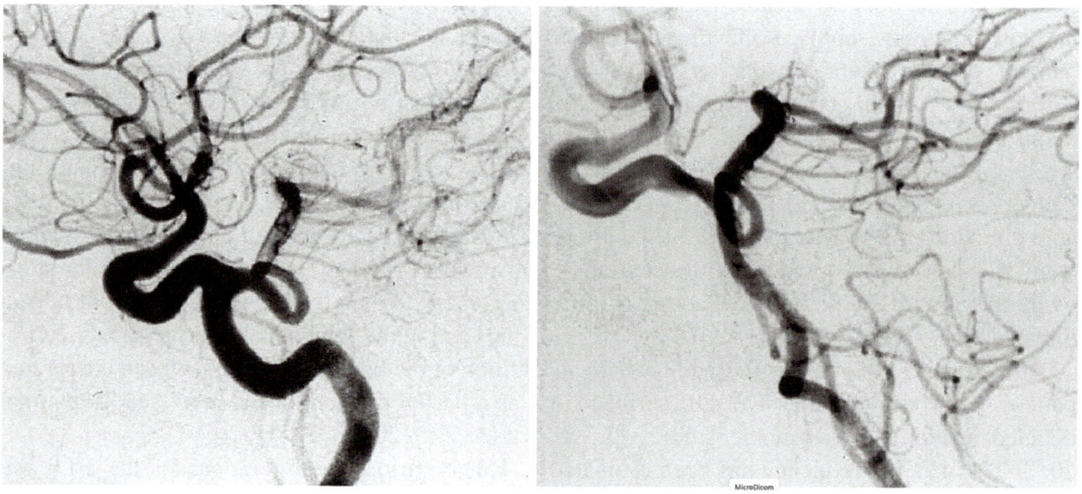

Fig. 5.2 Carotid angiogram. The PTR supplies PCA and SCA. Vertebral angiogram in the same patient. Normal developed VA joining distally the BA and the PTR. Indirect filling of the ICA with injection of the AchA. (Taken from Bradac [5])

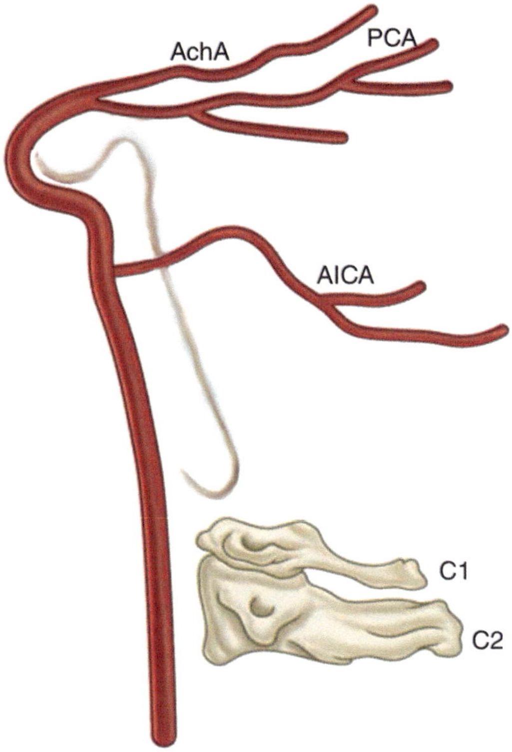

Fig. 5.3 Trigeminal Variant. Origin of the Anterior Inferior cerebellar artery (AICA) from ICA, at the level of origin of the PTR

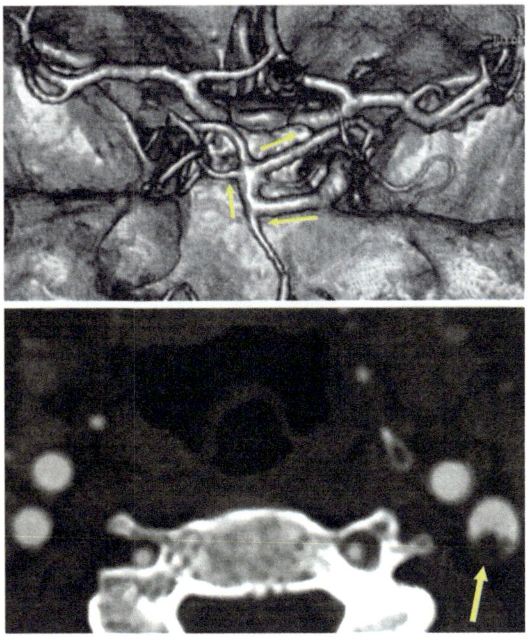

Fig. 5.4 Stroke in the vertebro basilar sector in patient with an atheromatic plaque (arrow) of the carotid artery (CT Angiography). Due to the persistent PTR, an embolus flew from the carotid in the BA and further in the PCA (arrows)

5.2 Mandybular Artery

Congdon [6] and later Padget [25] identified the artery at the embryo of 4 mm. It has been considered as remnant of the regressed first aortic arch. The artery is annexed by the new developed ICA arising from the third aortic arch. The mandibular artery develops connections with the distal branches of the ventral pharyngeal artery (future ECA). Both arteries supply the primitive maxillary process. The mandibular artery regresses rapidly. It is no longer recognizable at the embryo of 5–6 mm. It can rarely be identified on the angiogram in the adult, appearing as a fine branch arising from the horizontal portion of the petrous segment of ICA (Fig. 5.5).

On anatomic studies one can distinguish two branches [13]. The one is directly anteriorly joining at the level of the Pterygoid (Vidian) canal, the Vidian artery. This is a branch of the Internal Maxillary Artery (IMA) arising in the Pterygopalatine fossa running dorsally with a horizontal course joining the mandibular branch forming the Vidian-Mandibular artery. More about the Vidian Artery in Chap. 7.

The other branch of the mandibular artery courses infero-medially, passing through the cartilage of the foramen lacerum reaching the superior oropharyngeal area where it anastomoses with branches of IMA and AphA involved in the supply of the region. The above described connections can be an important collateral circulation between IMA and ICA (Fig. 5.6). They can be also a risk in cases of endovascular treatment of pathology in ECA area. The complex Vidian-Mandibular Artery can be involved in pathological condition, typically in juvenile angio-fibroma (Fig. 5.7).

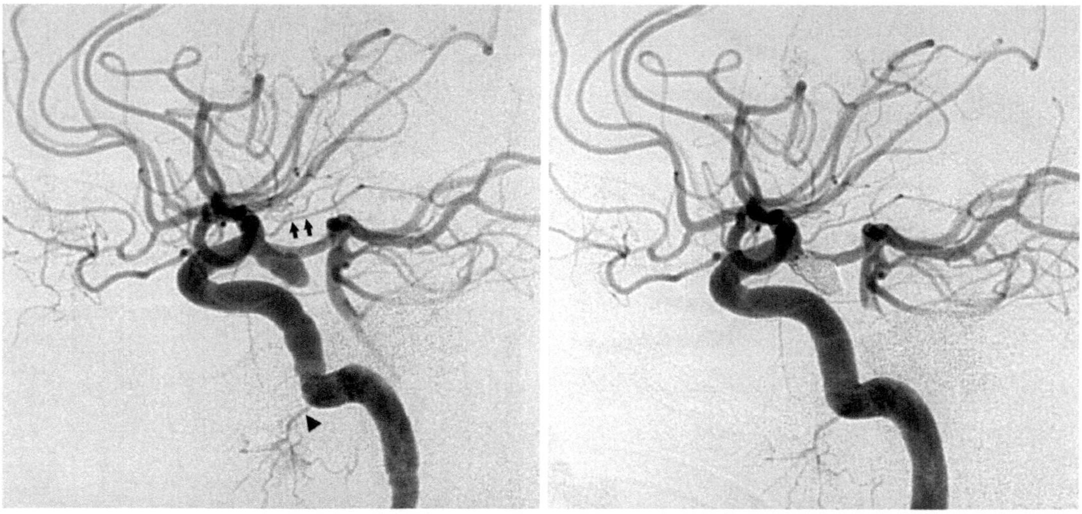

Fig. 5.5 Carotid angiogram. Persistent mandibular artery (arrow head). Patient with aneurysm of the PcomA treated endovascularly. AchA (arrows). (Taken from Bradac [5])

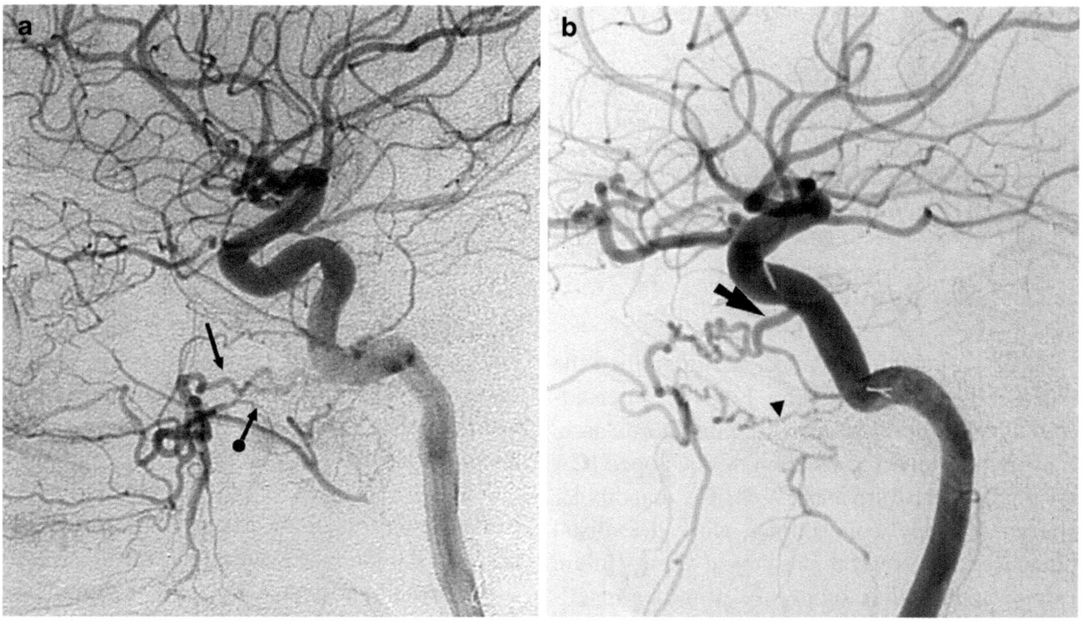

Fig. 5.6 Carotid angiogram in two patients treated with ligature of the external carotid artery. (**a**) Through the mandibular artery (arrow). Retrograde filling of IMA and of the peri-vaginal branch (arrow with dot). (**b**) Filling of the ILT (arrow). Retrograde injection of branches of IMA and retrograde filling of the Vidian artery (arrow head). (Taken from Bradac [5])

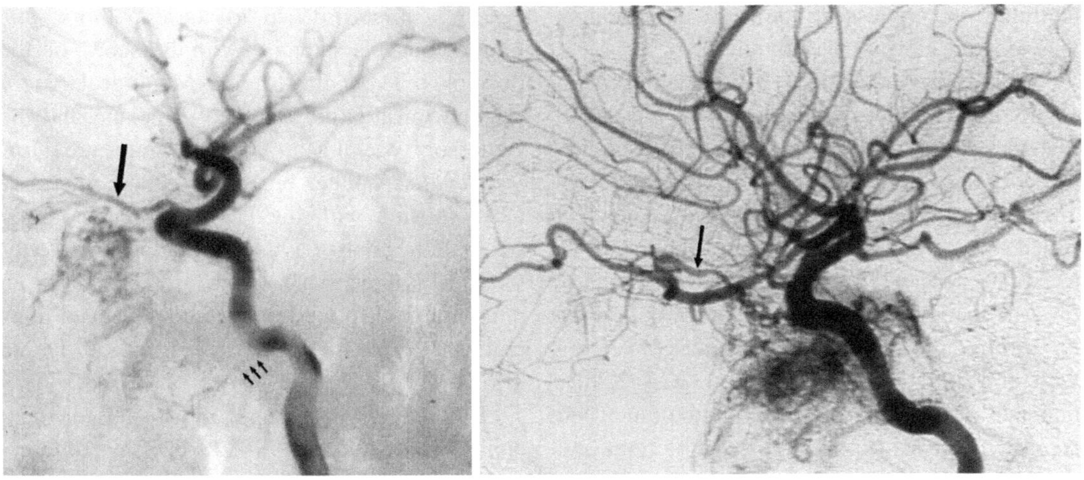

Fig. 5.7 Carotid angiogram in patient with juvenile angio-fibroma with intra-orbital and middle fossa extension. Involvement of the mandibular artery (three arrows). The tumor is supplied also by the recurrent meningeal branch (arrow) of the ophthalmic artery and ILT branches. (Taken from Bradac [5])

5.3 Hyoid Artery

The artery is a remnant of the regressed second aortic arch appearing at the embryo of 4 mm [6, 25]. It is annexed by the ICA. It gives off at the embryo of 12–14 mm, as important collateral, the stapedial artery. This runs cranially, enters the tympanic cavity, passes through the stapedial artery, and shortly after divides in the mandibular and supraorbital branches which play an important role in the development of the IMA (external carotid artery) and ophthalmic artery respectively (see Chaps. 6 and 7).

The mandibular artery runs extra-cranially through the *foramen spinosum* connecting with the maxillary branch of the ventral pharyngeal artery (future ECA). From the fusion of the mandibular and maxillary branches develops the internal maxillary artery (IMA). This gives off its branches, among them there is the basal part of the Middle Meningeal Artery (MMA) which runs cranially, passes through the *foramen spinosum* connecting intra-cranially with the distal part of the MMA developed from the supraorbital artery.

Attention: This mandibular artery should not be confused with the primordial mandibular artery remnant of the first aortic arch, described above, sometimes recognizable in the adult.

As far as it concerns the supraorbital artery, it is involved in the development of the orbital vascularization (see Chap. 6). One of its branches is the distal part of the MMA which is joined by the basal part developed from IMA forming together the final MMA.

At the embryo of 20 mm, the hyoid and the stapedial arteries have terminated their temporary function and regress. Remnants sometimes visible on the adult angiograms are branches supplying the tympanic cavity. One is the caroticotympanic branch arising from ICA being the remnant of the hyoid artery. The other is the superior tympanic branch arising from the MMA as remnant of the supraorbital artery.

A very rare anomaly is the persistence of the hyoid-stapedial artery, described in Chaps. 6 and 7.

5.4 Primary Maxillary Artery

As described by Padget, the artery appears at the 4 mm embryo arising from ICA immediately beyond the Rathke pouch short before the cranial and caudal division of ICA. It contributes to supply the optic vesicles, the basal prosencephalon, and partially the maxillary process. The artery dwindles and regresses rapidly. It is no longer visible at the embryo of 5–6 mm.

In a study performed at the embryo of 14–18 mm, Padget could identify a few small branches arising at the level of the future cavernous portion of ICA where the primitive maxillary artery had arisen and then disappeared. Padget called these branches "Remnant of the Primitive Maxillary Artery." These branches run medially towards the base of the *Sella Turcica* supplying the dura of the area, extending and connecting with those of the contro-lateral ICA. Other branches ran to the Infundibulum and Neurohypophysis supplying these structures and the adjacent dura.

A few years later, De la Torre and Netzky [7] in a study performed in injected human fetuses aged of 35–63 days confirmed the findings of Padget and identified another branch arising from cavernous portion of ICA directed laterally which the authors called "Persistent Primitive Maxillary Artery." In accordance to these authors, this artery connects laterally with branches of the developed IMA: the Middle Meningeal Artery passing towards the foramen spinosum and the Accessory Meningeal Artery through the *foramen ovale*. Another branch extended anteriorly anastomosing with the lacrimal branch of the ophthalmic artery passing through the Superior Orbital Fissure (SOF). In 1974, Kier [11] in an angiogram performed in injected advanced fetus confirmed the findings of Padget and De la Torre-Netzky.

In the following years, radio-anatomic and angiographic studies [8, 13, 20, 31] have progressively allowed a more precise demonstration of the branches arising from the cavernous ICA which are called today the "Infero-Lateral Trunk" (ILT) and the "Meningo-Hypophyseal Trunk" (MHT).

The ILT and MHT and the branches connected with them are shown in Fig. 5.8.

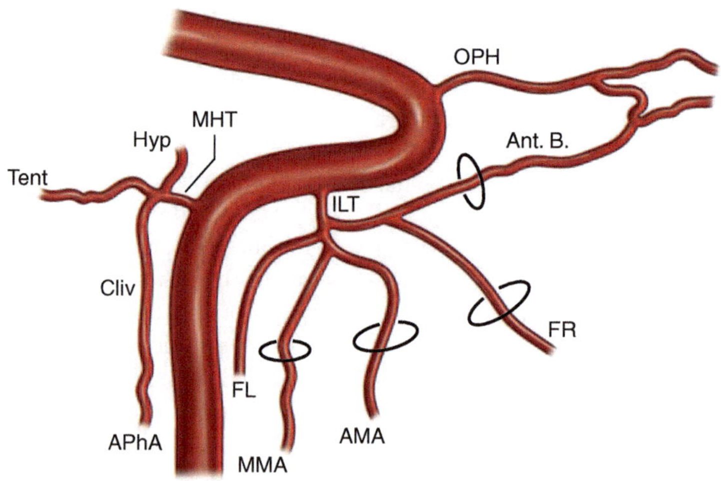

Fig. 5.8 Diagram showing the ILT and MHT of the cavernous portion of ICA and their branches
Branches of the ILT
– Lateral the ILT is connected with the MMA passing through the Foramen Spinosum and with the Accessory Meningeal Artery (AMA) passing through then Foramen Ovale
– Anterolateral with the Foramen rotundum artery passing through the corresponding Foramen
– Anterior with a branch running towards the orbita (Ant. B.), passing through the Superior Orbital Fissure, anastomosing with the Lacrimal branch of the Ophthalmic Artery (OPH)
– Posterior with a branch called "recurrent branch of the Foramen Lacerum" (FL) which runs along the petrous segment of ICA anastomosing at the level of the Foramen Lacerum with the carotid branch of the AphA
Branches of the MHT
These can arise as separate branches or as a common trunk dividing distally
Medial branches. These run on the base of the Sella supplying the dura of the region, anastomosing with the contro-lateral ICA. Other medial branches supply the infundibulum and Neurohypophysis (HYP)
Posterior branches extending along the tentorium supplying it
Posterior inferior branches extending along the clivus anastomosing with ascending branches of the AphA

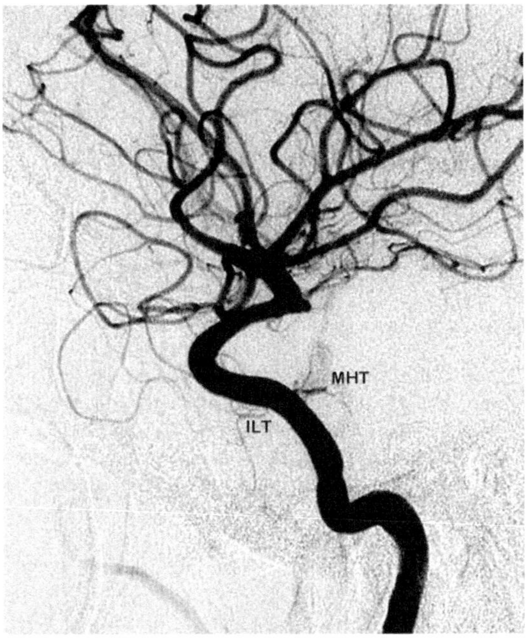

Fig. 5.9 Carotid angiogram showing the typical normal pattern of the ILT and MHT. (Taken from Bradac [5])

Through the above described connections, ILT and MHT can be a way of collateral circulation between ICA and ECA. On normal angiogram, these branches are commonly very small (Fig. 5.9), but can enlarge if involved in pathological conditions (Figs. 5.6b, 5.10, and 5.11).

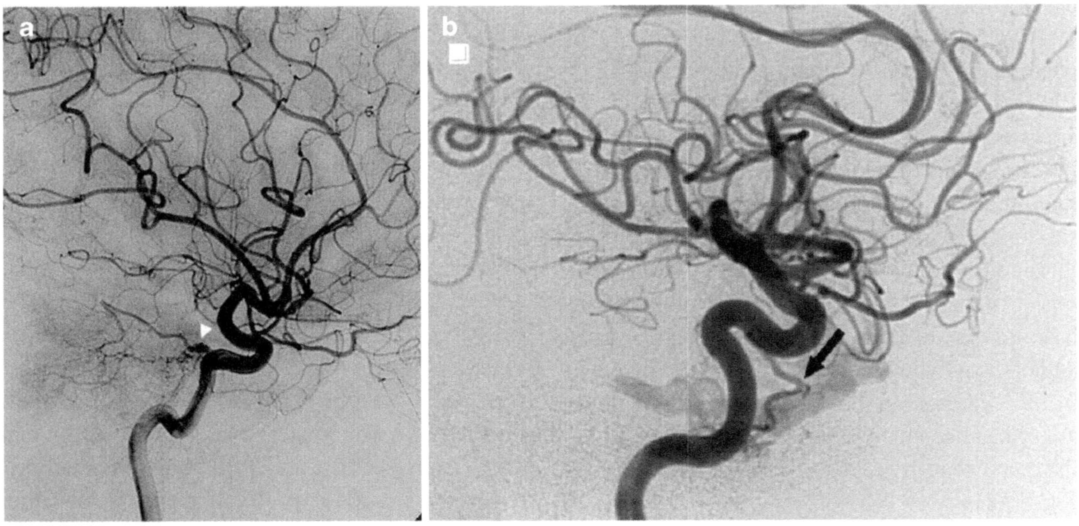

Fig. 5.10 Carotid angiograms in two different patients showing: (**a**) involvement of the MHT (arrow head) in a petroclival meningioma. (**b**) involvement of the ILT (arrow) in a DAVF of the middle cranial fossa. (Taken from Bradac [5])

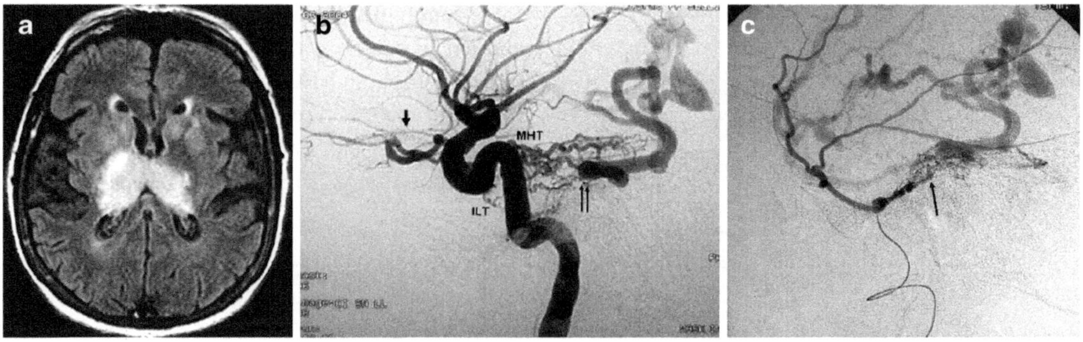

Fig. 5.11 Patient with petro-tentorial DAVF. (**a**) MR showing the bilateral impairment of thalamus and basal ganglia. (**b**) Carotid angiogram, dilated ILT, MHT, and recurrent meningeal branch of the lacrimal artery (arrow) involved in the supply of the fistula (three arrows). Venous drainage in the lateral mesencephalic vein, joining the Galen vein. The straight sinus is thrombosed. (**c**) Angiogram of the MMA showing involvement of its petro-squamous branch (arrow) and the drainage in the LMV. Due to the straight sinus thrombosis, there is a retrograde filling of the basal vein. (Taken from Bradac [5])

5.5 Hypoglossal Artery

This is the second more frequent anastomosis between ICA and BA persisting in the adult. It has been identified by Schmeidel [30] and later by Padget [25] at the embryo of 4–5 mm. At this phase, the hypoglossal connects the ICA with the BLC (Chap. 2). In the further evolution, the artery regresses but it can persist in the adult arising from the extracranial ICA, sometimes ECA, running cranially passing through the hypoglossal canal together with the hypoglossal nerve and the anterior condylar vein. The first angiographic report is that of Begg [2]. Several other studies have followed [21, 42]. According to these latter authors, the hypoglossal artery has a frequency of 0.29%. Cases of association with the proatlantal artery has been also reported [37]. The course of the persistent hypoglossal artery is shown in Fig. 5.12a.

The artery can appear with variants. One of these is the direct connection of the artery with the PICA [12, 42] without involvement of the vertebral artery (Fig. 5.12b).

An angiographic study has been reported by Andoh et al. [1]. This has been interpreted as a persistent connection of the hypoglossal artery with the Lateral Channel (LC) paralleling the BLC as described in Chap. 2. This hypothesis suggested by Schmeidel has been later more precisely described by Morris and Moffat [19].

Other explanation has been proposed, taking into consideration the possible various connections involving the Posterior Meningeal Artery (PMA), the PICA, and the Ascending Pharyngeal Artery (AphA). Origin of the PICA from the hypoglossal branch of the AphA [15] or from its jugular branch [40] as well as from the posterior meningeal artery [23] has been reported. Furthermore, the posterior meningeal artery can arise from the PICA [38]. These connections have been interpreted [15, 40, 42] as a condition favoring the origin of the PICA from the AphA through his hypoglossal or jugular branch.

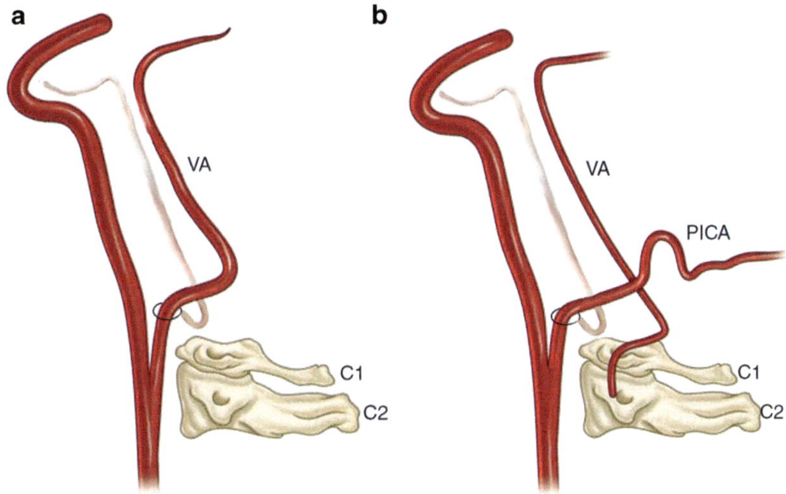

Fig. 5.12 Diagram showing the pattern of the hypoglossal artery connected with the VA (**a**) and the connection of the hypoglossal artery directly with the PICA (**b**)

5.6 Proatlantal Artery (PRA)

Arising from the dorsal aorta, appears at the 4–5 mm embryo an artery called by Padget "Proatlantal Artery," considering its course between the atlas and the occipital bone. It connects the Ductus Caroticus with the BLC and The LC.

Commonly regresses, but can sometimes persist in the adult as reported in anatomic-angiographic studies [10, 16, 37]. The artery arises from the extracranial ICA or sometimes from ECA, joining the horizontal part of the VA, continuing distally with a branch resembling in its course the occipital artery. The proximal part of the VA is absent or hypoplastic (Fig. 5.13).

Padget and later Bloch and Danziger [4] interpreted the horizontal part of the VA as remnant of the proatlantal artery. Another explanation of the persistent proatlantal artery has been proposed by Moffat [18, 19] and Haughton-Rosenbaum [9]. In accordance to these authors (see also Chap. 2), the fate of the PRA is linked with that of the *Ductus Caroticus* from which the PRA arises. If the *Ductus Caroticus* which normally disappears, does not regress, the PRA persists and in the further evolution can lead to the above described anomaly.

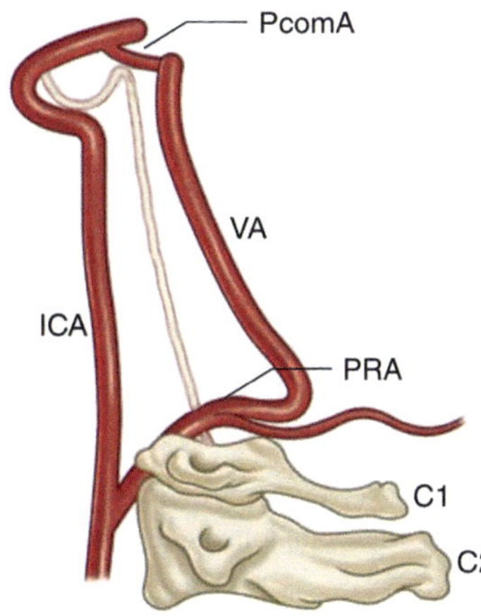

Fig. 5.13 Diagram showing the persistent Proatlantal Artery (PRA) connected with the VA. The artery continues in a distal branch similar in its course to the occipital artery

Other authors [14, 37], considering that the PRA has a course remembering that of the occipital artery and that the occipital artery (see chap. 7) can arise as variant from the ICA, have suggested that in both conditions we are dealing with the same artery: the PRA, which can acquire a different pattern depending on factors influencing the evolution.

5.7 Otic Artery

The artery appears early in the embryonic phase together with the trigeminal, hypoglossal, proatlantal arteries and regress together with them. Its persistence in the adult is extremely rare and difficult to demonstrate.

A case has been presented in an excellent anatomic-microangiographic study by Wollschlaeger and Wollschlaeger [43]. The artery appeared as a small branch arising from the petrous segment of the ICA, joining dorsally the anterior inferior cerebellar artery. Demonstration of its course through the auditory canal with CT or MR can be very useful for the diagnosis.

References

1. Andoh K, Tanohata K, Moriya N, Hagiwara H, Lee J, Sato M, et al. The posterior inferior cerebellar artery arising from the extracranial segment of the internal carotid artery via the hypoglossal canal without an interposed segment of the basilar artery: a persistent primitive hypoglossal artery variant. Clin Imaging. 2001;25(2):86–9.
2. Begg AC. Radiographic demonstration of the "hypoglossal artery": a rare type of persistent anomalous carotid-basilar anastomosis. Clin Radiol. 1961;12(3):187–9.
3. Bernasconi V, Cassinari V. Un segno carotidografico tipico di meningioma del tentorio. Chirurgia. 1956;11(3):586–8.
4. Bloch S, Danziger J. Proatlantal intersegmental artery. Neuroradiology. 1974;7(1):5–8.
5. Bradac GB. Applied cerebral angiography. Normal anatomy and vascular pathology. Cham: Springer; 2017. https://doi.org/10.1007/978-3-319-57228-4. 497 pages, ISBN 978-3-319-57227-7
6. Congdon ED. Transformation of the aortic-arch system during the development of the human embryo. Embryol Carneg Instn. 1922;14:47–110. Contributions to embryology.
7. De La Torre E, Netsky MG. Study of persistent primitive maxillary artery in human fetus: some homologies of cranial arteries in man and dog. Am J Anat. 1960;106(3):185–95.
8. Djindjian R, Merland JJ. Super-selective arteriography of the external carotid artery. Springer; 1978.
9. Haughton VM, Rosenbaum AE, Pearce J. Internal carotid artery origins of the inferior cerebellar arteries. AJR Am J Roentgenol. 1978;130(6):1191–2.
10. Hutchinson NA, Miller JD. Persistent proatlantal artery. J Neurol Neurosurg Psychiatry. 1970;33(4):524–7.
11. Kier EL. Development of cerebral vessels. In: Radiology of the skull and brain; 1974. p. 1089–130.
12. Kim JT, Heo SH, Lee SH, Choi SM, Park MS, Kim BC, et al. An uncommon anastomosis of the posterior inferior cerebellar artery and the external carotid artery with the patent vertebrobasilar system. Br J Radiol. 2009;82:e171–4.
13. Lasjaunias PL. Craniofacial and upper cervical arteries. In: Craniofacial and upper cervical arteries; 1981. p. 199.
14. Lasjaunias P, Doyon D. The ascending pharyngeal artery and the blood supply of the lower cranial nerves. J Neuroradiol. 1978;5(4):287–301.
15. Lasjaunias P, Guibert-Tranier F, Braun JP. The pharyngo-cerebellar artery or ascending pharyngeal artery origin of the posterior inferior cerebellar artery. J Neuroradiol. 1981;8(4):317–25.
16. Lie TA, Foundation EM. Congenital anomalies of the carotid arteries: including the carotid-basilar and carotid-vertebral anastomoses. An angiographic study and a review of the literature [Internet]. Excerpta Medica. 1968; Disponibile su: https://books.google.it/books?id=17tqAAAAMAAJ.
17. Meckel S, Spittau B, McAuliffe W. The persistent trigeminal artery: development, imaging anatomy, variants, and associated vascular pathologies. Neuroradiology. 2013;55(1):5–16.
18. Moffat DB. Developmental changes in the aortic arch system of the rat. Am J Anat. 1959;105:1–35.
19. Moffat DB, Morris ED. Abnormal origin of the basilar artery from the cervical part of the internal carotid and its embryological significance. Anat Rec. 1956;125(4):701–11.
20. Morris P. Practical neuroangiography. Philadelphia: Lippincott Williams & Wilkins; 1997.
21. Murayama Y, Fujimoto N, Matsumoto K. Bilateral persistent primitive hypoglossal arteries associated with a large ruptured aneurysm on one side. Surg Neurol. 1985;24(5):498–502.
22. O'uchi E, O'uchi T. Persistent primitive trigeminal arteries (PTA) and its variant (PTAV): analysis of 103 cases detected in 16,415 cases of MRA over 3 years. Neuroradiology. 2010;52(12):1111–9.
23. Ogawa T, Fujita H, Inugami A, Shishido F, Higano S, Uemura K. Anomalous origin of the posterior inferior cerebellar artery from the posterior meningeal artery. AJNR Am J Neuroradiol. 1991;12(1):186.
24. Ohshiro S, Inoue T, Hamada Y, Matsuno H. Branches of the persistent primitive trigeminal artery—an autopsy case. Neurosurgery. 1993;32(1):144–8.
25. Padget DH. The development of the cranial arteries in the human embryo. Washington, DC: Carnegie Institution of Washington; 1948. Contributions to embryology.
26. Parkinson D, Shields CB. Persistent trigeminal artery: its relationship to the normal branches of the cavernous carotid. J Neurosurg. 1974;40(2):244–8.
27. Piotin M, Miralbes S, Cattin F, et al. MR and MR angiography of persistent trigeminal artery. Neuroradiology. 1996;38:730.

28. Salas E, et al. Persistent trigeminal artery. An anatomical study. Neurosurgery. 1998;43:557.
29. Saltzman GF. Patent primitive trigeminal artery studied by cerebral angiography. Acta radiologica. 1959;51(5):329–36.
30. Schmeidel G. Die entwicklung der arteria vertebralis des menschen. Gegenbaur Morph Jahrbuch. 1932;71:315–435.
31. Schnürer LB, Stattin S. Vascular supply of intracranial dura from internal carotid artery with special reference to its angiographic significance. Acta Radiol Diagn. 1963;1(2):441–50.
32. Scotti G. Anterior inferior cerebellar artery originating from the cavernous portion of the internal carotid artery. Radiology. 1975;116(1):93–4.
33. Shin YS, Kim SY, Kim BM, Park SI. Ruptured aneurysm of the anomalous cerebellar artery originating from internal carotid artery presenting with carotid cavernous fistula: a case report. Am J Neuroradiol. 2005;26(7):1849–51.
34. Siqueira M, Piske R, Ono M, Marino JR. Cerebellar arteries originating from the internal carotid artery. AJNR Am J Neuroradiol. 1993;14(5):1229–35.
35. Suttner N, Mura J, Tedeschi H, et al. Persistent trigeminal artery: a unique anatomic specimen—analysis and therapeutic implications. Neurosurgery. 2000;47:428.
36. Sutton D. Anomalous carotid—basilar anastomosis. Br J Radiol. 1950;23(274):617–9.
37. Suzuki S, Nobechi T, Itoh I, Yakura M, Iwashita K. Persistent proatlantal intersegmental artery and occipital artery originating from internal carotid artery. Neuroradiology. 1979;17(2):105–9.
38. Tanohata K, Maehara T, Noda M, Katoh H, Sugiyama S, Okazaki A. Anomalous origin of the posterior meningeal artery from the lateral medullary segment of the posterior inferior cerebellar artery. Neuroradiology. 1987;29(1):89–92.
39. Teal JS, Rumbaugh CL, Bergeron RT, Scanlan RL, Segall HD. Persistent carotid-superior cerebellar artery anastomosis: a variant of persistent trigeminal artery. Radiology. 1972;103(2):335–41.
40. Uchino A, Suzuki C. Posterior inferior cerebellar artery supplied by the jugular branch of the ascending pharyngeal artery diagnosed by MR angiography: report of two cases. Cerebellum. 2011;10(2):204–7.
41. Uchino A, Kato A, Takase Y, Kudo S. Persistent trigeminal artery variants detected by MR angiography. Eur Radiol. 2000;10(11):1801–4.
42. Uchino A, Saito N, Okada Y, Kozawa E, Nishi N, Mizukoshi W, et al. Persistent hypoglossal artery and its variants diagnosed by CT and MR angiography. Neuroradiology. 2013;55(1):17–23.
43. Wollschlaeger PB, Wollschlaeger G. The circle of Willis. In: Newton TH, Potts DG, editors. Radiology of the skull and brain: angiography, vol. 2. St Louis: Mosby; 1974.

6 Ophthalmic Artery

At embryo of 4–5 mm, the already appeared optic vesicle is surrounded by a peri-ocular plexus, which supplies it. To the plexus converge branches of the Primary Maxillary Artery (PMA), arising from the distal ICA (its future Cavernous Portion), the Dorsal Ophthalmic Artery (DOA) arising from ICA, slightly cranial to the origin of the PMA, and the Olfactory Artery (OLF). This latter is the main branch of the Cranial Division of ICA. The artery, in its course toward the base of the Prosencephalon, to supply the Olfactory Lobe, runs close to the optic vesicle, optic vesicle, along the periocular plexus connection between these three artery develop [19, 22] (Fig. 6.1).

These connections in the further evolution, disappear, but in some cases as it is described further, can persist, explaining in the adult some anomalies of the ophthalmic arteries and other vessels.

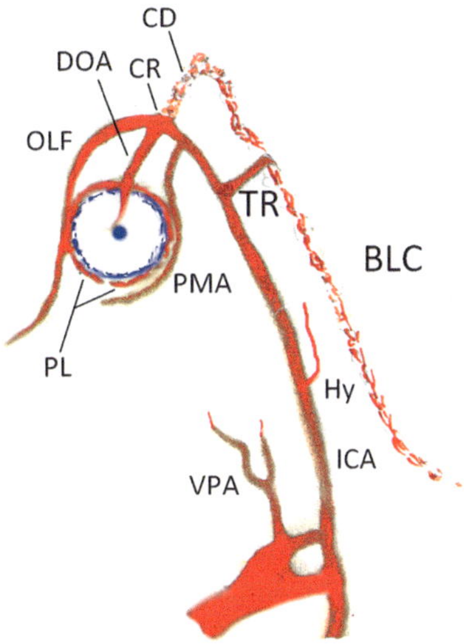

Fig. 6.1 Diagram showing the optic vesicle of the embryo of 4–5 mm. Peri-ocular plexus (PL). Olfactory Artery (OLF). Primary Maxillary Artery (PMA). Dorsal Ophthalmic Artery (DOA). Cranial (CR) and caudal (CD) division of ICA. Primary trigeminal Artery (TR). Bilateral Longitudinal Channel (BLC). Hyoid Artery (Hy). Mandibular Artery (MA). Ventral Pharyngeal Artery (VPA)

G. B. Bradac, *Origin and Development of Cerebral Vessels*,
https://doi.org/10.1007/978-3-031-78436-1_6

6.1 Evolution of the Ophthalmic Artery from 9 to 18 mm Embryo

The Primary Maxillary Artery (PMA) is regressed. At 9 mm embryo appears the Ventral Ophthalmic Artery (VOA) arising from ICA opposite the AchA. It gives off the Nasal Ciliary Arteries. The Temporal Ciliary Arteries and the Hyaloid Artery (future Central Retinal Artery) arise from the Dorsal Ophthalmic Artery. Both arteries form a ring around the Optic Nerve.

At 14 mm embryo, from the Hyoid artery, develops an important collateral, the Stapedial Artery. The artery runs cranially, passes through the Stape and shortly beyond divides in two branches: the *Mandibular (MA)* and the *Supra-Orbital (SUP) arteries.* The mandibular is the lower branch. It runs along the mandibular branch of the fifth nerve, passes through the Foramen Spinosum, becoming extracranial anastomosing with the Ascending Maxillary branch, of the VPA (Ventral Pharyngeal Artery, future External Carotid Artery) forming the mandibular—maxillary branch, from which develops the Internal Maxillary Artery (IMA, See Chap. 7). Among its branches there is the proximal part of the Middle Meningeal Artery (MMA). This later runs back toward the Intracranial Cavity, passes the Foramen Spinosum, anastomosing with the distal part of the MMA, developing from the Supra-Orbital branch. From the fusion of this segment develops the MMA.

As far it concerns the Supra-Orbital Artery, it contributes to the formation of the MMA and to the formation of all Intra-Orbital branches, with exception of that of Ocular bulbi, arising from the DOA and VOA (Fig. 6.2).

Following the regression of the Stapedial Artery, the SUP progressively dwindles and regresses. The Intra-Orbital branches are incorporated by the Ophthalmic Arteries. From its extra-ocular segments, the important remnant is the MMA, from which arises a branch extending anteriorly, entering the orbit to the Superior Orbital Fissure, anastomosing with the Lacrimal branch, remnant of the regressed SUP, now branch of the Ophthalmic arteries.

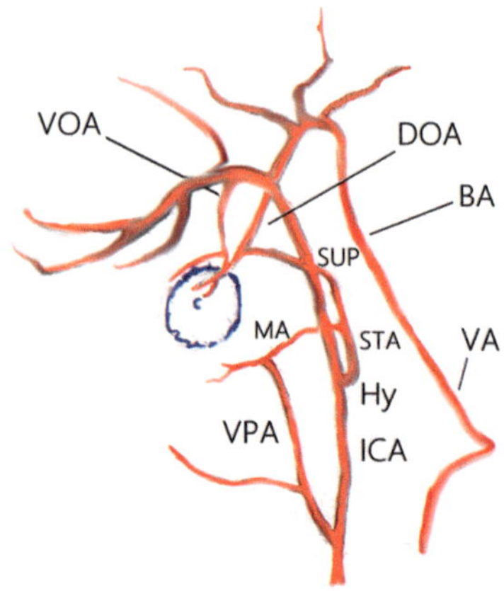

Fig. 6.2 Diagram of the embryo in evolution from 9 to 18 mm. From the Hyoid Artery arises the Stapedial Artery (STA). Mandibular Artery (MA). Supra-orbital Artery (SUP). Dorsal—Ventral Ophthalmic Arteries (DOA and VOA). Connections between VPA and MA. Branches of the cranial division of ICA (MCA, ACA, AchA). Vertebro-basilar system is formed (VA–BA)

Commonly this connection, called meningo-lacrimal branch, enters the orbital through the SOF, but in some cases through a small lateral foramen called "Hirtl foramen." In this context, it is useful to recall the studies of some authors [7, 16, 21], who demonstrated that in the early stages the great wing of the sphenoid bone is not ossified and so the artery, depending on its position can enter the orbit differently.

The VOA is annexed by the DOA, which is now the unique Ophthalmic Artery. Following the different growth in size and direction between the Frontal part of the brain and the orbital structures, the DOA becomes elongated and stretched. To compensate this condition, the artery moves along the ICA from its distal primordial origin to its more anterior final position. This process occurs by means of series of anastomotic loops, described by Streeter [30] who called it *Anastomotic Progression.*

At the embryo of 40–44 mm, the Ophthalmic Artery has reached the configuration comparable to that of the adult (Fig. 6.3).

There is a contemporaneous evolution of the cerebral branches of ICA, the evolution of the Vertebro-basilar system and the External Carotid Artery (see Chaps. 2, 3, and 7).

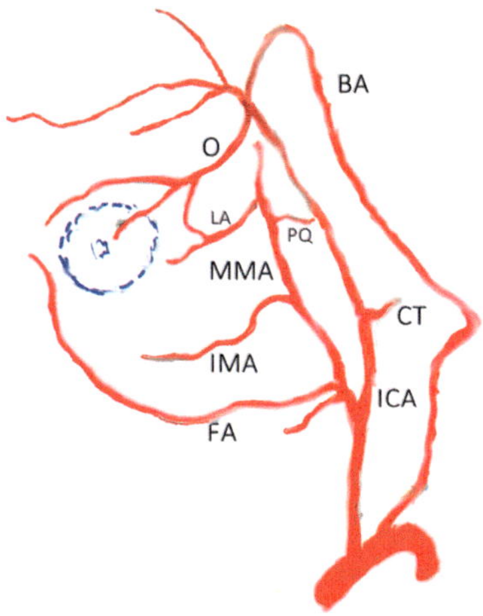

Fig. 6.3 Embryo at 44 mm. Ophthalmic Artery (O). Internal Maxillary Artery (IMA). Middle Meningeal Artery (MMA) connected with the Ophthalmic Artery (future Meningo-lacrimal branch, LA—Petro-squamous branch, PQ)

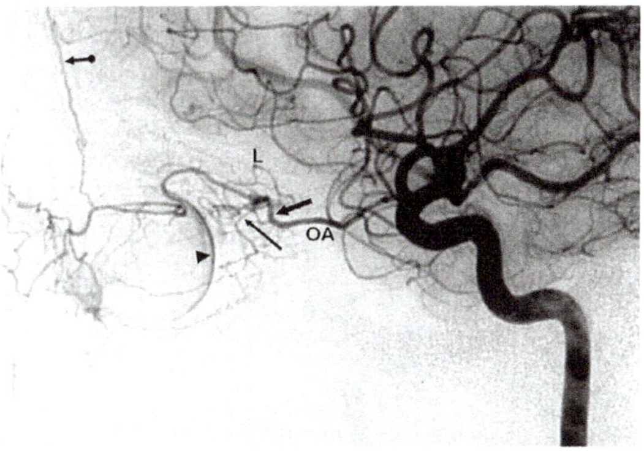

Fig. 6.4 Angiogram in the adult. Ophthalmic Artery (OA). Curve around the optic nerve (arrow). Ocular branches (small arrow). Lacrimal Artery (L). Choroid plexus (arrowhead). Anterior Falx Artery (Arrow with dot). (Taken from Bradac [2])

In the adult, in accordance to the studies of Hayreh [12–14], the Ophthalmic Artery arises commonly from the Superior Medial surface of ICA, close to the point where the ICA has perforated the Dura. The Ophthalmic Artery runs below the Optic Nerve, accompanying it through the Optic Canal. About 2 cm from its origin it forms a curve around the Optic Nerve, reaching his superior surface, continuing its course anteriorly, parallel and medial to the nerve. It gives off ocular, orbital, and extra-orbital branches. The ocular branches, including the Central Retinal Artery and the Ciliary Arteries, supply Optic Nerve, Retina, and Choroid. Among the orbital branches there are the Lacrimal branch and the Muscular branches for muscle and orbital periosteum. The extra-orbital branches include the Ethmoidal (Anterior and Posterior) which anastomose with Ethmoidal branches of the Spheno-palatine Arteries (branches of IMA). The Anterior Ethmoidal branch gives off the Anterior Falx Artery, anastomosing with the Falx Branches of MMA. Other extra-orbital branches are the frequent prominent Supra-Orbital branch, the Dorso-Nasal, the Medial Palpebral, and the Supra-Trochlear arteries, anastomosing with branches of ECA (Facial Artery, Infra-orbital branches of IMA) and frontal branches of the Superficial Temporal Artery.

On the Angiogram, the Ophthalmic Artery is better visible on the lateral view (Fig. 6.4). Typical in its course is the curve (remnant of the embryonic ring) from which arise the ocular branches. To identify this point is essential in cases of endovascular treatment involving the Ophthalmic Artery.

6.2 Variants

The most frequent is the origin of the Ophthalmic Artery from the MMA (Fig. 6.5).

This develops from an anastomosis between the anterior branch of MMA with the Lacrimal branch of the Ophthalmic Artery, both remnant of the Supra-Orbital Artery. This anastomosis, also called “Meningo Lacrimal” has been already identified in the embryo by Padget [22]. It can persist and dilate in the adult, associated with the regression of the Ophthalmic Artery, resulting in the anomaly [1–3, 6, 8, 17, 18, 31, 32].

This anomaly is typical configuration in lower vertebrates, as shown in the studies of comparative anatomy by some authors [4]. Progressively, in the higher scale of animals, this configuration changes. The Ophthalmic Artery acquires a double origin, partially from ECA and partially from

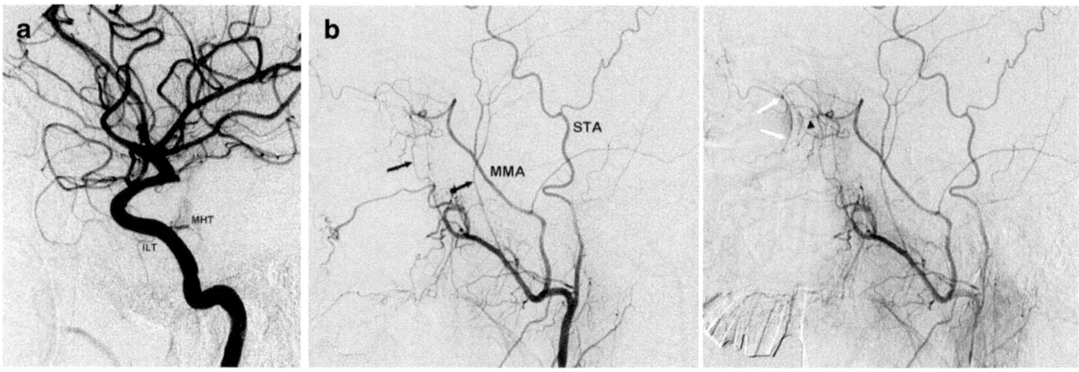

Fig. 6.5 (**a**) ICA angiogram. Absence of the Ophthalmic Artery. Note the presence of the ILT and MHT. (**b**) ECA angiogram (early and later phase). Middle Meningeal Artery (MMA). Through LA, connections with the Ophthalmic Artery filling of Choroid Plexus (white arrows). Deep temporal branches (arrow with dot). Superficial Temporal Artery (STA). (Taken from Bradac [2])

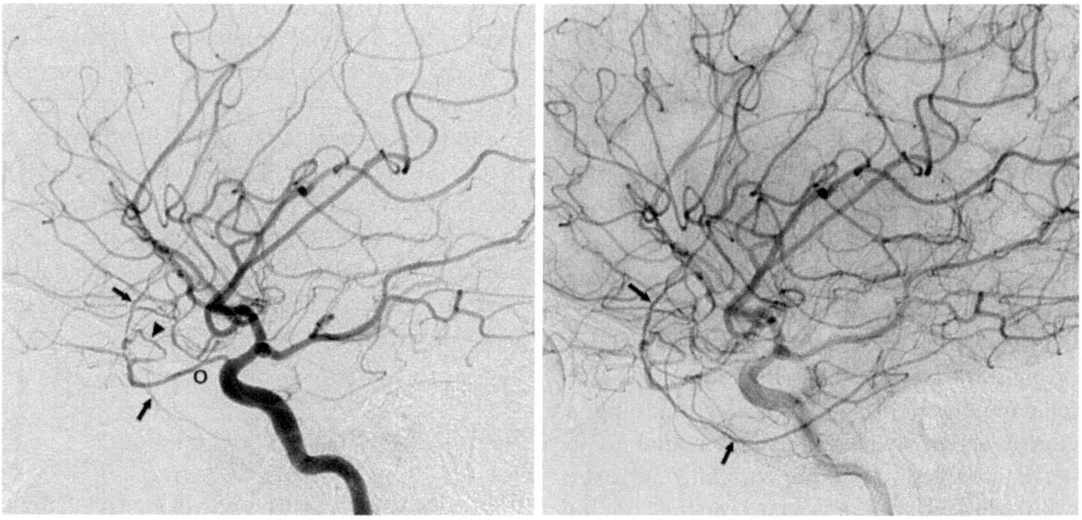

Fig. 6.6 Origin of the MMA (arrows) from Lacrimal branch (arrowhead) of the Ophthalmic Artery (O). (Taken from Bradac [2])

ICA. In the human, the Ophthalmic Artery arises commonly from ICA. In the cases of double contribution, frequently the Middle Meningeal Artery supplies the Orbital branches, while the ICA maintains the supply of the ocular structures.

Another variant involving the MMA is its origin from the OA. In these cases, from the lacrimal branch develops a recurrent branch running back through the SOF supplying the territory of the MMA, which is absent or hypoplastic (Fig. 6.6).

The second most common anomaly is the arising of the OA from cavernous ICA, occurring in about 0.42% of the cases [32] (Fig. 6.7).

Other authors have reported this variant [5, 9, 31].

The interpretation of this anomaly has not been unanimous. Taking into consideration the study of Padget, some authors [9, 31] to whom we agree have proposed that this anomaly is linked with the persistence of the primordial anastomoses between the PML, from which arises later the ILT, and the primordial Opthalmic Artery.

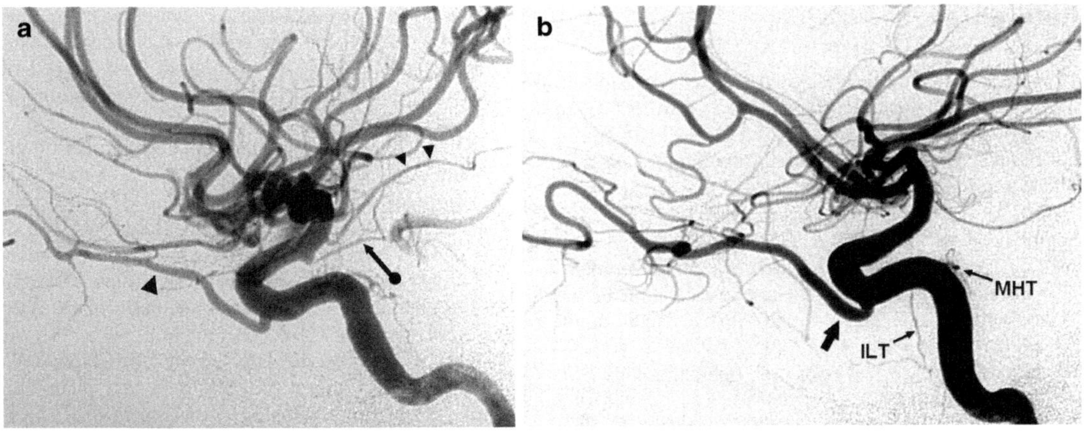

Fig. 6.7 Origin of the Ophthalmic Artery from Cavernous ICA. (**a**) Ophthalmic Artery (arrowhead). AchA (small arrowhead). PcomA (arrow with dot). (**b**) Another example of origin of the Ophthalmic artery from cavernous ICA (arrow). ILT and MHT. (Taken from Bradac [2])

6.3 Other Rarer Variants Can Develop

One is the origin of the OA from the supraclinoid segment of ICA at different levels [9, 11, 20, 23]. These can be interpreted due to persistence of the DOA or VOA. To this group belongs the variant of origin from the PcomA.

Another is the origin of the OA from the ACA. After the first report by Picard et al. [24], a few other cases have been described [9, 31]. These latter authors have related it to an anomalous evolution of the OLF. As already described above, this artery is involved in the supply of the optic vesicle making connections with the DOA. Persistence of these connections which can be taken over by the ACA which replaces the regressed OA, results in the anomaly.

6.4 Other Very Rare Anomalies

6.4.1 Origin of MMA from the Petrous Segment of ICA

In the normal evolution, the MMA develops from the fusion of its proximal and distal segments arising from the IMA and Supraorbital arteries respectively, both developing from the Stapedial Artery (collateral of the Hyoid artery, embryonic branch of the petrous segment of ICA). In the further evolution, the Stapedial Artery regresses. Its persistence can explain the origin of the MMA from the petrous segment of ICA. It can be associated with anomalous origin of IMA from petrous segment of ICA [10, 18, 26]. See also Chap. 7.

6.4.2 Origin of the OA from Basilar Artery

Another very rare variant is the origin of the OA from the BA [25, 27, 28]. This is difficult to explain considering the classical description of the embryogenesis: it has been proposed that this anomaly is due to the persistence of connections between the Stapedial Artery and BLA directly or through the PTA. However, these connections have never been demonstrated. Furthermore, Stapedial Artery and PTA appear in a different stage of the embryogenesis. Similar explanation has been used to explain another extremely rare variant represented by the origin of the MMA from the BA [15, 29].

References

1. Adachi B, Kihara T. Das Arteriensystem der Japaner, Verlag der Kaiserlich-Japanischen Universitat, zu Kyoto. Kommission bei Maruzen Co. 1928:26–46.
2. Bradac GB. Applied cerebral angiography. Normal anatomy and vascular pathology. Cham: Springer; 2017. https://doi.org/10.1007/978-3-319-57228-4. 497 pages, ISBN 978-3-319-57227-7.
3. Dilenge D, Ascherl GF. Variations of the ophthalmic and middle meningeal arteries: relation to the embryonic stapedial artery. Am J Neuroradiol. 1980;1(1):45–54.
4. Duke-Elder S. Text-book of ophthalmology. St. Louis: Mosby; 1932.
5. Fiore DL, Pardatscher K, Fiore D, Zuccarello M, Iraci G. Persistent dorsal ophthalmic artery: report of a case with associated fibromuscular hyperplasia of the extracranial internal carotid artery and multiple cerebral aneurysms. Neurochirurgia. 1981;24(03):106–8.
6. Gailloud P, Gregg L, Ruiz DSM. Developmental anatomy, angiography, and clinical implications of orbital arterial variations involving the stapedial artery. Neuroimaging Clin N Am. 2009;19(2):169–79.
7. Georgiou C, Cassell MD. The foramen meningo-orbitale and its relationship to the development of the ophthalmic artery. J Anat. 1992;180(Pt 1):119.
8. Gillilan LA. The collateral circulation of the human orbit. Arch Ophthalmol. 1961;65(5):684–94.
9. Gregg L, San Millán D, Tamargo RJ, Gailloud P. Ventral and dorsal persistent primitive ophthalmic arteries. Oper Neurosurg. 2016;12(2):141–52.
10. Guinto FCJ, Garrabrant EC, Radcliffe WB. Radiology of the persistent stapedial artery. Radiology. 1972;105(2):365–9.
11. Hamada J, Kitamura I, Kurino M, Sueyoshi N, Uemura S, Ushio Y. Abnormal origin of bilateral ophthalmic arteries: case report. J Neurosurg. 1991;74(2):287–9.
12. Hayreh SS. The ophthalmic artery: III. Branches. Br J Ophthalmol. 1962;46(4):212–47.
13. Hayreh SS, Dass R. The ophthalmic artery: I. Origin and intra-cranial and intra-canalicular course. Br J Ophthalmol. 1962a;46(2):65.
14. Hayreh SS, Dass R. The ophthalmic artery: II. Intra-orbital course. Br J Ophthalmol. 1962b;46(3):165.
15. Kumar S, Mishra NK. Middle meningeal artery arising from the basilar artery: report of a case and its probable embryological mechanism. J Neurointerven Surg. 2012;4(1):43–4.
16. Laine F, Nadel L, Braun IF. CT and MR imaging of the central skull base. Part 1: techniques, embryologic development, and anatomy. Radiographics. 1990;10(4):591–602.
17. Lombardi G. Ophthalmic artery anomalies. Ophthalmologica. 1969;157(5):321–7.
18. McLennan JE, Rosenbaum AE, Haughton V. Internal carotid origins of the middle meningeal artery: the ophthalmic-middle meningeal and stapedial-middle meningeal arteries. Neuroradiology. 1974;7(5):265–75.
19. Moffat DB. The embryology of the arteries of the brain: Arris and Gale lecture delivered at the Royal College of Surgeons of England on 27th February 1962. Ann R Coll Surg Engl. 1962;30(6):368.
20. N'da HA, Peltier J, Zunon-Kipré Y, Alsaiari S, Foulon P, Legars D, et al. An unusual superolateral origin of ophthalmic artery: an anatomic case report. Surg Radiol Anat. 2014;36:95–7.
21. Nemzek WR, Brodie HA, Hecht ST, Chong BW, Babcook CJ, Seibert JA. MR, CT, and plain film imaging of the developing skull base in fetal specimens. Am J Neuroradiol. 2000;21(9):1699–706.
22. Padget DH. The development of the cranial arteries in the human embryo. Washington, DC: Carnegie Institution of Washington; 1948. Contributions to embryology.
23. Parlato C, Di Nuzzo G, Luongo M, Tortora F, Briganti F. Anatomical variant of origin of ophthalmic artery: case report. Surg Radiol Anat. 2011;33:275–8.
24. Picard L. Radiological anatomy of the origin of the ophthalmic artery. Mod Probl Ophthalmol. 1975;14:164–9.
25. Rivera R, Choi IS, Sordo JG, Giacaman P, Badilla L, Bravo E, et al. Unusual origin of the left ophthalmic artery from the basilar trunk. Surg Radiol Anat. 2015;37:399–401.
26. Rodesch G, Choi IS, Lasjaunias P. Complete persistence of the hyoido-stapedial artery in man. Case report. Intra-petrous origin of the maxillary artery from ICA. Surg Radiol Anat. 1991;13(1):63–5.
27. Sade B, Tampieri D, Mohr G. Ophthalmic artery originating from basilar artery: a rare variant. Am J Neuroradiol. 2004;25(10):1730–1.
28. Schumacher M, Wakhloo AK. An orbital arteriovenous malformation in a patient with origin of the ophthalmic artery from the basilar artery. Am J Neuroradiol. 1994;15(3):550–3.
29. Seeger JF, Hemmer JF. Persistent basilar/middle meningeal artery anastomosis. Radiology. 1976;118(2):367–70.
30. Streeter GL. The developmental alterations in the vascular system of the brain of the human embryo. Contrib Embryol Carneg Inst. 1918;8:5–38.
31. Toma N. Anatomy of the ophthalmic artery: embryological consideration. Neurol Med Chir. 2016;56(10):585–91.
32. Uchino A, Saito N, Kurita H, Ishihara S. Double ophthalmic arteries arising from the internal carotid artery. Surg Radiol Anat. 2013;35:173–5.

External Carotid Artery 7

7.1 Early Evolution

At the embryo of 4–5 mm, from the Aortic Sac close to the origin of the third Arch arises the Primitive External Carotid Artery called by Congdon [3] *Ventral Pharyngeal Artery* (VPA). The first and second aortic arches disappeared. The mandibular and the hyoid arteries respectively are the remnants annexed by the ICA.

The distal branches of the VPA and Mandibular artery anastomose contributing to the supply of the developing maxillary process (Fig. 7.1). In the further evolution the Mandibular Artery, as described in Chap. 5, regresses. The artery sometimes persists in the adult as a small vessel arising from the petrous segment of ICA.

G. B. Bradac, *Origin and Development of Cerebral Vessels*,
https://doi.org/10.1007/978-3-031-78436-1_7

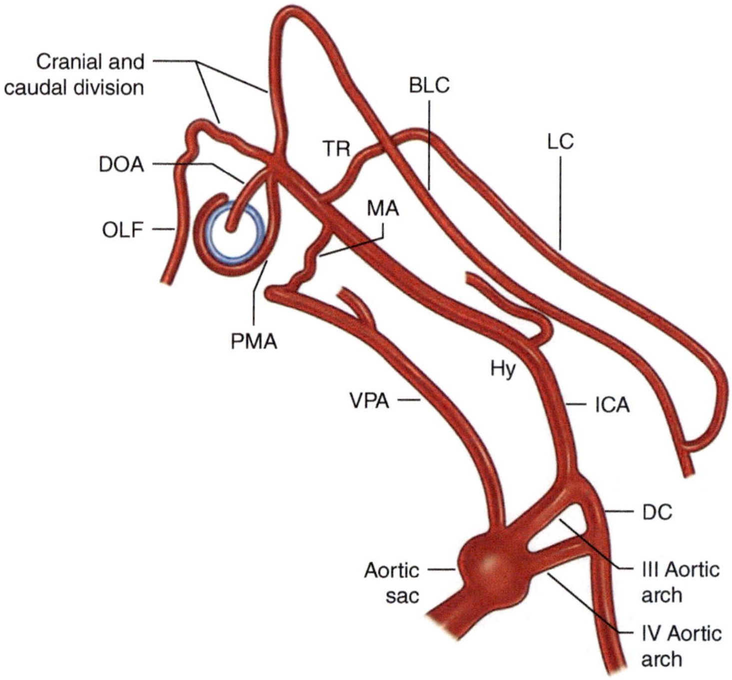

Fig. 7.1 The primitive ECA called *Ventral Pharyngeal Artery* (VPA) arises from the Aortic Sac. The Mandibular Artery (MA), remnant of the regressed first aortic arch, and the Hyoid artery (HY), remnant of the second aortic arch, are developed. Third and fourth aortic arches are present. Ductus Caroticus (DC). Internal carotid artery (ICA). Primary Maxillary Artery (PMA). Dorsal Ophthalmic Artery (DOA). Olfactory Artery (OLF). Cranial and caudal Division of ICA. Primary Trigeminal Artery (TR). Bilateral Longitudinal Channel (BLC), Lateral Longitudinal Channel (LC)

7.2 Evolution of the Embryo from 14 mm to 18mm

At the Embryo of 14 mm from the Hyoid artery arises an important collateral called "the Stapedial Artery" (see also Chap. 6). It runs cranially, enters the tympanic cavity, passes through the Stapedial Stapes, dividing then in two branches. The one is the *Mandibular* which should not be confused with the above described Mandibular Artery, already described in Chap. 5. The artery is directed extra-cranially, passes through the *Foramen Spinosum* connecting with the ascending branches of the VPA forming the Mandibular-Maxillary branch from which develops the Internal Maxillary Artery (IMA). From IMA arise progressively its branches. One of these is the proximal part of the Middle Meningeal Artery (MMA). This runs intra-cranially passing again through the *Foramen Spinosu*m joining its distal part developed from the *Supraorbital Artery*. This is the second branch of the Stapedial Artery, involved mainly in the development of the orbital vasculature (see Chap. 6). From it develops the distal segment of the MMA, joined by the proximal segment forming the complete MMA.

7.3 Evolution of the Embryo from 18 mm to 40–44 mm

At 18 mm embryo, the Stapedial Artery regresses. Its remnant, at its origin from the hyoid artery is the small Carotid Tympanic branch, arising now from the petrous segment of ICA.

The intra-orbital branches of the supra-orbital artery are annexed by the Ophthalmic Artery. From the MMA arises a branch directed to the orbita, as described in Chap. 6. Another small branch of the MMA directed posteriorly is the Superior tympanic branch, which becomes later a branch of the Petro-squamous branch of the MMA.

As far as it concerns the VPA, in this phase the artery regresses replaced by the new Linguo-Facial Thyroid trunk. The Facial artery extends cranially anastomosing distally with branches of the ophthalmic artery. Later appearing of the complex Ascending Pharingeal Artery - Occipital Artery and the Superficial Temporal Artery. The evolution of the last phases is shown in Fig. 7.2a, b.

At the embryo of 40–44 mm the External Carotid Artery has acquired the configuration comparable to that of the adult. It will reach its final pattern during the fetal phase.

A very rare deviation occurring in this phase of the evolution, identified in an interesting study by Rodesch et al. [12] is that in which the complex "Stapedial Hyoid" does not regress. The result is the origin of the Internal Maxillary Artery from the petrous segment of ICA. The evolution of the orbital vessels, as well of the other branches of the ECA, is commonly normal. In some cases, however, the persistence of the Stapedial Artery can be associated also with the anomalies involving the Middle Meningeal Artery (see Chap. 6).

The adult configuration of ECA has already been studied in detail by many authors [1, 2, 4, 7, 8, 10]. Only the most essential patterns of the single branches will be presented here.

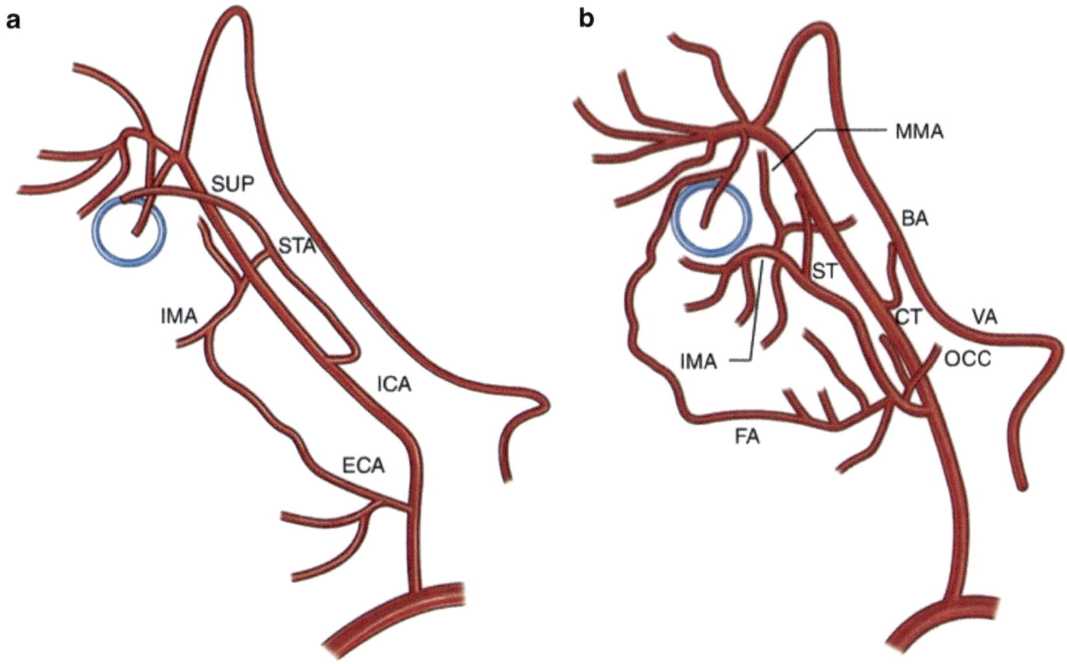

Fig. 7.2 Evolution of the embryo from 14–18 mm to the embryo of 40–44 mm. (**a**) Hyoid Artery (HY). Stapedial Artery (STA). Mandibular Artery (MA) joined by branches of the distal VPA. Formation of the Primary Maxillary Artery (IMA). Middle Meningeal artery (MMA). Supraorbital artery (SUP). (**b**) Appearing from VPA of the Linguo-facial trunk (LFT). The STA is regressed. Carotido-tympanic branch (CT) and future Petrous Squamous branch (PR) of Middle Meningeal Artery (MMA) appear. The IMA is in formation. The MMA is complete. The LFT is formed. The Facial Artery is developed, connected with the branches of the Ophthalmic Arteries. Progressive appearing also of the last branches. In (**a**) and (**b**) for completeness are shown the branches of the carotid system and the basilar and vertebral arteries, already described in Chap. 2 (Fig. 2.5a)

7.4 Internal Maxillary Artery (IMA)

The formed vessel develops rapidly becoming the largest and most important branch of ECA. The course of the IMA is shown in Fig 7.3a, b. It arises behind the neck of the mandibular, running anteriorly towards the masticator place, ending in the pterygopalatine fossa, where it divides in its terminal branches.

From its first segment arise the Inferior Alveolar Artery (Inf. A., supplying this area), the Middle Meningeal Artery (MMA), and the Accessory Meningeal Artery (AMA).

The MMA passes through the *Foramen spinosum*, becoming intra-cranial. It runs antero-laterally in the Middle Cranial fossa, towards the Pterion. Along its course, it gives off branches for the Dura of the middle and Anterior Cranial fossa. It runs further on the convexity, giving off branches for the Dura of the Fronto-parieto-temporo-occipital regions. Reached the midline, the branches connect, forming a longitudinal arcade, along the Dura covering laterally the Superior Sagittal Sinus. From the formed arcade develop descending branches for the falx cerebri, anastomosing anteriorly with the Ascending Falx branches of the Ethmoidal Arteries, branch of the Ophthalmic Artery and posteriorly with Falx Cerebellar Artery. On the convexity, the branches connect with those of the contralateral.

Short after its entering in the cranial cavity, the MMA send branches connecting medially with the ILT. Another branch is directed anteri-

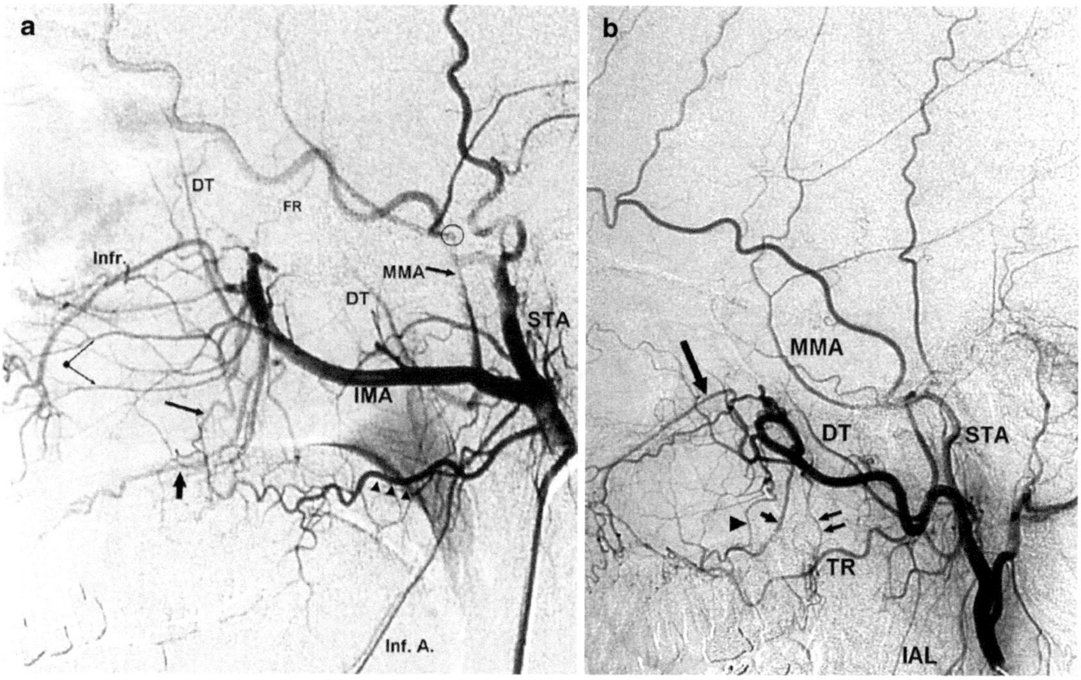

Fig. 7.3 Angiograms of the distal ECA. (**a**) Superficial Temporal Artery (STA). Internal Maxillary artery (IMA). Middle Meningeal artery (MMA). Inferior Alveolar Artery (Inf. A.). Deep temporal branches (DT). Infraorbital branch (infr.). Posterior superior Alveolar Artery (arrow). Descending Palatine Artery (great arrow). Sphenopalatine branches (arrow with angle). Transverse Facial Artery (arrow head). (**b**) The STA and the MMA are better shown. Posterior Superior Alveolar Artery (arrow head). Descending Palatine Artery (arrow). Inferior Alveolar Artery (IAL). Buccal Artery (arrows). Transverse Facial Artery (TR). (Taken from Bradac [2])

orly, becoming later the Anterior Branch of the ILT (see also Chap. 5) connected with the Lacrimal branch of the Ophthalmic Artery. Another branch, sometimes well-developed called the Petro-squamous Artery is directed dorsally to the region of the Petrous bone, supplying the Dura of the region. There are connections with a branch of the Anterior Inferior Cerebellar Artery (Chap. 3). The Petro-Squamous Artery is involved in the supply of the tympanic cavity (Superior Tympanic Artery) and in the supply of the Facial Nerve, in its course, in the facial canal, being in a balance with the Stylo-Mastoid branch of the Occipital Artery. The MMA can be involved as an important supplying branch in many pathological conditions, typically meningioma and dura artero-venous fistulas. Examples are presented in Figs. 5.11, 7.4a–c, and 7.5.

As far as it concerns the AMA (Accessory Meningeal Artery), it arises as single or a common branch with the MMA. Differently from the MMA, devoted to the supply of meninges, the AMA in his proximal extracranial segment, gives off branches supplying the Superior oropharyngeal region anastomosing with other branches of the IMA and Ascending Pharyngeal Artery. The AMA enters the cranial cavity passing through the *foramen ovale*, anastomosing with the ILT (see also Chap. 5). The AMA can be involved in intra-cranial pathologies, commonly together with the MMA and extra-cranially in pathologies of the superior oropharyngeal areas, such the juvenile angio-fibroma.

The IMA runs further anteriorly in the "Masticator Space" where it gives descending branches for the Pterygoid, Buccal, Masseter muscles and ascending branches for the Deep Temporal muscles. These latter can anastomose with the lacrimal branch of the Ophthalmic Artery.

The artery ends in the Pterygopalatine fossa where it gives off the Posterior Superior Alveolar artery for the superior alveolar area, the Infraorbital branch entering the orbit through the inferior orbital fissure, running in the infraorbital canal supplying the adjacent bone and muscles anastomosing distally with branches of the ophthalmic artery (Fig. 7.3) and the Descending palatine artery supplying palate and the superior.

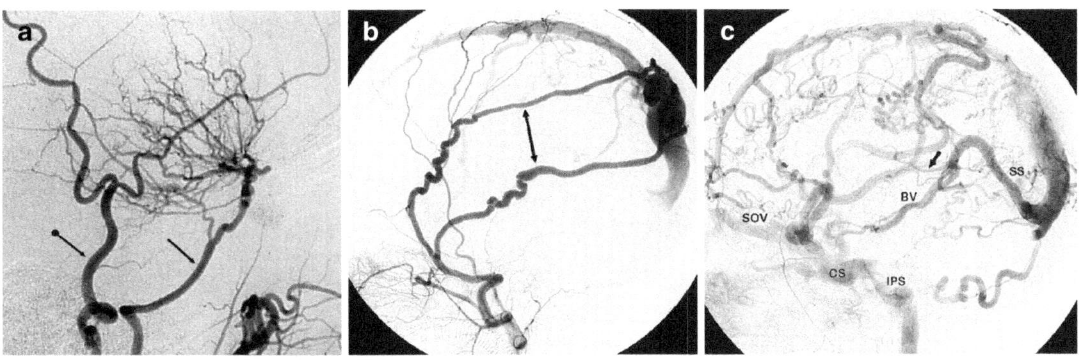

Fig. 7.4 (**a**) Temporo-basal meningioma, richly vascularized by distal branches of the middle meningeal artery. Middle Meningeal Artery (arrow) supplying the tumor. Superficial Temporal Artery (arrow with dot). (**b**) Dural arteriovenous fistula at the level of the SSS in a child. Angiogram of the right external carotid artery (lateral view). Dilated branches of the middle meningeal artery (MMA) (arrow), supplying the fistula in the middle portion of the enlarged SSS. (**c**) Late venous phase. The SSS is distally occluded at the level of the Torcular Herophili. There is a venous congestion, with rerouting of the venous drainage partially in the straight sinus (SS) and further in the superficial and deep venous system (arrow). Basal Vein (BV), continuing to its anterior tributaries. The superficial venous system drains mainly into the cavernous sinus (CS) and further to the inferior petrosal sinus (IPS) and Superior Ophthalmic Vein (SOV). (Taken from Bradac [2])

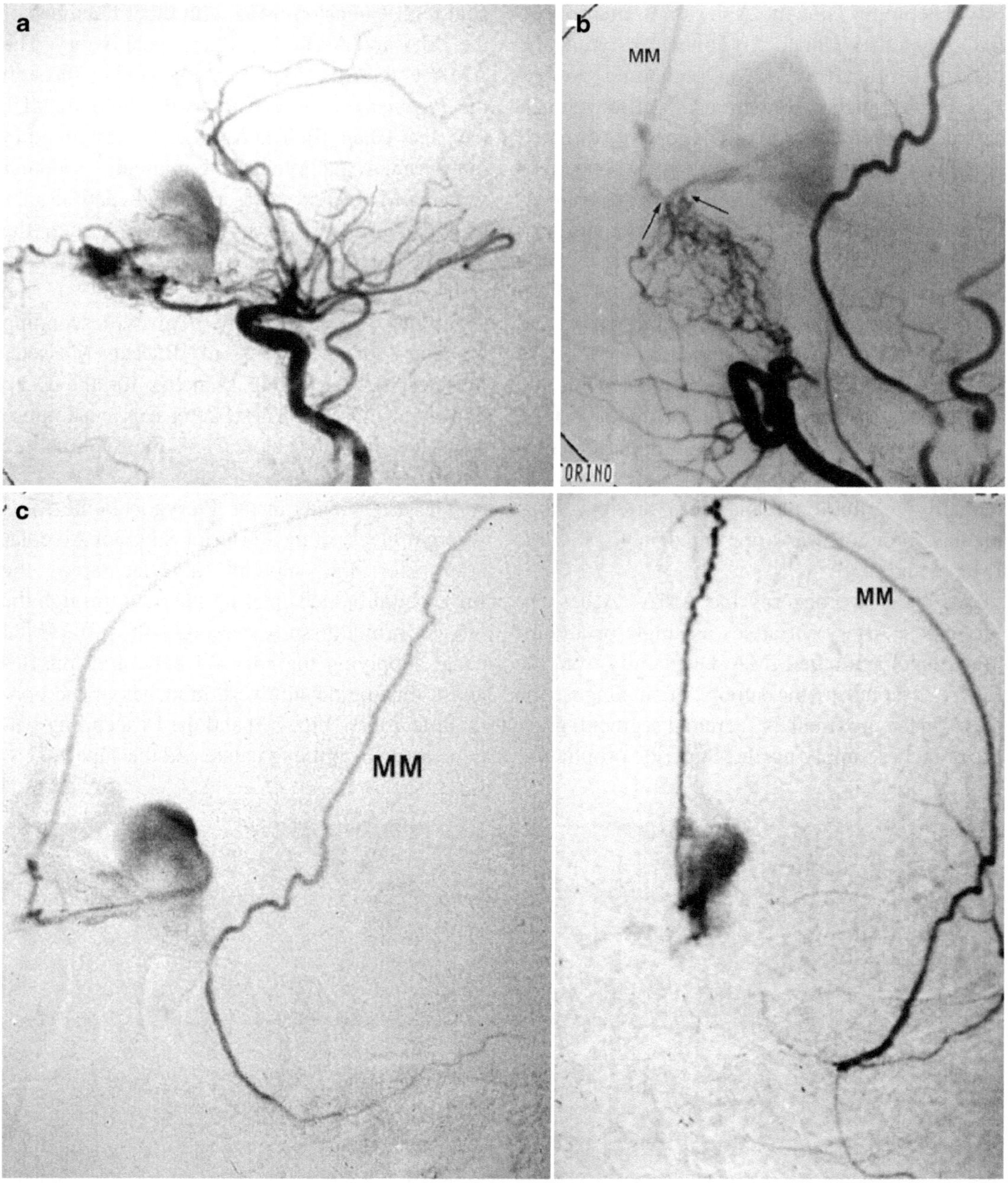

Fig. 7.5 Fronto basal DAVF. (**a**) ICA angiogram showing involvement of the ethmoidal branches of the ophthalmic artery. (**b**) ECA angiogram. Involvement of the Sphenopalatine branches of IMA (arrow). (**c**) The fistula is also supplied by the Falx artery of the MMA. (Taken from Bradac [2])

Other branches arising in the Pterygopalatine fossa are the Pterygo-vaginal artery, passing through the Pterygo-vaginal canal involved in the supply of the oropharyngeal area, the *Foramen Rotundum* artery, passing through the *Foramen Rotundum* anastomosing with the ILT, and the Vidian artery, anastomosing with the persisting Mandibular Artery (See also Chap. 5), which along its course can give also branches for the oropharyngeal region (Fig. 7.3).

As already described in Chap. 5, all these connections can be useful as a collateral way between

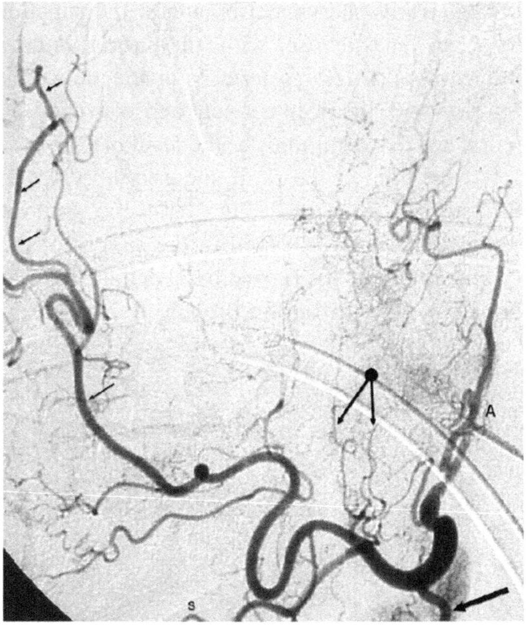

Fig. 7.6 Selective angiographic study of the Facial Artery. Ascending palatine artery (A), branches for the submandibular gland (arrow) and masseter muscle (arrow with dot). Submental artery (S). Distal branches (small arrows) ending in the angular artery. (Taken from Bradac [2])

ICA and ECA. They can also favoring the involvement of both sectors in pathological conditions (Figs. 5.6 and 5.7).

The terminal branch of IMA is the Spheno-Palatine Artery (Fig. 7.3) entering the nasal cavity through the Spheno-Palatine Foramen, giving off branches for the nasal mucosa which anastomose with the descending vessels arising from the Ethmoidal branches of the ophthalmic artery.

7.5 Facial Artery

It arises from the regressing VPA frequently as a common trunk with the lingual artery devoted to the lingual structures. The facial artery extends progressively cranially ending as the angular artery anastomosing with extra-orbital branches of the ophthalmic artery. It gives off many branches for the mental and facial region. One branch sometimes well-developed is the ascending palatine artery anastomosing with other branches of IMA and AphA artery at the superior oropharyngeal area. Examples are presented in Figs. 7.6 and 7.7.

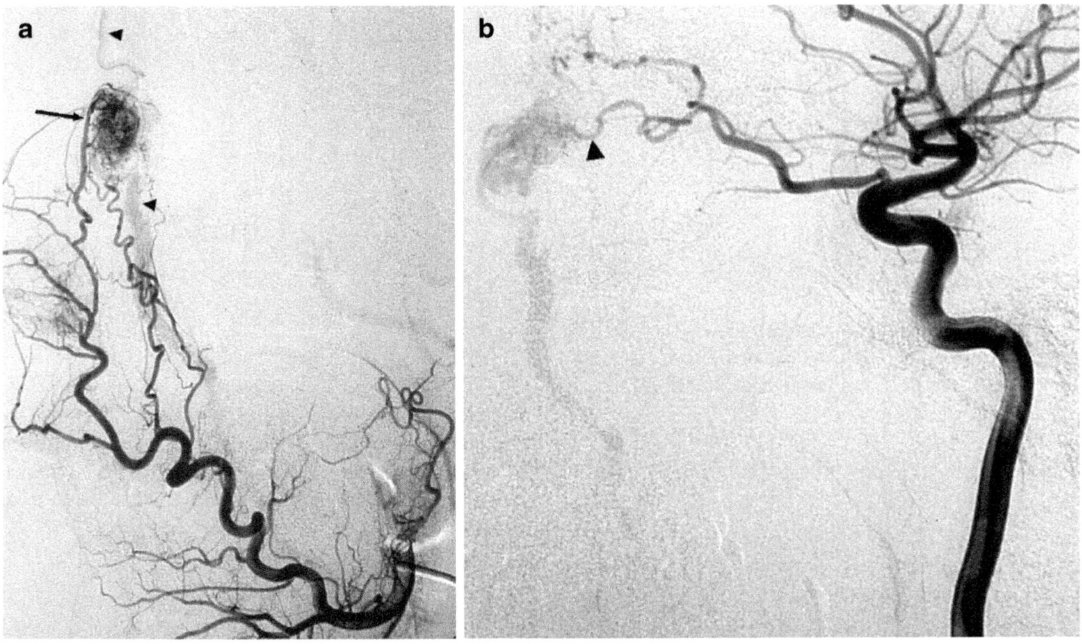

Fig. 7.7 Arteriovenous angioma of the right ala of the nose supplied by branches of the facial artery. (**a**) Lateral angiogram of the Facial Artery. The arteriovenous angioma is supplied by the angular artery (arrow). Early drainage in the facial and frontal veins (arrowhead). (**b**) Distal branches of the Ophthalmic Artery (arrow head) supplying the malformation. (Taken from Bradac [2])

7.6 Ascending Pharyngeal Artery (AphA)

It can be assumed that it arises at the embryo of 18–44 mm from the posterior wall of the formed ECA probably together with the developing occipital artery, maintaining sometimes these connections in the adult (Fig. 7.8). Origin from ICA can also occur, as shown, sometimes in the adult [13]. In its course cranially the artery gives off anteriorly pharyngeal branches, the superior of them anastomose with the corresponding branches of IMA, posteriorly connections can develop with the deep cervical and with the vertebral arteries commonly at the level of C2–C4.

At the base of the skull, the artery divides in its terminal branches (Fig. 7.9): the Inferior Tympanic Artery, involved in the supply of the tympanic cavity, the Hypoglossal and the Jugular branches, and the Carotid Branch.

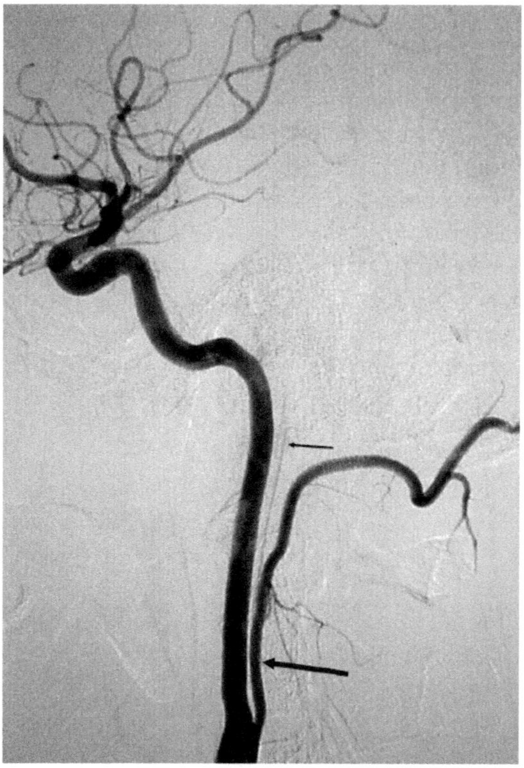

Fig. 7.8 ICA angiogram, lateral view. The occipital artery (arrow) and the AphA (small arrow) arise as a common trunk from the ICA. (Taken from Bradac [2])

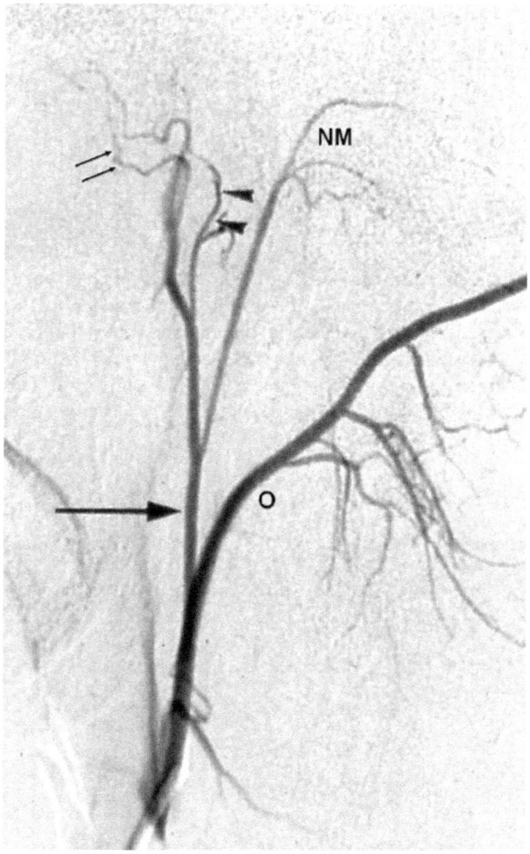

Fig. 7.9 Selective angiogram of the AphA arising as a common trunk from the Occipital Artery (O). Superior Pharyngeal branches (arrows). Inferior Tympanic branch (arrow head). Neuromeningeal trunk (NM). (Taken from Bradac [2])

7.6.1 The Hypoglossal Branch

The hypoglossal branch runs in the hypoglossal canal together with the XII nerve, the Anterior Condylar Vein, and when present with the persistent Hypoglossal artery. It gives off descending and ascending branches, the first anastomoses with the ascending Radiculo-Menigeal branch arising from VA at the C3–C4 level. It anastomoses with a branch running on the dorsal surface of the odontoid process with the contralateral branch, contributing to the formation of the so-called Odontoid Arch (Figs. 7.10 and 7.11). The ascending branch runs on the medial surface of *clivus* connecting with descending branches of MHT, as described in Chap. 5.

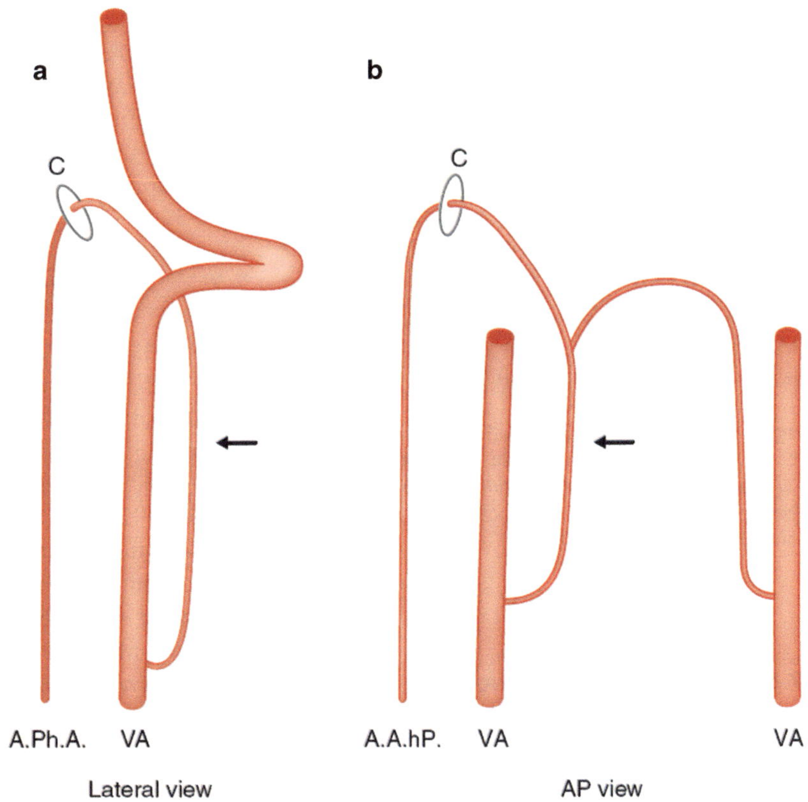

Fig. 7.10 Drawing. (**a**) Lateral view showing the connection of the Hypoglossal artery with the vertebral artery formed by the hypoglossal branch passing through the Hypoglossal canal taking a descending course connecting with the ascending radiculo-meningeal branch of the VA (arrow). (**b**) AP view showing the connections through a branch running on the dorsal surface of the odontoid process with the contralateral. (Taken from Bradac [2])

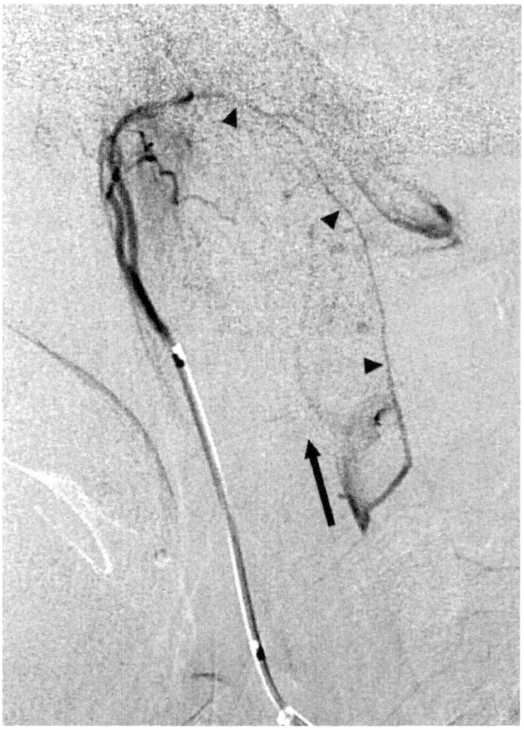

Fig. 7.11 Selective study of the Hypoglossal branch of the AphA in a patient with a Tympano-jugular Paraganglioma. Dangerous anastomosis with the radiculo-meningeal branch (arrow head) of the Vertebral Artery (arrow). (Taken from Bradac [2])

7.6.2 The Jugular Branch

The Jugular Branch runs through the jugular foramen together with the IX, X, XI nerves. It gives off an ascending branch extending on the lateral surface of clivus anastomosing with descending branches of the MHT (see also Chap. 5).

Both the Hypoglossal and the Jugular branches can also give branches supplying the dura of the posterior fossa.

7.6.3 The Carotid Ramus

It arises from the distal AphA, accompanies the ICA in its petrous course anastomosing at the level of the Foramen Lacerum with a recurrent branch of the ILT.

Due to its course and connection, the AphA can be involved in many pathological processes, such as tumors, typically paraganglioma and juvenile angiofibroma and DAVFs of the skull basis and of the cervico-occipital regions. Examples are shown in Figs. 7.12a–c and 9.23.

It can play an important role in the supply of the *rete mirabile* (Chap. 3) and in the anomaly involving the hypoglossal artery and the PICA (see Chap. 5).

7.7 Occipital Artery

Padget [11] described the artery arising from ECA at the embryo of 18–44 mm. It can sometimes arise from ICA, as reports first by Newton and Young [9] on an angiographic study in the adult (Fig. 7.8). Also a rarer origin from the VA can occur [2].

Along the course of the artery, three segments can be identified (Fig. 7.13a). The first is ascending giving off the Stylo-mastoid artery, entering the Stylo-Mastoid Foramen, accompanying the Facial nerve, and anastomosing with the Petro-Squamous branch of the MMA (see also Chap. 3). Sometimes the Stylo-Mastoid Artery arises from the Posterior auricular artery, a small branch developing frequently in common with the occipital artery, devoted to the supply of the pinna of the ear. From the second more horizontal segment arises the Mastoid branch, entering the mastoid foramen together with the emissary vein. It gives off meningeal branches for the pos-

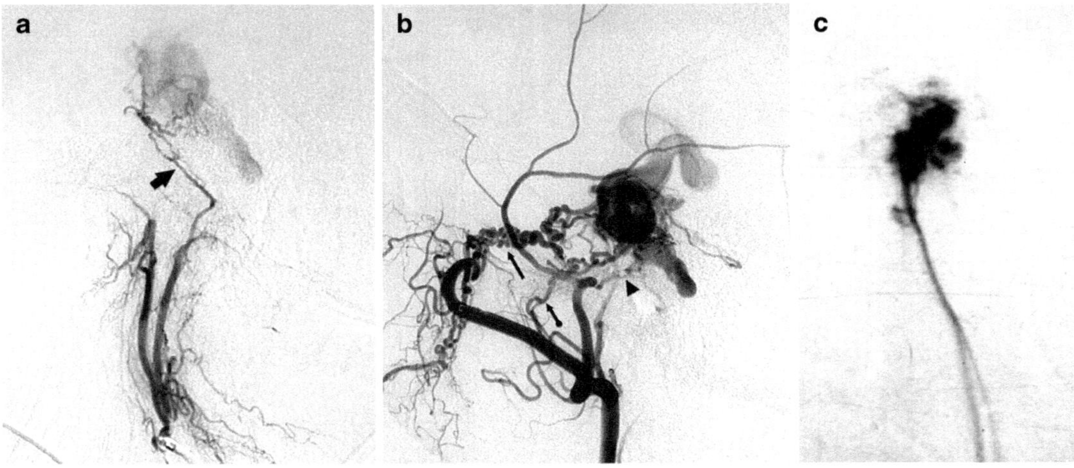

Fig. 7.12 (**a**) Angiogram of the AphA showing the supply through the clival branch (arrow). (**b**) There is also involvement of many branches of IMA. Foramen Rotundum Artery (arrow). Accessory Meningeal Artery (arrow with dot). Middle Meningeal Artery (arrow head). (**c**) Small paraganglioma in another patient supplied only by the tympanic branch of the AphA. (Taken from Bradac [2])

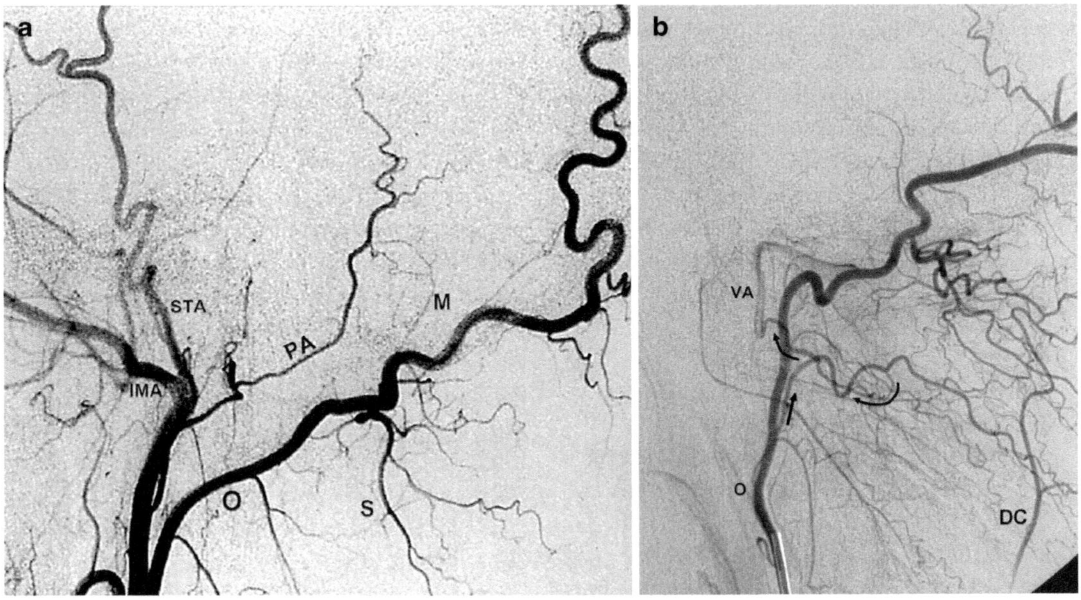

Fig. 7.13 (**a**) Angiogram of the distal ECA. Internal maxillary Artery (IMA). Superficial Temporal Artery (STA). Posterior Auricular Artery (PA). Occipital Artery (O). Splenial branch (S). Mastoid branch (M). (**b**) Selective angiogram of the occipital artery (O) in another patient. There is a clear anastomosis (arrows) between the cutaneous-muscular branch of the ascending segment of the occipital artery with the VA. There are other anastomoses between the horizontal segment of the occipital artery and the deep cervical artery (DC). This latter is retrograde injected and partially also connected to the VA. (Taken from Bradac [2])

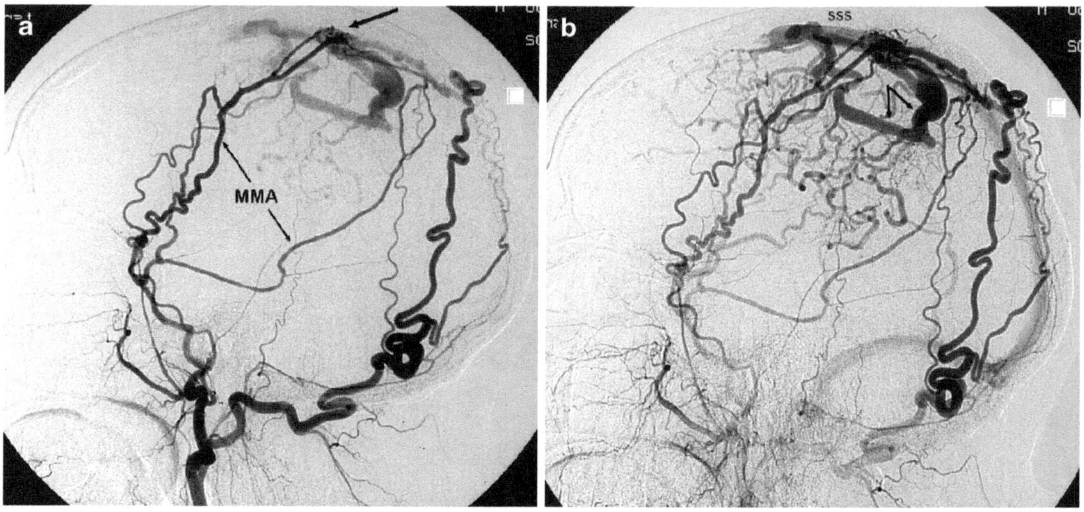

Fig. 7.14 Angiogram of ECA in patient with DAVF (arrow) at the level of the Superior Sagital Sinus (SSS). (**a**) Supplied by branches of the Middle Meningeal artery (MMA) and Transosseous branches of the occipital artery (O). (**b**) There is a retrograde filling of the parietal cortical veins. (Taken from Bradac [2])

terior fossa in balance with branches arising from AphA, VA, MMA. From the first and second segments arise Muscolo-Cutaneous branches which have connections with the VA and the Deep Cervical Arteries at the C1–C2 level (Fig. 7.13b). The terminal segment is again ascending. It can give trans-osseous branches anastomosing with the MMA involved in DAVFs (Fig. 7.14a–b).

7.7.1 Considerations About Anomalous Origin and Pattern of Occipital Artery and AphA

Comparative studies in mammals [5, 6] (see also Chap. 3) have shown, in some of these, the presence of a network (RETE MIRABILE) replacing the aplastic cervical segment of the Internal carotid artery (ICA). Typically, from the common carotid artery arises a trunk formed by the proximal segment of the aplastic ICA, from the occipital artery and from ascending pharyngeal artery. This latter is greatly involved in the supply of the Rete Mirabile, and can sometimes be so hypertrophied to be mistaken for the ICA. From the Common carotid artery arise the other branches of ECA. Among them the Internal Maxillary artery is also involved in the supply of the Rete.

This pattern can be present exceptionally in the adult human replacing the aplastic ICA. Other anomalies in the adult not so rare, as described above, are the origin of the occipital and ascending pharyngeal arteries from ICA. Therefore, it seems conceivable that some aspects of the early embryogenesis in the human are not so greatly different from that of some animals. This could favor, in particular conditions, the developing of the above described anomalies.

As far as it concerns the relationship between the Occipital and the Vertebral Artery, the above described studies have shown that connections between these arteries are a typical pattern in many mammals. The same connection can be present in the human and become active if the flow in one of the two vascular sectors is impaired. It is therefore not surprising that a deviation of the normal evolution could result in the origin of the Occipital from the VA.

7.8 Superficial Temporal Artery (STA)

It is with the IMA the second terminal branch of ECA. The artery arises in the parotid gland, crosses the zygomatic process, extending cranially, giving off branches supplying the scalp in the temporo-parietal and partial frontal regions (Figs. 7.3 and 7.13). It can give off the transverse facial artery. This latter arises directly from the distal ECA or as a branch of the IMA. It can be well developed if the Facial Artery is hypoplastic. The STA can give off trans-osseous branches anastomosing with the MMA, and with its anterior frontal branches can anastomose with the distal branches of the ophthalmic artery.

References

1. Allen WF III, Kier EL, Rothman SL. The maxillary artery: normal arteriographic anatomy. Am J Roentgenol. 1973;118(3):517–27.
2. Bradac GB. Applied cerebral angiography: normal anatomy and vascular pathology. Cham: Springer; 2017. https://doi.org/10.1007/978-3-319-57228-4. 497 pages, ISBN 978-3-319-57227-7
3. Congdon ED. Transformation of the aortic-arch system during the development of the human embryo. Embryol Carneg Instn. 1922;14:47–110. Contributions to embryology.
4. Djindjian R, Merland JJ. Super-selective arteriography of the external carotid artery. Berlin: Springer; 1978.
5. Du Boulay GH. Comparative neuroradiologic vascular anatomy of experimental animals. Radiology of the skull and brain, vol. 2763. St. Louis: Mosby; 1974. p. 2786.
6. Du Boulay GH, Verity PM. The cranial arteries of mammals. (No Title). London: Williams Heinemann; 1973.
7. Lasjaunias PL. Craniofacial and upper cervical arteries. Baltimore/London: Williams & Wilkins; 1981.
8. Morris P. Practical neuroangiography. Lippincott Williams & Wilkins; 1997.
9. Newton TH, Young DA. Anomalous origin of the occipital artery from the internal carotid artery. Radiology. 1968;90(3):550–2.
10. Osborn AG. Diagnostic cerebral angiography. Philadelphia: Lippincott Williams & Wilkins; 1999.
11. Padget DH. The development of the cranial arteries in the human embryo. Washington, DC: Carnegie Institution of Washington; 1948. Contributions to embryology
12. Rodesch G, Choi IS, Lasjaunias P. Complete persistence of the hyoido-stapedial artery in man. Case report. Intra-petrous origin of the maxillary artery from ICA. Surg Radiol Anat. 1991;13(1):63–5.
13. Teal JS, Rumbaugh CL, Segall HD, Bergeron RT. Anomalous branches of the internal cartoid artery. Radiology. 1973;106(3):567–73.

8 Considerations About Meninges and Their Vascularization

In accordance with the studies of Streeter, described in Chap. 2, from the Meninx Primitiva, a mesenchymal tissue, covering the developing brain, develop the extra-cerebral tissues, including the Meninges, bone, and scalp. The consequence of this process is the separation of cerebrum from the extra-cranial tissues, as well as the corresponding vessels.

As far as it concerns the meninges, they progressively cover all part of the brain, including the convexity and the base.

From the primordial meninges, in the further evolution, develop two important segments: the *Falx Cerebri* and the *tentorium.*

As far as it concerns the Falx, it develops from the meninges of the cerebral convexity, growing inside the fissure separating the cerebral hemispheres. It extends through the whole cranial cavity, attached anteriorly to the *Crista Galli* and posteriorly to the occipital protuberance.

Caudally, the Falx has a free margin, lying anteriorly commonly at the level of the cingulate sulcus. Posteriorly is more inferiorly located, close to the Splenium of Corpus Callosum. The peri-callosal artery, running in the peri-callosal sulcus above the corpus callosum lies below the free margin of the Falx, with exception of his segment around the splenium. Differently, the calloso-marginal artery, which runs in the cingulate sulcus, lies in the most part of its course above the free margin of the Falx.

At the origin of the dura of the convexity, the Falx divides in two folls, forming a triangular space, in which runs the developing Superior Sagittal Sinus. Along the free margin of the Falx, can develop the Small Inferior Sagittal Sinus, connected through the Galen vein with the Straight Sinus. In the anatomical study of Oka et al. [7], it was absent in 10% of the cases.

The tentorium is a horizontal dural segment with a slightly downward course, attached medially to the Falx Cerebri and laterally to the dura of the convexity of the occipital bone at its squamous segment. Antero-lateral, the tentorium joins at the superior border of the petrous bone the dura, covering the middle cranial fossa. It extends further anteriorly connecting with the petro-clinoid ligament of the posterior clinoid process. Antero-medial, the tentorium has a free margin surrounding an opening space (*Tentorial Incisura*) forming a kind of collar around the brainstem [8]. The space contains many important vascular structures, including arteries (AchA, PCA, and SCA) and veins (BV). These have been described in detail in Chaps. 3 and 9. The tentorial incisura communicates anteriorly with the optic chiasm, optic nerve, and subcallosal area, the optic tract extends dorsally. Laterally it communicates with the Sylvian Fissure.

The consequence of this evolution is that the cranial cavity is divided by the tentorium in supra-tentorial (containing the cerebral hemi-

G. B. Bradac, *Origin and Development of Cerebral Vessels*,
https://doi.org/10.1007/978-3-031-78436-1_8

spheres) and infra-tentorial (containing the structures of the posterior fossa) part. At the posterior part of the junction of the Falx Cerebri and tentorium, grows caudally a similar smaller structure called the *Falx Cerebelli,* separating the posterior-superior part of the cerebellar hemispheres.

Along the junction of the Falx Cerebri, with the tentorium, develops the straight sinus. At the attachment of the tentorium with the dura covering the occipital bone, develops the Transverse Sinus and the Superior Petrosal Sinus, develops along the attachment of the tentorium at the superior border of the Petrous bone.

At the junction of the Falx Cerebri, tentorium, and the smaller Falx Cerebelli develops the Occipital Sinus, which extends anteriorly along the margin of the Occipital Foramen.

8.1 Considerations About Meningeal Arteries

All these meningeal segments request for their supply, the development of many meningeal vessels, which take a different origin and extent. The main contribution is through the External carotid artery, but many other branches arise from the Ophthalmic artery, from the extracerebral Internal carotid and Vertebral arteries and a few from cerebral vessels (Anterior Cerebral Artery, Posterior Cerebral, and Cerebellar Arteries). Branches with different origin converge to the same meningeal territories where they anastomose and together supply the area. This anatomic condition can be a useful way of collateral circulation, but can also favor the involvement of branches with different origin in the supply of pathologies such as meningiomas and Dural Arterio-venous Fistulae related to the meninges of the area involved.

Meningeal branches can rarely be also involved in the supply of pathologies of the brain such Arterio-venous malformation (see also Chap. 9). This could be due to an anomalous evolution in the early phases of embryogenesis in which the separation of cerebral from extracerebral vessels occurs (Chap. 2).

The middle meningeal artery is the vessel which has the greatest extension, supplying the dura of the convexity and base in the supratentorial area. As described in detail in Chap. 7, the artery is formed by the fusion of branches developing from the primordial internal maxillary artery with branches of supra-orbital artery, both derivatives of the Stapedial Artery. Along its course in the Middle Cranial fossa and further to the convexity, the Middle Meningeal Artery develops many connections involving the Internal Carotid Artery, through the ILT, the Ophthalmic Artery, and the Anterior Inferior Cerebellar Artery through its petrosal segment.

Due to its great extension and rich connections, the artery can be involved in many pathological processes. An example is shown in a case of temporo-basal Meningioma (Fig. 7.4a). Other examples showing the involvement of the MMA in DAVF are in Figs. 7.4b, c, 7.5, and 7.12. Fistulae can occur directly following a traumatic tear of MMA and accompanying MMV along their course in the middle cranial fossa, spheno-parietal sinus, and convexity. In this context, it is interesting to describe a pathologic condition which has appeared in patients with cranio-cerebral trauma. A fistula developed between the MMA and the Middle meningeal vein, which drained in the Superior Ophthalmic vein without involvement of the Cavernous sinus as reported by a few Authors [2, 9, 10, 12, 13]. It can be assumed that the fistula developed on the basis of a persistent early embryogenesis condition, in which the cavernous sinus was still not developed and the Superior Ophthalmic vein drained directly in the Meningeal vein deriving from the regressing Pro-Otic sinus (Chap. 9). The anomalous Fistula is shown in the Diagram (Fig. 8.1).

As far as it concerns the dura of the sellar and clival regions several vessels are involved. The ones arise from the Meningo Hypophyseal Trunk (MHT) and from the Infero lateral trunk(ILT), others from clival branched of the AphA (see Chaps. 5 and 7).

The tentorium is supplied by a few groups of arteries. One group is made by branches arising from the MHT. Another group is formed by

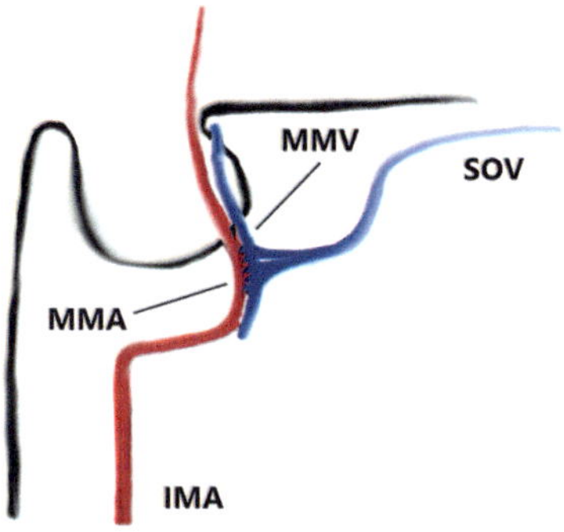

Fig. 8.1 Diagram showing the connections of the Middle Meningeal Artery (MMA) with the Superior Ophthalmic Vein (SOV). Cavernous Sinus (CS) not involved. Internal Maxillary Artery (IMA)

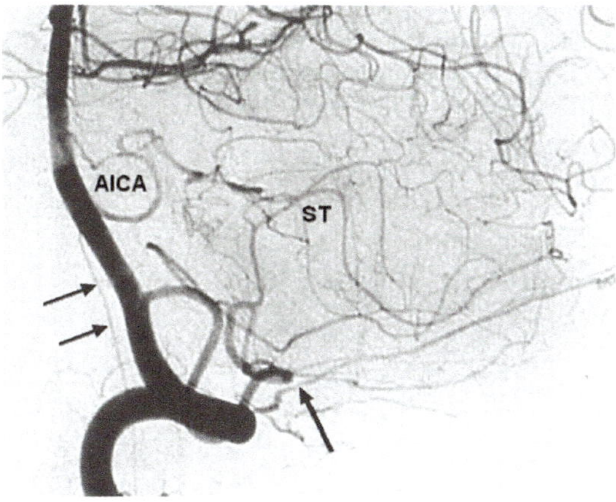

Fig. 8.2 Vertebral angiogram, lateral view. Origin of the Posterior Meningeal Artery from the VA at C1 level (arrow). Note the presence of the Anterior Spinal Artery (small arrows). Typical pattern of the supra-tentorial segment (ST) of the PICA

branches arising from the first segment of the Superior Cerebellar Artery. In the study of Ono et al. [8], the contribution of the SCA was about 28%. Another artery is the so-called "Davidoff-Scheckter artery," arising from the P1 segment of PCA, described in detail in Chap. 3. All these branches run along the free margin of the tentorium towards the falco-tentorial region, where they anastomose with the other meningeal branches of the area.

As far as it concerns the dura of the posterior fossa, it is supplied by the so-called Posterior Meningeal Artery [5, 6]. It arises commonly from the extra-cranial vertebral artery, just below the

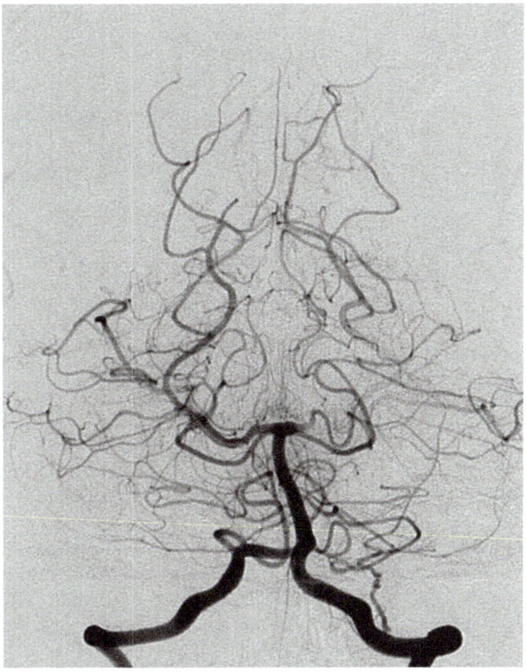

Fig. 8.3 Vertebral angiogram (AP view). Origin of the Meningeal branch (arrow) from the VA, having a lateral origin and course. (Taken from Bradac [1])

Foramen Magnum. A rarer origin from the posterior-inferior cerebellar artery has been also reported [3, 11]. The artery runs on the midline, close to the Falx Cerebelli, towards the Torcular Herophili, giving off branches for the Falx and for the dura covering the cerebellar hemispheres. Due to its course, is also called "Falx Cerebellar Artery." It can sometimes extend along the dura close to the SS, anastomosing with the other branches of the falco-tentorial area. Examples are shown in Figs. 8.2 and 8.3.

The Posterior Meningeal branches can be involved in pathologies involving the dura of the posterior fossa, such as meningiomas and DAVF. Examples are presented in Figs. 8.4 and 8.5.

In the supply of the dura of the posterior fossa, an important contribution can originate sometimes from branches of occipital artery, especially from Mastoid branch, or from the Hypoglossal branch of the Ascending Pharyngeal artery [4]. There is a balance in the supplied area between all these branches.

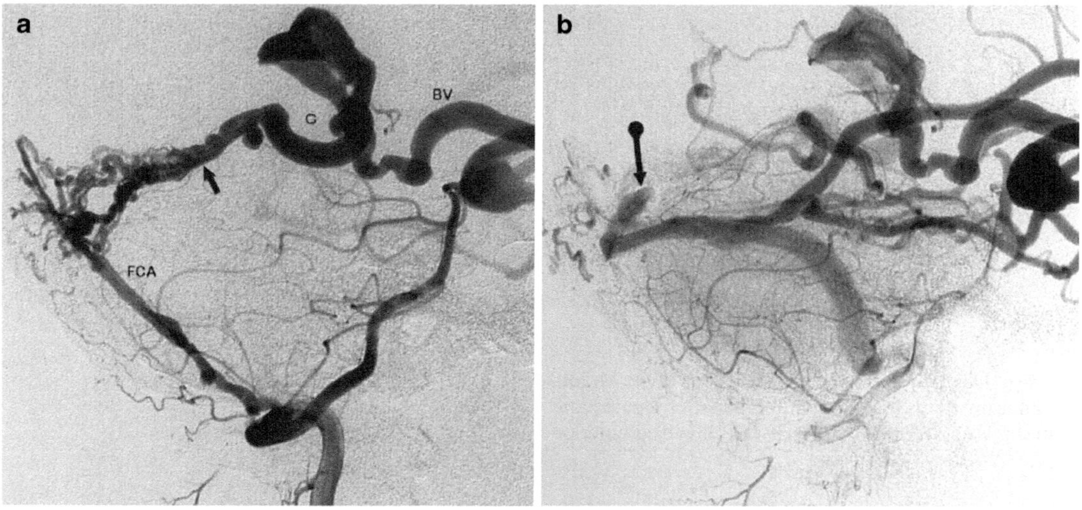

Fig. 8.4 DAVF at the level of the Straight Sinus (SS). (**a**) Vertebral angiogram, lateral view. Dilated meningeal branch (Falcine Artery, FCA) supplying the fistula. The Straight Sinus (arrow) was occluded. Rerouting of the drainage towards the Galen Vein (G) and Basal Vein (BV). (**b**) Late phase showing the occlusion of the Straight Sinus (arrow with dot). (Taken from Bradac [1])

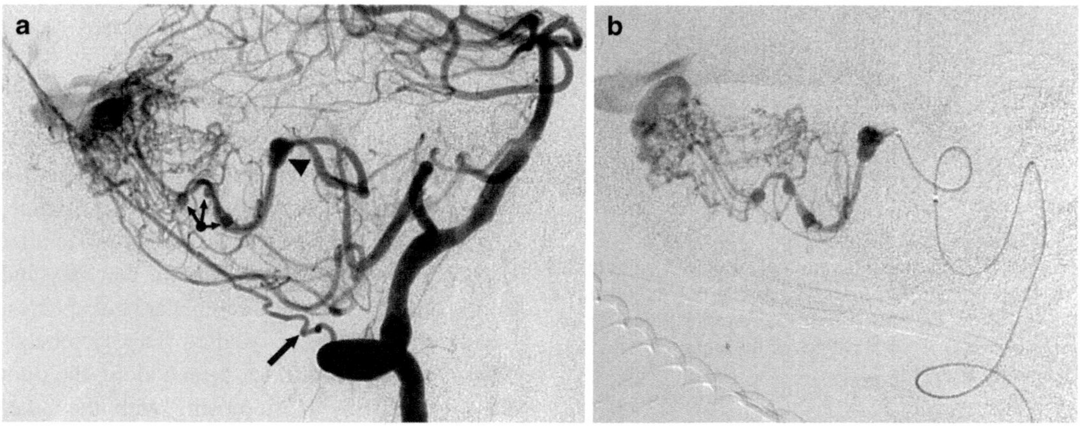

Fig. 8.5 (**a**) Another patient presenting with an Artero-Venous Malformation. Vertebral angiogram, lateral view. The malformation is supplied by branches of the PICA, where "stress aneurysms" were present (arrowhead, small arrow with angle). The meningeal branch (arrow) is not involved. (**b**) Selective study of the PICA, preceding the occlusion of the AVM and aneurysms. (Taken from Bradac [1])

As far as it concerns the venous drainage, this occurs through the Meningeal veins accompanying the Middle meningeal arteries. The greater is the Middle meningeal vein associated with the Middle Meningeal artery. The vein runs cranially accompanying the artery, draining in the SSS and TS running above or through the Lacunae. Caudally it can run through the foramina of the Middle cranial fossa reaching the Pterygoid plexus. The meningeal vein contributes to the formation of the so-called Sphenoparietal sinus also known as Brechet sinus from the French anatomist who described it in the 1829. In accordance to the reports of Padget in 1956 and later of Hacker in 1974 (see also Sect. 9.11), the sinus is formed by two components. The one is the

Parietal branch of the Meningeal vein, the other is the Superficial Middle cerebral vein running below the lesser wing of the sphenoid wing towards the Cavernous sinus, being the Sphenoidal part of the sinus. The two components can sometimes anastomose, leading to the formation of the Sphenoparietal sinus.

References

1. Bradac GB. Applied cerebral angiography. Normal anatomy and vascular pathology. Cham: Springer; 2017. https://doi.org/10.1007/978-3-319-57228-4. 497 pages, ISBN 978-3-319-57227-7.
2. Bradač GB, Schramm J, Kaernbach A. Traumatic exophthalmos due to an uncommon arteriovenous fistula without involvement of the cavernous sinus: case report. J Neurosurg. 1981;55(6):993–6.
3. Lang J. Skull base and related structures: atlas of clinical anatomy. New York: Schattauer Verlag; 1995.
4. Lasjaunias P, Merland JJ, Theron J, Moret J. Dural vascularization of the middle fossa (author's transl). J Neuroradiol = Journal de neuroradiologie. 1977;4(4):361–84.
5. Newton TH, Mani RL. In: Newton TH, Potts DG, editors. Radiol of skull and brain. St. Louis: Mosby; 1974.
6. Newton TH, Weidner W, Greitz T. Dural arteriovenous malformation in the posterior fossa. Radiology. 1968;90(1):27–35.
7. Oka K, Rhoton AL Jr, Barry M, Rodriguez R. Microsurgical anatomy of the superficial veins of the cerebrum. Neurosurgery. 1985;17(5):711–48.
8. Ono M, Rhoton AL Jr, Peace D, Rodriguez RJ. Microsurgical anatomy of the deep venous system of the brain. Neurosurgery. 1984;15(5):621–57.
9. Pakarinen S. Arteriovenous fistula between the middle meningeal artery and the sphenoparietal sinus: a case report. J Neurosurg. 1965;23(4):438–9.
10. Shi ZS, Ziegler J, Feng L, Gonzalez NR, Tateshima S, Jahan R, et al. Middle cranial fossa sphenoidal region dural arteriovenous fistulas: anatomic and treatment considerations. Am J Neuroradiol. 2013;34(2):373–80.
11. Tanohata K, Maehara T, Noda M, Katoh H, Sugiyama S, Okazaki A. Anomalous origin of the posterior meningeal artery from the lateral medullary segment of the posterior inferior cerebellar artery. Neuroradiology. 1987;29(1):89–92.
12. Theron J, Clay C, Djindjian R. Etude Angiographique et embolisation d'une fistule arterio-veineuse durale paracaverneux d'un type anatomique particulier. Ann Radiol; FR. 1975;18:739–46.
13. Unterhofer C, Chemelli A, Waldenberger P, Bauer R, Ortler M. Traumatic fistula between the middle meningeal artery and the sphenoparietal sinus. Acta Neurochir. 2009;151:1301–4.

9 Embryogenesis of the Cerebral Veins

Basically, the venous development in every embryonic phase lags behind that of the arteries, and so while the configuration of the arteries, even if not complete, is similar to that of the adult at the embryo of 40–44 mm, aged of 52–56 days, that of the veins reaches this result, only later, at the embryo of 80 mm at the age of 70–80 days (Padget 1956–1957).

9.1 Embryo of 5 mm

At the embryo of 5 mm the Neural Tube is covered by a primitive capillary plexus which drains at the dorsal lateral surface in the superficial located venous plexus, which in turn drains in bilateral three dural channels. These already described by Evans [11], Sabin [54], and Streeter [63] have been called by Padget: the Anterior (AD), (for Telencephalon, Diencephalon, and Mesencephalon), the (MD) for Pons and Cerebellum), and the Posterior (PD) (for medulla). All three channels drain in bilateral lateral dural channel called *Primary Head Sinus* (PHS) continuing caudally in the bilateral Anterior Cardinal Vein (Future internal Jugular Vein, IJV). One can already mention here, as described by Streeter (Chap. 2) that following the formation of DURA at about the embryo of 12–14 mm a clear separation appears between the Dural channels and the pial veins which drain in the dural channels, but are intra-dural.

Another important tributary of the PHS, entering the Anterior dural channel, is the Primitive Maxillary Vein draining the blood of the optic vesicle and partially also the basal Prosencephalon and the developing maxillary process.

Each PHS continues in bilateral Anterior Cardinal Vein (future IJV). This meets caudally the ascending Posterior Cardinal vein, draining the blood of Body. Together contribute to the formation of the Common Cardinal Vein (Ductus of Cuvier), entering the venous part of the primordial Heart.

Appearing of the Ventral Pharyngeal Vein (VPV), draining the blood of the inferior facial area. This can be considered as the primordial external venous drainage.

This evolution is shown in Fig. 9.1.

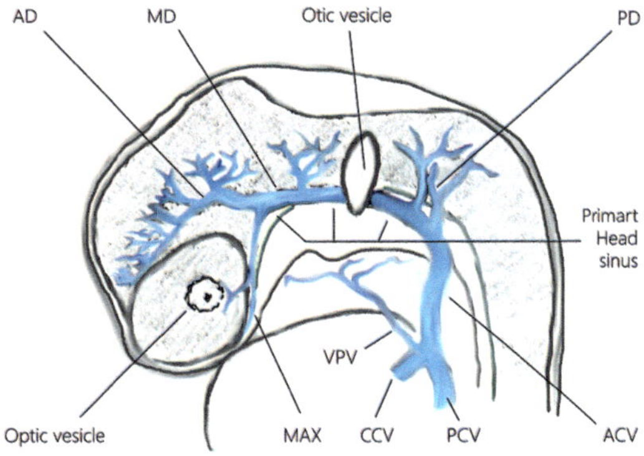

Fig. 9.1 Diagram (modified from [46]) showing the venous drainage at the embryo of 5 mm. Anterior (AD), Middle (MD), Posterior (PD) dural channels. Primary Head Sinus (PHS). Primary Maxillary Vein (MAX). Anterior Cardinal Vein (ACV), Posterior Cardinal Vein (PCV), Common Cardinal Vein (CAV). Ventral Pharyngeal Vein (VPV). Otic and Optic Vesicle

G. B. Bradac, *Origin and Development of Cerebral Vessels*,
https://doi.org/10.1007/978-3-031-78436-1_9

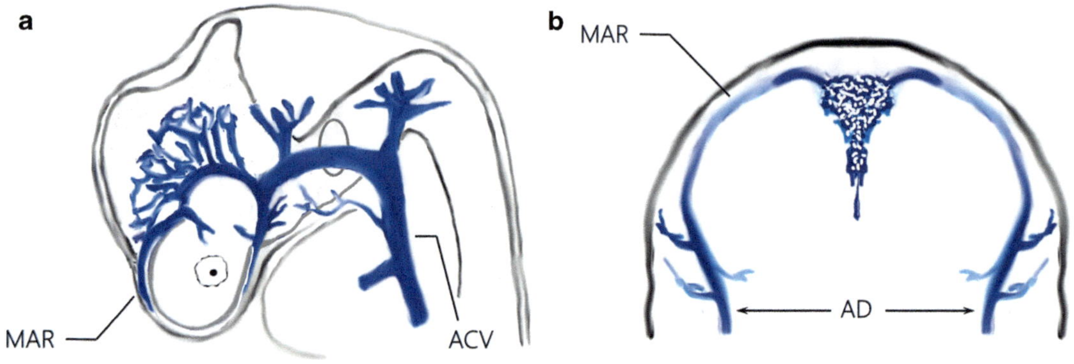

Fig. 9.2 (**a**) Diagram (modified from [46]) showing the appearing of the Marginal sinus (MAR). (**b**) On the AP view the Marginal sinus, with that of the contralateral, forms a plexural structure from which develops later the Superior Sagittal Sinus. Note the cranial displacement of the IPV now draining in the ACV

9.2 Embryo of 10–12 mm

At the embryo of 10–12 mm (30 days of age), following the growth of Telencephalon and Diencephalon with increasing of their arterial supply, the present venous drainage through the Anterior Dural Channel (AD) is no longer sufficient. To compensate this new situation from the AD, a new complementary channel develops. This channel already described by Markowski [38] who called it "the Primary Marginal vein," has been later defined by Padget [46, 47] "The Primary Marginal Sinus." This is a paired dural vascular structure running on the lateral surface of the anterior Telencephalon connected on the midline with the contralateral forming a plexiform Structure from which develops later the Superior Sagittal Sinus (Fig. 9.2).

9.3 Embryo of 18–24 mm

At embryo of 18–24 mm, many changes occur characterized mainly by:

- *Appearing of the primordial deep venous system*
- *Regression of the Primary Head sinus*
- *Appearing of new dural channels*
- *Evolution of the extra-cranial venous drainage*

Following the development of the Choroid Plexus, with its rapid growth, there is involvement of the Choroidal Arteries and appearing of the first deep venous channels, draining it. These are the superior and inferior choroid vein.

As far as it concerns the superior it has been called by Padget, for convenience "The Primitive Internal Cerebral vein" (the future internal cerebral vein). Actually the vein has been identified in earlier studies by Markowski in 1922 [38] and Hoechstetter in 1942 [22] who called the vessel "The Prosencephalic Vein," a term which will be used in the present work. This is a single median trunk formed, in accordance to Padget, by two components: choroid and diencephalic. The vein drains in the right Marginal Sinus, by the way of a new developed venous trunk (the future Straight sinus).

As far as it concerns the Inferior choroid vein, it is a bilateral channel also with a diencephalic component, draining in the temporary Marginal Sinus. Following the regression of the Sinus, the Inferior Choroid Vein drains in the Tentorial Sinus (Figs. 9.3 and 9.4).

At the embryo of 18 mm, due to the growth of the Otic Vesicle, the Primary Head Sinus (PHS) is compressed and displaced caudally. It progressively dwindles and regresses, replaced by a new channel. This develops dorsally to the Otic vesicle connecting the Middle with the Posterior dural channel. From the new dural channel develops the Transverse sinus which continues dorsally in the formed Sigmoid Sinus derived from the posterior dural channel. In this process, the Anterior dural channel is not involved. It progressively regresses replaced temporary by the Marginal sinus.

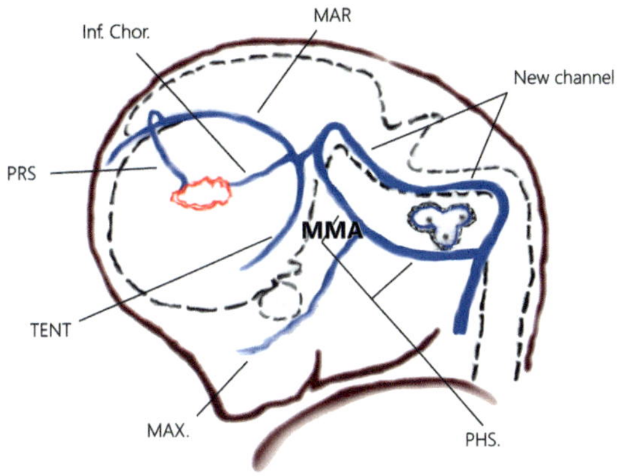

Fig. 9.3 Diagram modified from [46]. The Marginal sinus is regressing. The Tentorial Sinus (TENT) is appearing. The Primary Head Sinus (PHS) is regressing. Appearing of a new channel (the future Transverse Sinus). Primary Maxillary Vein (MAX) is in regression. Appearing of the Superior (Prosencephalic) and Inferior Choroidal Veins draining the small-developed Choroid Plexus

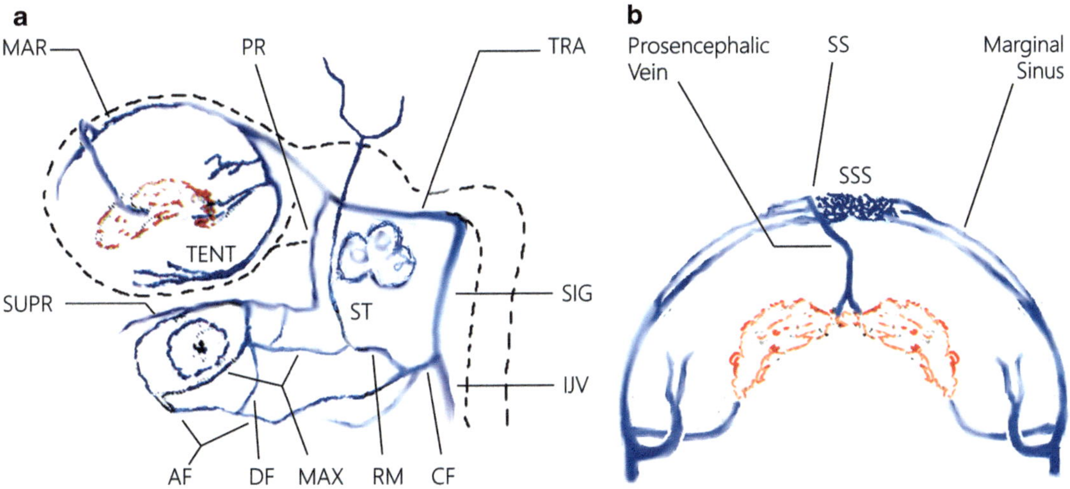

Fig. 9.4 (**a**) Modified from [46]. The regression of the Marginal sinus continues. Growing of the Tentorial sinus (TENT). Appearing of the Pro-otic sinus (PR). Transverse sinus (TRA). Supraorbital vein (SUPR). Maxillary vein (MAX) in regression. Developing of the extra-cranial venous drainage. Anterior Facial Vein (AF). Its connections with the orbital vein. The Primary Maxillary Vein (MAX) extends dorsally joining the Superficial Temporal Vein (ST) forming the retromandibular vein (RM). AF and RM join, forming the Common Facial Vein (CF), entering the IJV. (**b**) AP view. Connection on the midline of both Marginal Sinuses. Appearing of the Primordial Superior Sagittal Sinus, in form of a plexus. The drainage of the Prosencephalic vein in the right Marginal sinus by the way of appeared Primordial Straight sinus is shown. The Inferior Choroidal Veins drain in the Marginal Sinus Later in the Tentorial sinus

At the embryo of around 20 mm two new channels appear. One is the so-called *Tentorial sinus.* The developing of this new channel depends on the fact that following the continuous growth of the Telencephalon, Diencephalon, and Mesencephalon, at the embryo of 18–24 mm the Marginal sinus is no longer sufficient to receive the increased number of venous tributaries and progressively regressed replaced by the Tentorial sinus. To the new sinus, now drain the Telencephalic veins (the future superficial and deep middle cerebral), the Diencephalic and Mesencephalic veins. The other new channel is the *Pro-otic* sinus arising from remnants of the regressing PHS and from partially regressed Middle dural Channel involved in the formation of the Transverse sinus. The new channel extends medially and anteriorly in the middle cranial fossa towards the Sella area, where it receives the blood of the orbital veins, in a phase in which the cavernous sinus is not developed.

The Primary Maxillary vein is no longer involved as the main drainage of the orbital structures. Its main function is now the drainage of the Maxillary process and adjacent structures. Its intra-orbital segment dwindles, becoming in the future the Inferior Ophthalmic vein. The main drainage of the orbital structures is taken over by the appearing of the Supra-Orbital Vein (future Superior Ophthalmic vein), draining as described above in the Pro-otic Sinus.

It should be taken into consideration that from the Pro-otic sinus develop as its derivatives the Middle Meningeal Veins (MMV), which can be considered as remnant in the further evolution of the regressed Sinus. Therefore, it is thinkable that connections between the MMV and the orbital veins develop in this phase in which the orbital veins drain in the Pro-otic. These connections can persist in some cases in the adult favoring the formation of the Fistula described in Chap. 8.

In the meantime, there is a further evolution of the structures of the facial area. From the primordial Ventral Pharyngeal Vein (VPV) develops the facial lingual trunk. The facial vein (anterior facial) extends along the face, towards the orbita, where, through the angular branch, anastomoses with the orbital channels. Furthermore, a new connection (Deep Facial Vein) develops between the Anterior Facial vein with a new Maxillary vein, draining the region of the Maxillary process.

A new vein appears: the Retro-mandibular channel, developing from the junction of the Superficial Temporal Vein, draining the scalp of the Temporo-parietal area, with the persistence of segment of the Maxillary vein. The Retro-mandibular vein joins the Anterior Facial vein, forming the Common Facial vein, tributary of the Internal Jugular vein.

The above described evolution, involving the intra-cranial and extra-cranial venous sector is shown in the diagrams (Figs. 9.3 and 9.4).

9.4 Evolution of the Embryo from 24 mm to 80 mm

In this phase the Intra-cranial and Extra-cranial venous systems undergo many changes. The primordial veins disappear, replaced progressively by new channels, which at embryo of 80 mm present with a pattern basically comparable to that of the adult. The evolution of the embryo toward the 80 mm, is shown in the diagrams (Fig. 9.5a–c).

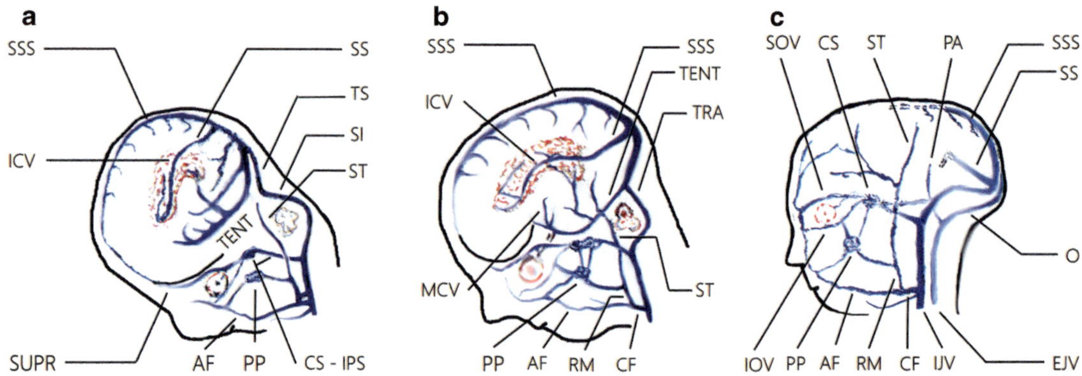

Fig. 9.5 Modified from [46]. (**a**) The Pro-otic sinus is regressed. Its remnants are the Cavernous Sinus (CS) receiving the blood of the orbital veins, mainly through the Supraorbital Vein. The further drainage of the CS continues in the Inferior Petrosal Sinus. Superior Sagittal Sinus continuing in the Transverse Sinus (TS) and Sigmoid Sinus (SI). Straight Sinus (SS). It has in this phase a higher position, becoming progressively lower in the evolution. Appearing of the Internal Cerebral Vein (ICV) draining directly in the SS. (**b**) The Tentorial sinus (TENT) due to its new connection with the TS is stretched and progressively dwindles. From it arise new channels (Middle Cerebral, Diencephalic, and Mesencephalic veins). (**c**) Details of the previous figure showing better the evolution of the extracerebral venous drainage. The Pterygoid Plexus is developed (PP). It receives many tributaries (see text). Vesalius Vein (V) connecting CS and PP. Connection with the Inferior Ophthalmic Vein (IOV). Frontal Vein (F) draining partially in the Superior Ophthalmic vein (SOV) continuing in the CS and partially in the AF. Superficial Temporal Vein. Late appearing of the External Jugular Vein, receiving the blood of the Occipital (O) and Posterior Auricolar (PA) Veins. Not the now more typical course of the Straight Sinus

9.5 Evolution to the Final Configuration

This develops progressively in the further fetal phase, continuing in the first early years after the birth. It is described in the following sections, in which the evolution of single group of vein is considered separately:

- Regression of the Pro-Otic sinus and the Tentorial sinus
- Appearing of the Cavernous sinus and Dural sinuses
- Appearing of the Superficial Venous System
- Appearing of the Deep Venous System
- The veins of the posterior fossa
- Final evolution of extra-cranial venous drainage
- The cranio-cervical region

9.6 Regression of the Pro-otic Sinus and the Tentorial Sinus

At the embryo of 40 mm, the Pro-otic sinus begins to dwindle and finally disappears completely. Its remnant is anteriorly the Cavernous sinus (CS) receiving the blood of the orbital region mainly through the developed Supraorbital vein. The CS continues posteriorly in the Inferior Petrosal sinus entering caudally in the sigmoid sinus. In accordance to Padget, in this phase, the main function of the CS is the drainage of the orbital veins. As far as it concerns, two other channels which in the adult are connected with the CS, represented by the Superior petrosal sinus (SPS) and the Superficial Middle cerebral vein are still in evolution and at this time have not connection with the CS. As far as it concerns the SPS, in accordance to Markowski [38] and Padget [46, 47], the sinus in this phase is still in formation. To the caudal end of the progressively regressing Pro-otic sinus drains the Anterior Metencephalic vein (future Petrosal vein) which is in this phase the most important vein of the structures of the Posterior fossa, receiving the blood from part of cerebellum and Pons.

In the further evolution towards the embryo of 80 mm, from the Anterior Metencephalic vein, as its dural extension along the crest of the temporal bone, where now the tentorium is attached, develops the Superior petrous sinus. Its connection, however, with the CS does not develop before the end of the feta phase and sometimes after the birth. Until this time, the primary function of the sinus is to drain the blood of cerebellum and pons. To complete the consideration about the evolution of the CS and SPS, we add the interpretation of Streeter. This author has considered that the CS and the SPS develop together as remnants of the regressed Primary Head sinus. The CS receives the blood of the orbital veins draining dorsally to the SPS.

Back to the Pro-otic sinus, other remnant of it in accordance to Padget [46] is the meningeal vein as already described in Chap. 8. The vein contributes with the Superficial middle cerebral vein to the formation of the Sphenoparietal sinus.

As far as it concerns the Tentorial sinus, at about the embryo of 40 mm, it undergoes great changes. Following the growth and extension dorsally of the cerebral hemispheres, the tentorial sinus is pushed dorsally connecting with the Transverse sinus. In the meantime, the temporal lobe has developed. The Tentorial sinus is forced to take a more medial course anteriorly and more lateral course dorsally due to the connections with the Transverse sinus. The consequences are that the sinus is elongated, stretched, and later regresses. The remnants are the developing Superficial Middle Cerebral Vein which will be an important venous channel for the superficial venous system, and Deep Middle cerebral veins, the Diencephalic and Mesencephalic channels from which develops the Basal vein.

The evolution of both the Pro-otic and the Tentorial sinuses is shown in the diagram (Fig. 9.5).

9.7 Appearing of the Cavernous Sinus and Dural Sinuses

Appearing as remnant of the Pro-otic sinus, the Cavernous Sinus develops rapidly and it is well recognizable at embryo of 80 mm. Its evolution is completed towards the advanced fetal phase. It has been studied in details in the adult by several authors [7, 20, 27]. It is formed in the para-sellar area by a fold of the Dura of the Middle Cranial fossa, dividing in two layers: one medial, adherent to the periosteum of the sphenoid, the other lateral, forming the medial wall of the middle cranial fossa. The lateral layer forms also the roof of the sinus continuing medially in the *diaphragma sellae*.

The CS is not a typical venous sinus, but a space containing the ICA surrounded by a network of veins and nervous elements (sympathetic plexus, cranial nerves III, IV, V, and first and second branch of the trigeminal nerves). Taking into consideration this findings, some authors [48, 65] have proposed to call the CS as "Space of cavernous sinus." The venous plexus of each side communicate each other through anterior and posterior channels running in the dura of the *diaphragma sellae* forming the so-called Coronal Sinus.

Due to his position in the central part of the base of the cranial cavity, it develops as a cross-road to which converge several venous channels (Fig. 9.6).

Anteriorly, the CS is connected with ophthalmic veins, reaching the Sinus passing through the Superior Orbital fissure. Laterally, it can receive the blood of the SMCV and uncal vein, when these channels have not taken a different way of drainage. Posteriorly, it drains in the IPS and as described above in the further evolution in the SPS. Bridging veins connected with the CS with the Ponto-mesencephalic vein and with the Clival venous plexus.

Other connections are with the Pterygoid Plexus and with the Anterior Condylar confluence. This latter will be described in detail in the section in which the extracranial venous drainage and that of the Cranio-cervical region are considered.

A typical angiographic example of CS is shown in Fig. 9.6.

Due to these several connections, the CS is involved as a way of venous drainage in many pathological conditions. These can affect directly

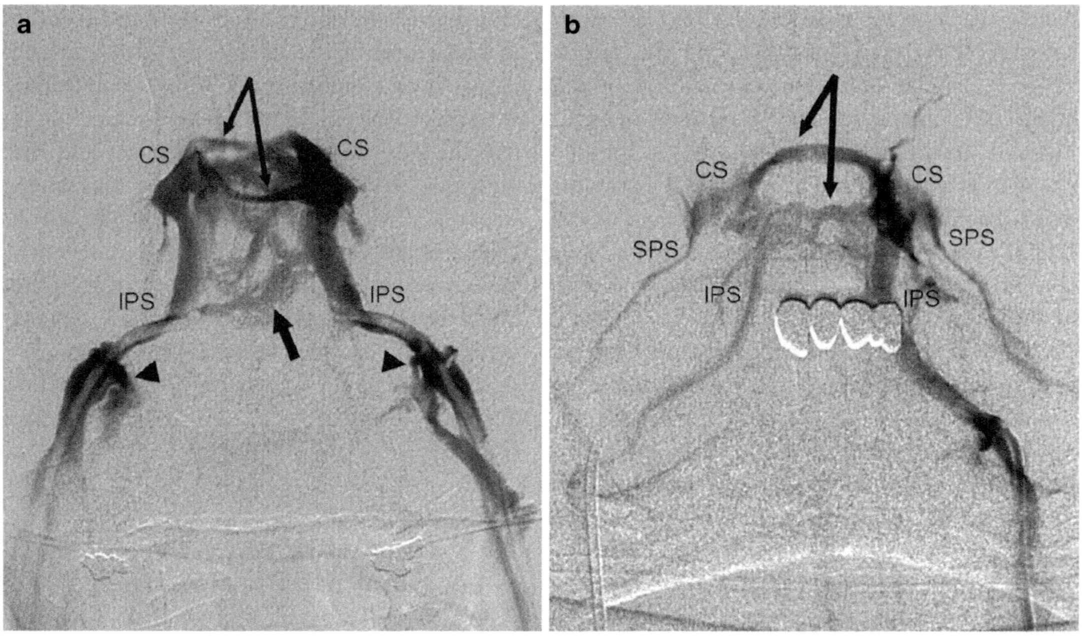

Fig. 9.6 Adult carotidogram. (**a**) Selective catheterization of both the Inferior Petrosal Sinuses. Cavernous Sinus (CS) Coronary Sinus (arrow with angle). Clival Venous Plexus (arrow). Anterior Condylar Confluence (arrowhead) connected with the Lateral Condylar Vein. (**b**) Another patient. Selective injection of the Left Inferior Petrosal Sinus (IPS). Cavernous Sinus (CS). Coronary Sinus (arrow with angle). Superior Petrosal Sinus (SPS)

the sinus such as in the direct carotido-cavernous shunt or in indirect shunt, as in the DAVF. The CS is also frequently involved in pathologies developing far from it, intra-cranially and extra-cranially (intraorbital, cranio-facial, and cranio-cervical regions).

9.8 Development of Dural Sinuses

9.8.1 Superior Sagittal Sinus (SSS)

It has first appeared as a plexus formed on the mid-line by the fusion of both Primitive Marginal sinuses at the embryo of 10–12 mm. At the embryo of 20 mm the evolution of the SSS progresses more rapidly. Following the growth of the cerebral hemispheres. In the longitudinal fissure, between the cerebral hemisphere, grows a mesenchymal tissue, originating from the Dura of the Convexity, forming the *Falx Cerebri*. It is at the junction of the Falx with the convexity Dura that the SSS develops.

From the initial plexus appear longitudinal channels, which extend dorsally. The channels progressively fuse together in a unique vessel. In accordance with Streeter, the formation of the sinus is almost complete at the embryo of 50 mm. The evolution continues up to the birth and after it. Indeed, it is nor rare in young children [21] to see more than one channel. In accordance with Streeter in the growth of the SSS two processes are involved. One is the so-called Passive Progression, in which the sinus extends due to the traction made by the growing parenchyma. The other is an active process called "Anastomotic Progression" in which from the initial plexus new loops develop, while the older loops regress. Dorsally the SSS reaches the Transverse sinus. It joins the Transverse sinus not on the midline, but on its right segment. That means that in this phase of evolution the joining area of SSS and TS called *Torcular Herophili* is located more on the right.

Padget explained this pattern with the difference in the evolution of the extra-cranial venous drainage especially of the Innominate Trunk. In the embryo, the right Jugular vein drains directly with a vertical course in the right relatively short Innominate trunk draining the blood in the Superior Cava vein and further in the right Atrium. In contrast, the left innominate develops later and has a longer, transverse course to reach the Superior Cava vein. In the further evolution during the fetal phase, and in the adult life a certain grade of equalization occurs due to the progressively symmetrical growth in length of both innominate trunks resulting in the adult a frequent symmetrical draining of the SSS in both Transverse sinuses.

In the diagram (Fig. 9.5) and in the angiograms (Fig. 9.7) the evolution of the SSS with its variable configuration in the adult is shown.

There are some anatomic aspects of the SSS which should be considered, even if they are not recognizable on the angiogram. Close to the SSS there are enlarged dural venous pouch called "Lacunae" connected with the SSS more frequently located in the fronto-parietal regions. They drain the blood of the Meningeal veins accompanying the Meningeal arteries. There are no connections with the cortical veins which commonly reach the SSS passing beneath the Lacunae [43].

The Arachnoid villi (Arachnoid Granulations), also called Pacchionian granulations from Italian pathologist Antonio Pacchioni, who first described them in the 1705, play an important role in the returning of cerebrospinal fluid in the vascular system. They are formed by the protrusion in the sinus of the arachnoid space surrounding the cortical veins entering the sinus especially abundant in the Transverse sinus [16, 35]. They can Also develop and invade the Dura matter, far from the sinuses, extending towards the Calvarium producing bone defects typically in the fronto-parietal regions. They are commonly absent in the early childhood, appearing progressively in the adult life [16, 35].

9.8.2 Transverse Sinus (TS)

The TS develops at the embryo of about 20 mm from a new channel connecting the Primordial Middle Dural Sinus with the Posterior dural channels. Beginning at the embryo of 35–50 mm following the growth of the cerebral hemispheres associated with the formation of the

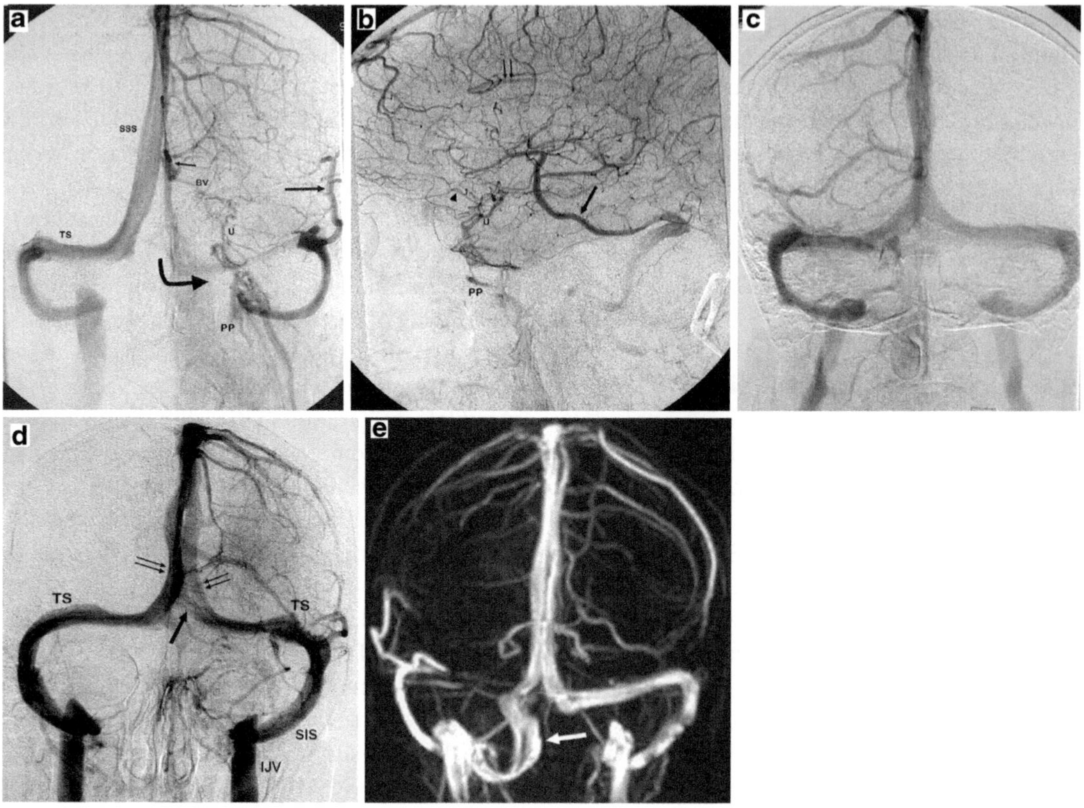

Fig. 9.7 (**a**) Venous Carotid Angiogram, AP view. Drainage of the SSS in the right Transverse Sinus (TS). The distal segment of the Left TS is filled through a large Labbé Vein (arrow). Its proximal segment is hypoplastic, partially filled by the Straight Sinus (arrow with angle) receiving the blood from the Basal Vein (BV) and Internal Cerebral Vein (arrow). Note that the BV is small. Its predominant drainage is directed anteriorly in the uncal vein (U) draining in the Pterygoid Plexus (PP). The Superficial Middle Cerebral Vein is absent. (**b**) Lateral view, same indications. (**c**) Other venous angiogram, AP view. Equalization of the drainage of the SSS symmetrical in both Transverses Sinuses. (**d**) Other venous angiogram, AP view. Anomalous drainage of the SSS due to its duplication. There are two channels of the SSS (arrows) each draining separately, one in the right and the other in the left TS. Small connection at Torcular Herophili. (**e**) Venous angio-MR, AP view. Duplication of the SSS. One channel drains in the well-developed right occipital sinus (arrow), the other in the left TS. (Taken from Bradac [4])

Tentorium, the TS acquires progressively its typical configuration, with an horizontal part connected with the contralateral if developed. It bends anteriorly continuing in the Sigmoid sinus, passing further through the jugular Foramen, continuing in the Intenal Jugular Vein. As described above, it receives the SSS which drains in its right segment. Following the progressively equalization of the drainage of SSS, the joining point (Torcular Herophili) of the SSS and TS is displaced frequently on the midline.

About the variations of the TS visible on the adult angiograms, the relatively frequent, is the hypo-aplasia of its proximal segment, while the distal part is filled receiving the blood from the temporo-occipital region and from the cerebellar veins shown on the vertebral angiogram.

9.8.3 Straight Sinus (SS)

It appears at the 18 mm embryo as a drainage way of the Prosencephalic vein to the Right Marginal sinus. Following the formation of the SSS, the Straight Sinus is annexed by it and in the further evolution it follows the SSS in its dorsal migration. At the embryo of 40 mm the

Prosencephalic vein regressed replaced by the Internal Cerebral Vein (ICV) draining in the SS. The sinus is now well recognizable. In its course towards the SSS, it has a slight relative high position which becomes lower at the 80 mm. It acquires its typical course obliquely upward directed, only late in the fetal phase and in the young children [21] (Fig. 9.5). Similarly, to the SSS it drains in the embryo-fetal phases in the right TS. Following the progressively equalization of drainage of the SSS and TS, the way of drainage of the Straight Sinus changes following that of the SSS and TS. Due to equalization of drainage, as described above of SSS and TS, the SS reach the SSS and TS in the median located *Torcular Herophili*. In the cases of persistent predominance of drainage of the SSS in the right TS, differently from the embryonic phase, in the adult the SS drains in the left TS, probably as a compensation. The typical adult course of SS is shown in Figs. 9.9, 9.10, and 9.18 and in the Figs. 9.11, 9.12, and 9.16.

The Straight sinus can be Hypo-Aplastic and its drainage can be replaced by the Falcine sinus. This is an embryonic vessel running in the Falx connecting the Galen vein or Straight sinus with the SSS. This normally regresses, but in some cases persists in the adult together with the Straight Sinus or replaces it [5, 53]. An example is shown in Fig. 9.8a.

The SS is typically involved as the main venous drainage in the Galen Vein malformation, appearing dilated not rarely duplicated, associated with other anomalies of the sinuses. Frequent is its association with the Falcine sinus which can replace the SS (Fig. 9.14).

9.8.4 Occipital Sinus (OS)

It develops at the embryo aged of 80–90 days arising from plexiform structures arising in the Dura at the junction of the formed SSS, TS, and SS. It extends anteriorly continuing along the internal margin of the *Foramen Magnum*, entering anteriorly the Sigmoid Sinus draining in the IJV: It has connections with the medial located Marginal Sinus (not to be confused with the *primordial* Marginal Sinus), which drains anteriorly into the Anterior Vertebral Basilar plexus. Therefore, the OS is involved in the venous drainage of the IJV and also in the drainage of vertebral venous system. In the fetal and young children is relatively large, in advancing age it becomes smaller and can also completely disappear [33, 58]. Some authors [75] have interpreted this evolution as due to the acquired upright position of the child learning to walk. It should be considered that in this position the venous drainage is directed preferentially in the vertebral system. It can be assumed that in the adult the preferential venous drainage in the vertebral system occurs through the development of new channels, making the way through the occipital sinus no longer necessary. This important aspect will be described further in this section.

Normal Anatomy of the sinus is shown in Fig. 9.8b.

Anomalies of the sinus can rarely occur (Fig. 9.7e).

9.8.5 Marginal Sinus

The growth and evolution of the sinus is tightly linked with that of the OS [69], especially considering its connections with the OS as described above.

In this context, interesting are the observations performed by some authors [12, 66] *studying the skulls of Australopithecines (Primordial Hominoid). These authors have shown indirectly a very large Occipital-Marginal sinus which they interpreted as an adaptation of the cranial venous drainage preferentially directed in the Vertebral Venous System, following the acquired upright position, linked to the bipedalism.*

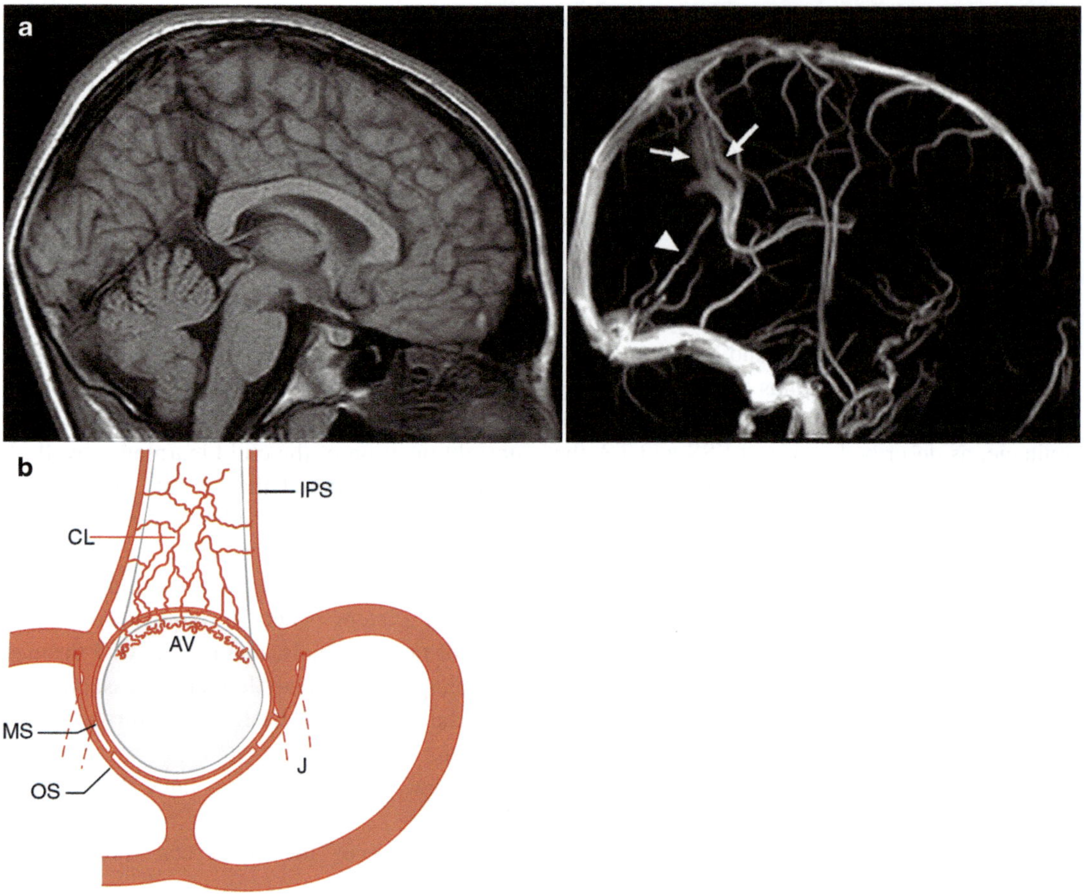

Fig. 9.8 (**a**) MR and Venous angio-MR showing an hypoplastic Straight Sinus (arrowhead). Replaced by a persistent Falcine Sinus (arrows) formed by several segments. (**b**) Diagram showing the Occipital (OS) and Marginal (MS) Sinuses and their connections. The OS, arising at the junction of the SS, SSS and runs from the Torcular Herophili around the Foramen Magnum entering the Sigmoid Sinus and the IJV. Medially, the OS has many connections with MS. This latter is connected with the Sigmoid Sinus with the Clival Plexus (CL) and with the Anterior Epidural Vertebral Plexus (AV). Inferior Petrosal Sinus (IPS). (Taken from Bradac [4])

9.9 Superficial Venous System

The earlier veins at the embryo od 4–5 mm are the pial veins, developing from the primary network, lying on the surface of the brain. From these veins which, in accordance to Padget lie beneath the arteries, develop numerous veins draining in the primary dural channels. Following the growth of the brain with separation of Dural layers from cerebral Parenchyma as described by Streeter (Chap. 2), the superficial dural collectors are displaced laterally. The tributary veins arising from the pial layer to reach the dural collectors are elongated and some dwindle and regress. The pial veins maintain their position on the surface of the brain; the tributaries (arachnoidal) to the sinuses have a long course in the subarachnoid space lying now superficial to the arteries. These veins, which receive the blood from cortex and adjacent developed white matter, runs on the surface of the cortex (cortical veins) in the subarachnoid space for a short or long course, entering the sinuses. Some of these veins, called *bridging veins* [32, 33, 43] before entering the sinuses fuse partially or completely with the superficial dura.

The veins, named depending on the cerebral lobe from which receive the blood [19, 43, 56] have been divided in a few groups (Figs. 9.9, 9.10, and 9.18).

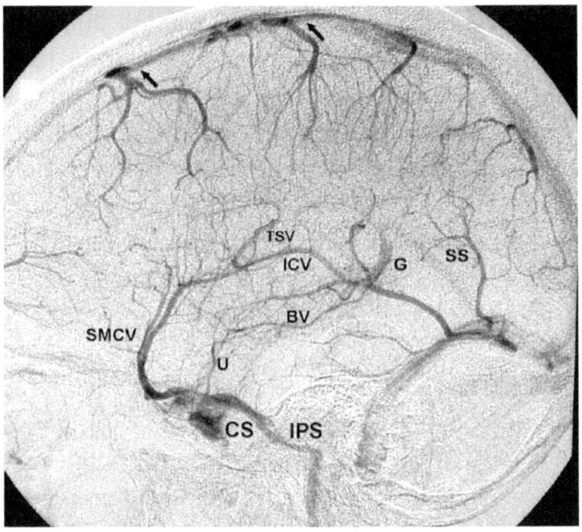

Fig. 9.9 Lateral Carotid Angiogram, showing the Superior group of Cerebral Cortical veins with their typical course (arrows). The Anterior Inferior group is represented by a large Superficial Middle Cerebral Vein (SMCV) draining in the Cavernous Sinus (CS) continuing in the Inferior Petrosal Sinus (IPS). There are two Labbé veins. Note the well-developed Internal Cerebral Vein (ICV) receiving blood from the Thalamo Striate Vein (TSV). The Basal Vein (BV) is small. Some of its tributaries drain in the Uncal Vein (U). Galen Vein (G). Straight Sinus (SS). (Taken from Bradac [4])

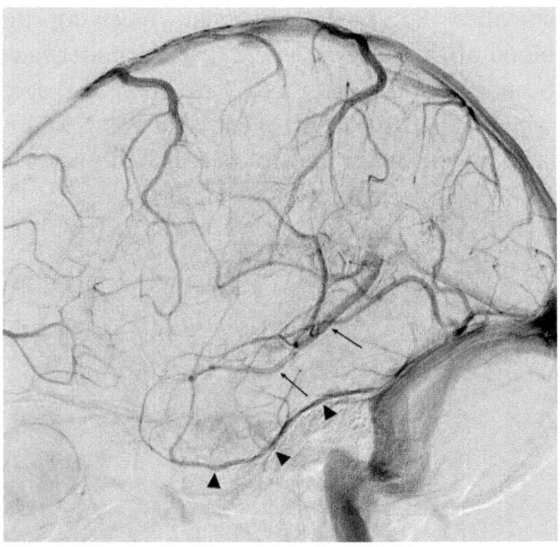

Fig. 9.10 Lateral carotid angiogram. A small SMCV runs along the base of the Middle Cranial fossa (arrow) reaching the Superior Petrosal Sinus and entering the TS. There is a large Labbé vein. The Basal Vein is well-developed

9.10 The Superior Group

The veins of this group drain and, run on the surface of then Fronto-parietal-occipital regions, as well as the anterior part of the fronto-basal area (the dorsal part belong to the system of the Basal vein), draining in the SSS. Sometimes a great vein described by Trolard (French anatomist) in the 1868 connected the Superior with the anterior-inferior group. In the frontal area, the veins enter the SSS at a right angle. The most posterior join the sinus forming progressively a more oblique angle in the direction against the blood of the sinus.

9.11 The Anterior-Inferior Group

The main vein is the Superficial Middle cerebral vein (SMCV) draining the inferior fronto-parietal lobes and the supero-lateral temporal lobe. The SMCV runs on the surface of the Silvian fissure, it turns then medially continuing along the inferior border of the Sphenoid wing in the so-called Sphenoidal part of the Sphenoparietal sinus, ending in the Cavernous sinus (see also Chap. 8). The drainage in the CS occurs in about 20%. In other cases, the SMCV can take a different way of drainage. The channel can run on the floor of the Middle Cranial Fossa, reaching the Pterygoid plexus having passed through the foramina of the base (*Foramen Ovale* and *Spinosum*). This kind of drainage has been called "Para-cavernous." The vein can also continue its course dorsally entering the Superior petrosal sinus and further the TS (Fig. 9.10) forming the so-called Petrosphenoidal sinus, considered as a remnant of the Tentorial sinus.

An interesting pattern of the drainage has been described by some authors [15, 57], who identified the presence of a second venous space, they called "The Lateral Cavernous Sinus" developed by the division of two sheets of the lateral wall of the CS. In according to these authors, in about 20% the SMCV drains in the Lateral Cavernous Sinus, continuing in the Para-cavernous Sinus or later in the Superior petrosal sinus or TS.

The SMCV can be absent and so the drainage is directed towards the Labbé Vein or can have a drainage partially directed in the CS and partially in the Labbé vein.

9.12 The Posterior-Inferior Group

These veins drain the lower-lateral part of the temporal-occipital lobe, frequently through a Labbé vein or several small channels entering the TS directly or by the way of a tentorial channels.

The veins of the basal-medial surface of the temporo-occipital lobes drain in the Basal vein and in the TS respectively.

9.13 Veins of the Medial Group

The veins of the superior group of the fronto-parietal area run upwards, curve over the superior margin of the surface connecting with ascending branches of the Lateral group, before they together enter the SSS. The lower part of the Medial surface draining mainly the Cingulate gyrus and Corpus Callosum drain in the Anterior and Posterior peri-callosal veins [43] respectively in the frontal, parietal regions. The Anterior peri-callosal vein is a paired channel coursing around the Genu of Corpus Callosum, further in the cisterna of the *Lamina Terminalis* reaching the Anterior Cerebral vein tributary of the Basal vein. In rarer cases, it can drain in the Inferior Sagittal sinus. The Posterior Cerebral vein is a paired channel, runs dorsally around the Splenium, entering the Galen vein or Internal cerebral or the Basal vein [43]. As far as it concerns the veins of the medial surface of the occipital lobe, they drain partially in the anterior Calcarine vein directed anteriorly in the Posterior peri-callosal or Basal Vein and partially in the Posterior Calcarine vein running towards the SSS.

9.14 Development of Deep Venous System

The growth of Basal Ganglia, Thalamus, and formed White Matter, including Corpus Callosum and Fornix, requests more specific venous channels replacing the regressing primordial. The new developed veins drain basically into two collectors: the internal cerebral vein(ICV) and the Basal vein(BA), both draining in the Galen Vein continuing in the Straight sinus (Fig. 9.11). Many authors have been involved in these studies, starting in the fifties [13, 28, 76] continuing and becoming progressively more precise in the subsequent years [23, 29, 44, 56, 61, 62].

The ICV is the first channel of the Deep System, appearing at the embryo of 40–44 mm at the end of the embryonic phase, while the Prosencephalic vein which has played an important role in the primordial evolution is dwindling and finally disappears. The ICV in this first phase drains directly in the SS (Fig. 9.5a, b). This condition changes with the developing of the Galen Vein. The distal part of the Prosencephalic vein plays a last role contributing to the formation with the ICV of the Galen vein. This new channel runs around the splenium of Corpus Callosum, entering the SS, having a flow commonly opposite to that of it.

The ICV receives the blood mainly from the so-called Sub-Ependimal vein, receiving the blood of medullary veins [23]. These latter have been subdivided in "deep," draining the deep white matter in the sub-ependymal veins, and in "superficial" white matter draining in the superficial venous system.

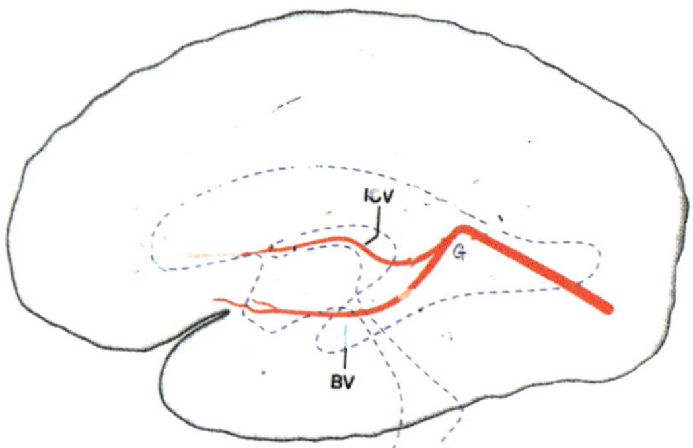

Fig. 9.11 Diagram showing the two main collectors of the Deep venous system. The Internal cerebral vein (ICV) and the Basal vein (BV), draining in the Galen Vein, continuing in the Straight Sinus, designed on a background of Brain and Ventricle system

The ICV, is a paired channel running in the *Tela Choroidea* in the roof of the third ventricle, arisen from fusion at the level of Foramen of Monro of the Thalamo-striate vein (TSV) with the Septal vein (SV). The TSV is a paired vein, which in spite of its name, is not involved in venous drainage of thalamus. The vein following the growth of the Internal capsule has been displaced medially running between the Thalamus medially (Diencephalon) and the *Nucleus Caudatus* laterally (Telencephalon). It is formed by the so-called Terminal vein running in the *Stria Terminalis* and a few Caudate veins draining the blood of body and head of the Caudate nucleus. The Caudate vein can also drain directly more dorsally in the ICV.

The Septal vein (SV) is formed by several deep medullary veins, converging bilaterally to the anterior lateral corner of the frontal horn. It runs first medially, then dorsally in the sleeve of the *Septum Pellucidum* joining the TS, continuing in the ICV. It can have an anomalous course reaching the ICV more dorsally.

There are other tributaries of the ICV:

The Medial Atrial (MAV) and the Lateral Atrial (LAV) veins run on the medial, lateral wall of the atrium and lateral wall of the occipital horn, respectively. They receive the blood of the medullary veins of the parietal and occipital regions. They drain sometimes as a common trunk in the ICV and lateral LAV can sometimes reach the BV.

The Choroid veins. They appear following the development of the Choroid Plexus. The one group is the Anterior-superior, component of the Prosencephalic vein, late annexed by each ICV, the other is the Posterior-inferior, draining first in the Marginal Sinus, later in the Tentorial Sinus, becoming tributary of each Basal Vein.

As far as the Striate Veins are concerned, the Superior group drains the blood of the Superior part of the Basal Ganglia, part of the Internal Capsula and Claustrum, entering directly the ICV or first in the Thalamo-striate veins. The Inferior group drains the inferior part of the Basal Ganglia, becoming tributary of the Basal vein.

The Thalamic veins [17, 64]. The superiors are the first to appear at about the embryo of 18–20 mm. They drain the supero-medial part of the thalamus, entering the ICV. The inferior group drains in the later developed Basal vein. They receive the blood mainly from the infero-lateral Thalamus.

The typical course of the ICV and its tributaries is shown on the Diagram (Figs. 9.11 and 9.12) and on the Carotid angiograms (Figs. 9.9, 9.10, and 9.13).

An anomalous evolution involving the formation of the ICV is the so-called Galen Vein Malformation. The causes of this anomaly are not completely clear. In accordance to the studies of Raybaud et al. [49], the essential factor is thought to be the persistence of the Prosencephalic vein, while the ICVs and the Galen vein do not develop. The Prosencephalic vein develops as a huge venous pouch to which converge many feeding arteries, mainly the persistent choroidal branch of the Peri-callosal Artery and the Posterior Choroidal branches of the PCA. As far as it concerns the appearance and evolution of these branches in the embryonic phase, see Chap. 3. The further venous drainage occurs through a dilated Straight sinus and through the often present Falcine sinus which rarely cannot replace the SS. Other anomalies involving the transverse sinus and occipital sinus can be present consequence of the malformation or indicating a more extensive pathology involving the venous sector. Examples are presented in Fig. 9.14a, b.

Among the anomalies, involving the deep venous system, there is the so-called Development

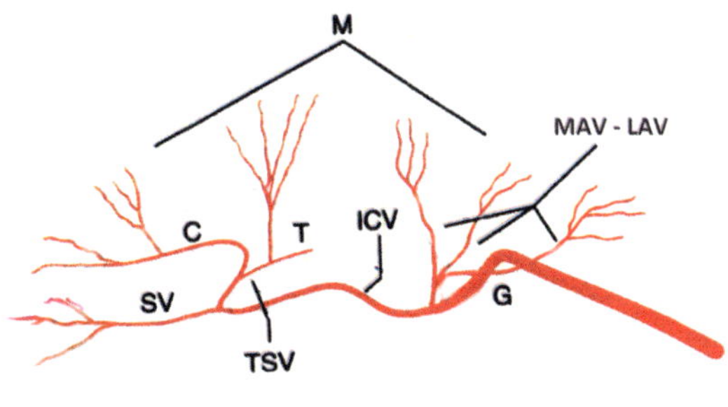

Fig. 9.12 Diagram showing the ICV and its tributaries. Terminal vein (T), Thalamo-striate vein (TSV), Vein of Nucleus Caudatus (C), Septum Pellucidum Vein (SV). Lateral Middle Atrial Vein (MAV), Deep Medullary Veins (M)

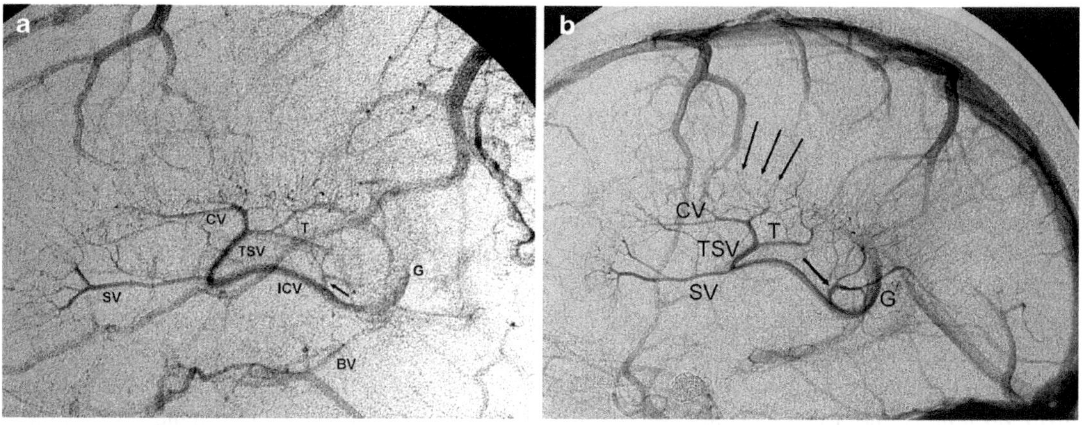

Fig. 9.13 (**a**) Lateral Carotid Angiogram. Terminal vein (T), Thalamo-Striate Vein (TSV). Caudate Vein (CV), Septal vein (SV). Fainted filled Medullary Veins. Galen Vein (G). Small Basal Vein (BV). Lateral Middle Atrial vein (arrow). (**b**) Other patient. The indications are the same. Note an SV reaching the ICV more dorsally. There is a large Atrial Medullary vein (arrow). (Taken from Bradac [4])

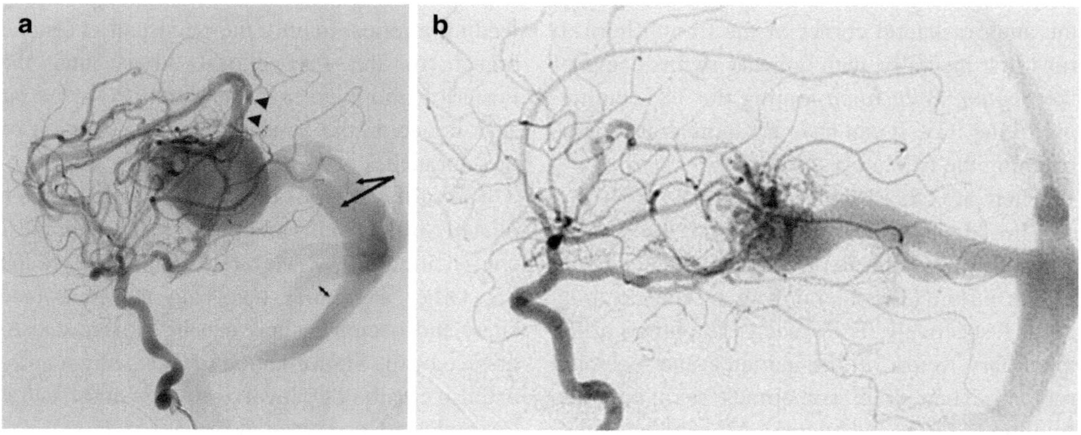

Fig. 9.14 (**a**) Galen Vein malformation. To the persistent dilated Prosencephalic Vein converge the distal choroidal branches of the Pericallosal Artery (arrowhead) and the Posterior Choroidal branches of the PCA. Dilated and Duplicated Straight sinus (arrow with angle) continuing in the dilated occipital sinus (arrow). (**b**) Galen Vein malformation, other example. The main supply of the Prosencephalic vein is through the posterior choroidal branches of the PCA Drainage in the duplicated Falcine Sinus. (Taken from Bradac [4])

Venous Anomaly (DVA). In accordance to the studies of Saito and Kobayashi [55] and Lasjaunias et al. [34], the DVA is considered to be the result of an anomalous evolution of the Medullary veins (Superficial-Deep cerebral and cerebellar). In this anomaly, the medullary veins do not drain each separately in their collectors. Instead a group of Medullary veins converge together in a unique large collector (Fig. 9.15a, b). Differently from capillary malformations (Telangiectasia) the interposed parenchyma is normal. The DVA are commonly an incidental discovery. They can sometimes present with hemorrhage which are thought to be due to the frequent associated Cavernous angiomas or thrombosis of the great collector [45]. The DVA differ from real malformation such the cavernous or capillary angiomas, already well described in previous work. [4].

Another very rare anomaly is the so-called Sturge-Weber syndrome, which belongs to the complex group of cranio-encephalic malforma-

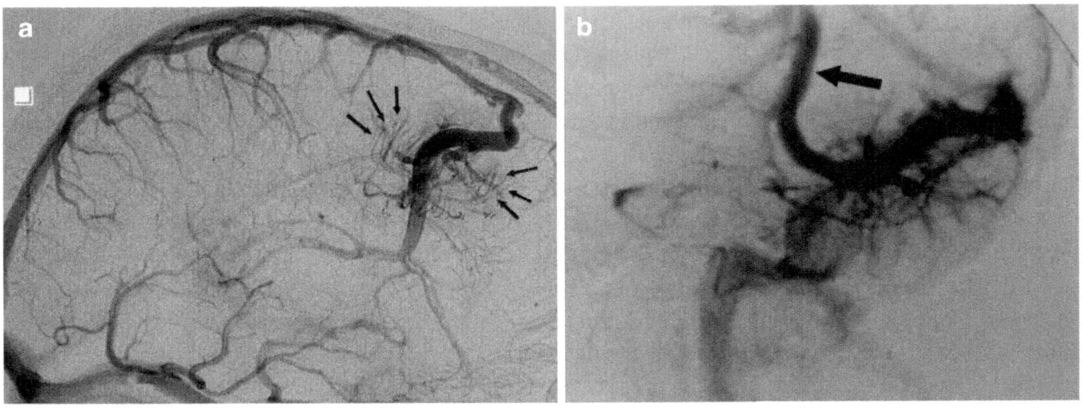

Fig. 9.15 Two different patients with a DVA. (**a**) Carotid venous angiogram. Many medullary veins (arrows) converge to a unique collector draining in the SSS. (**b**) Vertebral venous angiogram. The cerebellar medullary veins converge to a dilated Precentral vein (arrow) draining in the Galen vein. (Taken from Bradac [4])

tions such as the Rendu-Osler and the Wyburn-Mason syndromes, involving variably the head, neck, and cerebrum. The Sturge-Weber is a familial disease characterized, when complete, by a facial nevus, in the trigeminal distribution mainly in the first branch, a retinal angioma and a leptomeningeal angiomatosis. This latter is formed by a rich network of capillaries and venules involving the pial and subarachnoidal membranes. In accordance to some authors [6], it is considered as due to an anomalous development of the superficial venous drainage involving the cortical and the superficial medullary veins. The drainage is redirected to the deep venous system involving the deep medullary veins, and further the subependymal veins and choroid plexus.

In this context, I think it is useful to mention the Cerebral Arterio-venous malformations. Only short considerations are made, since they have been already described in detail in a previous work [4]. They have been first described as a particular pathology by Rokitansky [74] and Virchow [73], pathologists respectively in Wien and Berlin. In the following years, the malformations have been progressively identified as a special entity [40, 52].

They appear with an area called "NIDUS" to which converge several arteries connected directly without interposition of capillaries with draining veins. Progressively changes of the involved vessels develop with formation of arterial aneurysms and great dilatation and sometimes thrombosis of the veins. Degenerative alterations occur in the interposed and sometimes surrounding parenchyma.

They differ from the Galen vein malformation which develops in the fetal phase, involving a specific vascular sector. The AVMs can appear in different parts of the brain involving the supplying arteries and draining veins of the affected region. They commonly develop in the adult and children age. Cases, however appearing in the fetal phase or in the advanced age, have been reported. They can be diagnosed presenting with epileptic seizures or acutely with hemorrhage. Spontaneous disappearing following thrombosis, as well as their reappearance can occur [42].

The association with other pathologies of the brain such as Eterotopia or non-specific brain insult such as radiotherapy, as well as with other vascular malformations (Rendu-Osler syndrome, Wyburn-Mason syndrome), pathologies of vessels (Coarctation of Aorta, Fibromuscular Hyperplasia), and other complex pathologies such Neurofibromatosis have been reported and considered by some authors [31] as factors favoring the developing of AVM.

In conclusion: Many doubts remain about the pathogenesis and evolution of the AVM. In this context, it is useful to reconsider the phases of the evolution in which the cerebral vessels appear and progressively develop, described by Streeter [63] presented in Chaps. 2 and 3. In the early phases of embryogenesis, the primordial vascular plexus differentiates in arteries, capillaries, and veins. Deviation in this process would engender predisposing conditions, being in the further evolution factors favoring the formation of AVM. Furthermore, in this early phase, the veins and the artery run very close to each other and so the possibility of an anomalous communication is great [47, 68]. Another important aspect which should be considered, is the complex process of adaptation of the developing vessels to the continuous changes and growing of the brain. It could be that in some preferential brain sectors, the vessels take an anomalous way of evolution, probably on the influence of hemodynamic factors leading to the formation of the AVM.

Later immunohistochemical studies [59, 70] have emphasized the important role in the formation of AVM played by an alternate balance of growth factors (VEGR1-2) and a group of Cytokine (Angioopoietine 1–2) probably on the basis of gene mutations. In this context, it is interesting to recall that AVM can develop in some cases of "Hereditary Hemodynamic Telangiectasia" (Rendu-Osler syndrome) in which a known gene mutation has been demonstrated [36].

9.14.1 Basal Vein

The vein first described by the German pathologist Rosenthal [51] appears as an entity, later in the evolution, not before the embryo of 80 mm. It develops from many tributaries of the regressed Tentorial Sinus through longitudinal anastomoses forming the BV.

In its typical final pattern, the vein is characterized by a very long course which has been subdivided in a few segments.

The vein is formed at the level of the Anterior Perforated Substance (APS) by the fusion of a few vessels. The larger is frequently [8] the Deep Middle Cerebral vein (DMCV), draining the veins of the Insula. The DMCV runs medially in the deep of the Sylvian fissure receiving at the level of the APS the Inferior Striate veins, veins of the fronto-basal area (olfactory and Fronto-basal) and the Anterior cerebral vein draining mainly the Corpus Callosum.

The formed trunk of the BV runs first anterior then lateral to the cerebral peduncles, continuing around it, taking a slightly upwards course entering the Galen Vein. The PCA lies inferiorly and the AchA crosses the BV superiorly from medial to lateral. Along its course the BV receives many tributaries. The ones are the Peduncular veins draining the anterior-inferior Thalamic veins, passing through the Posterior Perforated Substance (PPS), connected medially with the median and lateral Ponto-mesencephalic veins. Other tributaries are: the Uncal vein, draining the Uncal region (this can be sometimes an important anomalous drainage way of the Basal vein) and other veins come from the temporal region (the Hippocampal vein, and Cortical veins of the infero-medial lobe). Another tributary, frequently prominent is the Inferior Ventricular vein which arises in the body of the lateral ventricle. It runs in the Atrium, continuing in the temporal horn, leaving it ending in the BV.

The typical course of the BV and of its tributaries is shown in the Diagram (Fig. 9.16a, b) and on the angiograms in Figs. 9.9, 9.10, and 9.16c.

Considering the complexity of the process leading to the formation of the Basal vein, it is not surprising that some connections do not develop or develop differently resulting in many anomalies [25, 56].

Among the most frequent is the preferential drainage of the anterior tributaries in the so-called Uncal vein. In other cases, the drainage of the anterior tributaries occurs in the Ponto-mesencephalic veins (Anterior or Lateral). At the level of the lateral Mesencephalic Sulcus, from the BV, can arise the vein running in the sulcus (Lateral Mesencephalic Vein) which has connection with Petrosal vein and Superior Petrosal sinus. The vein can be a preferential drainage of the BV. In other cases, the BV does not run towards the Galen Vein. Instead, it takes a more lateral course entering the TS, frequently after having a short segment in the tentorium. This pattern is considered as expression of remnant of the Tentorial Sinus. Examples of anomalous configuration are shown in the Figs. 9.17 and 9.18.

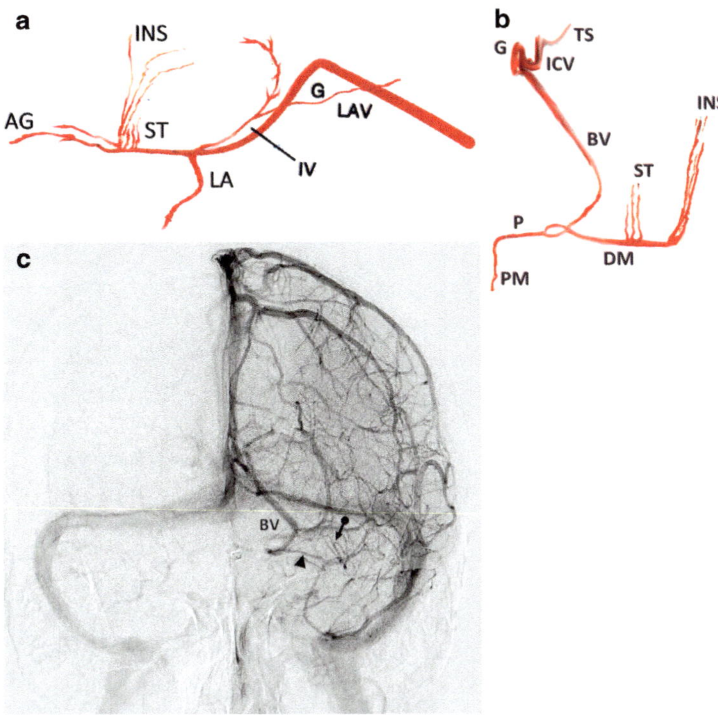

Fig. 9.16 (**a**) Diagram showing the typical course of the Basal Vein and its tributaries. Anterior tributaries (AG). Insula (INS). Inferior Striate Vein (ST). Lateral Mesencephalic Vein (LA). Lateral Atrial vein (LAV) joining the Inferior Ventricular Vein (IV). Galen vein (G) draining the Straight Sinus. (**b**) Diagram, AP view, showing the course of the Basal Vein (BV) around the cerebral peduncle. Deep Middle Cerebral Vein (DM) receiving the blood from the Insular Vein (INS) and Inferior Striate Vein (ST). The anterior tributaries are not shown. The connection with the peduncular vein (P) joining the Ponto-mesencephalic Vein (PM) is also shown. These are however commonly not recognizable on the angiogram. Galen Vein (G) to which drains also the Internal Cerebral Vein (ICV) receiving the Thalamo-Striate Veins (TS). (**c**) Carotid Venous Angiogram (AP view). Basal Vein (arrows). Deep Middle Cerebral Vein (arrow head). Inferior Striate Veins (arrow with dot)

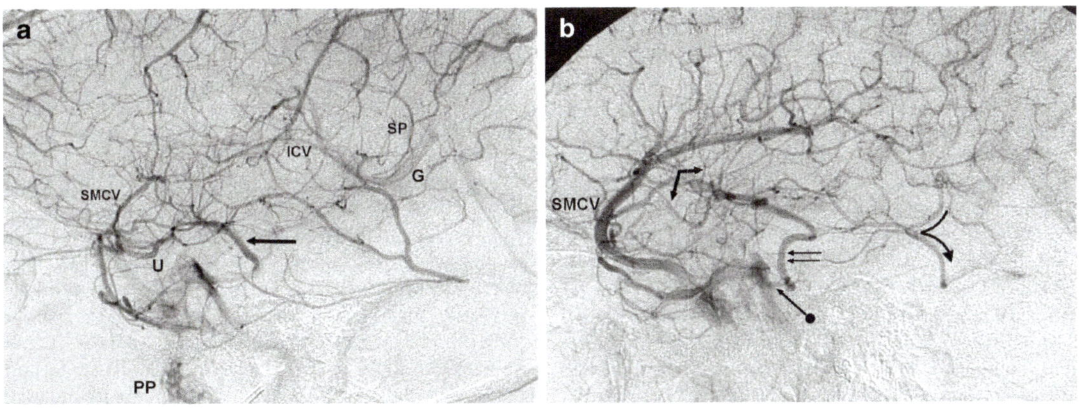

Fig. 9.17 (**a**) Only the posterior segment of the BV is present. It connects with the Lateral Mesencephalic vein (arrow with angle). The anterior tributaries of the BV drain partially in the Ponto-mesencephalic Vein (arrows) and partially in a small Uncal Vein (arrow with angle) which joins a large Superficial Middle Cerebral Vein (SMCV) draining in the Cavernous Sinus. Note the presence of Bridging veins (arrow wit dot) with the Cavernous Sinus. (**b**) The BV is absent. The Anterior tributaries drain in the Uncal Vein (U) which is connected with the SMCV. Both drain in the Pterygoid Plexus (PP). Partially, the drainage of the Anterior tributaries is in the Lateral Ponto-mesencephalic Vein (arrow). Galen Vein (G) receiving the blood of the Internal Cerebral Vein (ICV). Note the well-developed splenial vein entering the Galen Vein. (Taken from Bradac [4])

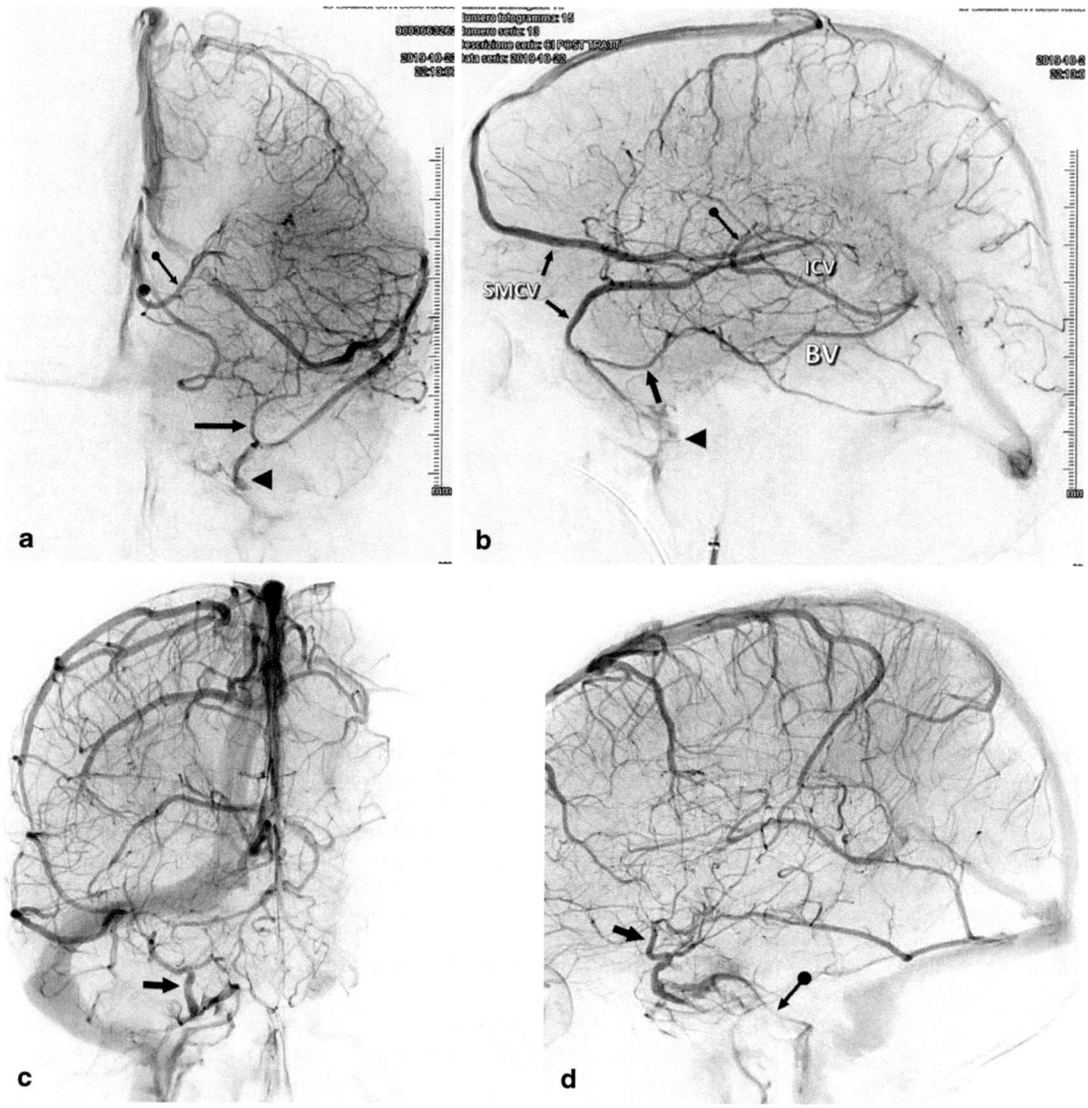

Fig. 9.18 (**a**) Carotid angiogram, AP view. There is a well-developed BV, with its typical course draining in the Galen Vein. Thalamo-Striate Veins (arrow with dot) continuing in the ICV. The anterior tributaries of BV drain in the Uncal vein (arrow). This joins the Superficial Middle Cerebral Vein (SMCV). Both draining in the Pterygoid Plexus (arrowhead). (**b**) Lateral view. Basal Vein (arrows). Uncal Vein (great arrow). Pterygoid Plexus (arrowhead). The two components of the SMCV (arrow with angle), one joining the Uncal Vein, the other draining in the SSS are well demonstrated. Internal Cerebral Vein (ICV) receiving the blood of the Thalamo-Striate Vein (arrow with dot). Galen Vein continuing in the SSS. (**c**) AP view. Another patient with anomalous BV. The distal BV is not developed. Its anterior tributaries join the dilated Uncal Vein (arrow) draining in the Pterygoid plexus. There are connections of the Uncal Vein with the Cavernous Sinus, continuing in the IPS. (**d**) Lateral view. The connections of the Uncal Vein (arrow) with the Cavernous Sinus as well as is drainage in the Pterygoid Plexus are better shown. Inferior Petrosal Sinus (small arrow). Labbé Veins. One of the branches runs first in the tentorium, before entering in the TS. Note the preferential drainage of the SSS in the right TS

9.15 Veins of the Posterior Fossa

In accordance to Padget [46], the first vein developing in the Posterior Fossa, as described above, is the so-called Anterior Metencephalic Vein (AM) developing as remnant of the regressed Pro-otic vein. The vein drains the blood of Brainstem and Anterior part of cerebellum. In the further evolution, the AM becomes the Petrous vein draining in the Superior Petrosal sinus. The Posterior part of the veins mainly involved in the drainage of Cerebellum develop later, following the development of the Cerebellar Hemispheres. The veins of this group called Posterior Metencephalic (PM) drain mainly in the Transverse and Straight sinuses and part in the Galen vein sharing their drainage with the veins of the deep cerebral system.

In the adult, the veins of the Posterior fossa have been subdivided considering their drainage in three groups [3, 4, 8, 24, 26, 39, 50, 56]. The Anterior Petrosal group draining in the Petrosal Vein, the Superior group draining in the Galen Vein, and the Posterior group draining in the Transverse and Straight sinuses.

It should be noted, however, that through the numerous connections of the veins of the different groups, the way of drainage can change.

To the Anterior group belong the anterior Ponto-mesencephalic vein (APM). This is a longitudinal channel running on the surface of Pons on the midline or adjacent to it. Superiorly the APM is connected with the Interpeduncular veins which as already described are tributaries of the BV, and so making a link of the APM with the BV or Posterior Mesencephalic vein (PM).

Inferiorly, the APM are connected with the Anterior Medullary vein (AM), continuing in the Anterior Spinal vein. Laterally to the APM, bilaterally, there is another longitudinal channel, running on the dorso-lateral surface of the pons, continuing caudally in the Lateral Medullary vein. This latter at the level of the Restiform body runs more medially, joining the contro-lateral forming the Posterior Medullary vein, continuing in the Posterior Spinal vein.

Transverse channel, on the surface of the pons and medulla, connect the Median with the Lateral channel, and more lateral with the anterior cerebellar vein, draining in the petrosal vein, tributary of the Superior Petrosal Sinus.

A vein of this group, sometimes very large, is the Lateral Mesencephalic vein (LM). It connects the BV or Posterior Mesencephalic vein with the Petrosal vein, by the way of the Brachial Veins.

Another small vein of this group is the vein of the Lateral Recess of the fourth ventricle. It receives blood from plexus and partially from tonsilla. It reaches the Petrosal Vein.

To the superior group, belong the Superior Vermian veins, running on the midline on the surface of the Superior Vermis, entering the Galen Vein. Another venous channel is the Precentral Vein, running in the Precentral Cerebellar Fissure, draining in the Galen Vein. It is formed by few branches running on the surface of the Brachium Pontis, called Brachial Vein (BR), which are connected along their course with the Lateral Mesencephalic Vein and caudally with the Petrosal Vein. Another important channel of this group is the Posterior Mesencephalic vein (PM). On the vertebral angiogram, the pattern of the PM is that of the Basal vein, differently from it the tributaries (Insula channels, Inferior Striate vein and the other veins of the anterior group) filled in the drainage of the structures, supplied by the ICA are not involved on the vertebral angiogram. This explains the only posterior segment of the vein on the vertebral angiogram. It drains in the Galen Vein and has anteriorly connection with the APM, through the Interpeduncular veins.

In the posterior group, there are the Hemispheric Cerebellar veins, draining in the Transverse Sinuses, frequently, after a short course in the Tentorium as bridging veins, and the Inferior Vermis veins. These latter are paired veins formed by the union of superior and inferior retro-tonsillary tributaries. Each runs in the Inferior Vermian Sulcus, entering commonly the Straight Sinus.

The veins of the posterior fossa are shown in the diagram (Fig. 9.19) and on the angiogram (Figs. 9.20 and 9.21).

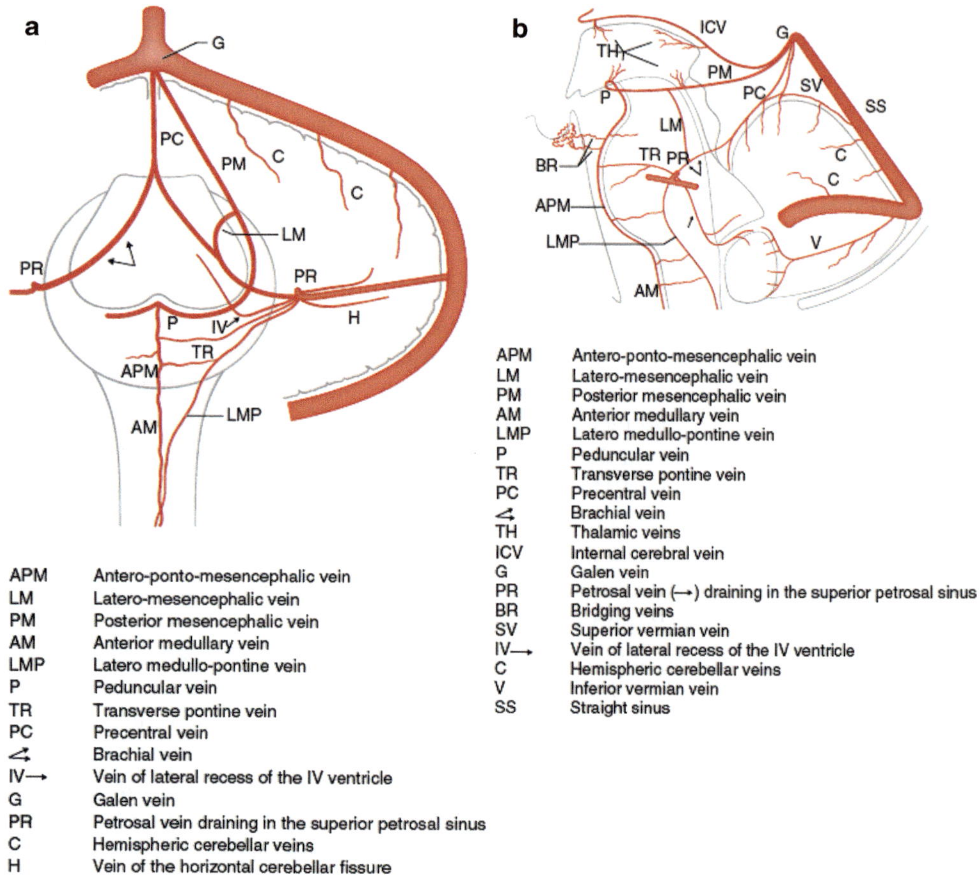

Fig. 9.19 (**a**) Posterior fossa veins seen in the AP view. (**b**) Lateral view of the posterior fossa veins. (Taken from Bradac [4])

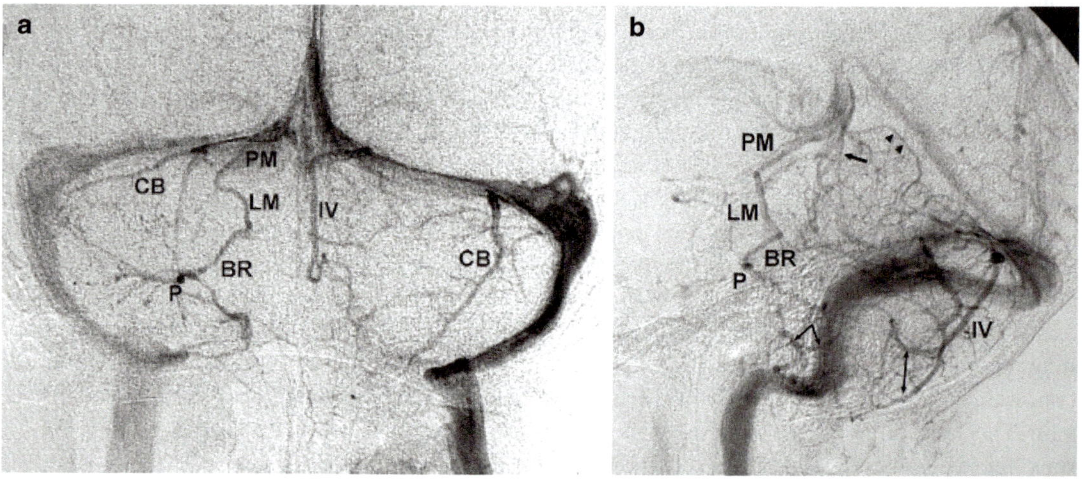

Fig. 9.20 (**a**) Vertebral Angiogram, lateral view. Only the posterior segment of the Posterior mesencephalic vein (PM) is present. It drains in the Galen vein. There is a large Lateral Mesencephalic vein (LM) draining in the Petrosal vein (P) through the Brachial vein (BR). Other veins of the Posterior fossa are recognizable. Precentral vein (arrow), Superior vermian vein (arrowhead). Inferior vermian vein (IV). Retro-tonsillar branches (arrow). (**b**) AP view, same indications. (Taken from Bradac [4])

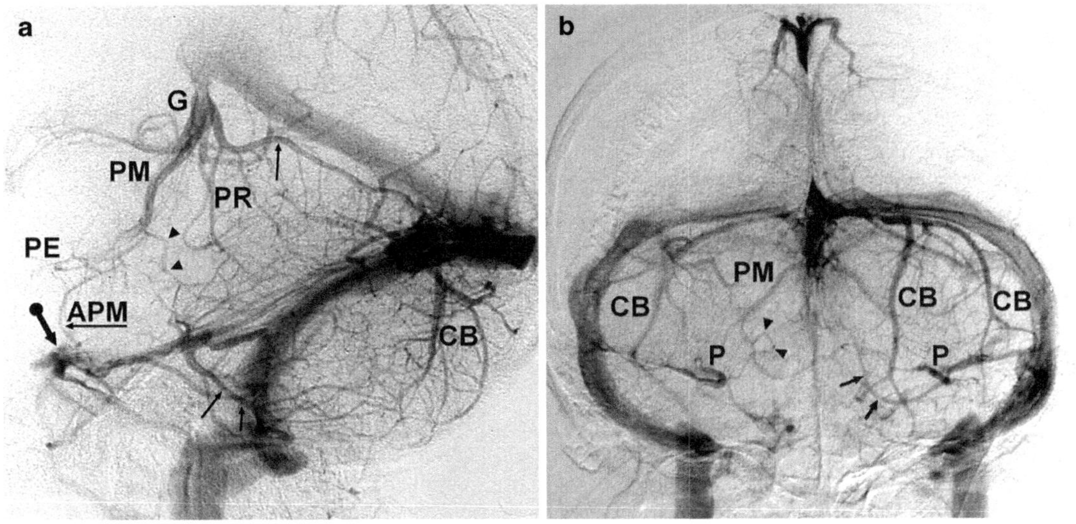

Fig. 9.21 (**a**) Vertebral angiogram, lateral view. Posterior Mesencephalic vein (PM), entering the Galen Vein (G), to which flow also the blood of the Precentral (PR) and Superior vermian (arrow) veins. Connections of the PM with the Anterior Ponto-mesencephalic vein (APM) through the Interpeduncular veins (PE). There is a small Lateral Mesencephalic (arrows head) connecting the PM with the petrosal vein (P), better identified in (**b**). Note the presence of bridging veins, connecting the APM with the Cavernous Sinus (arrow with dot). (**b**) AP view. The Petrosal Vein enters the Superior Petrosal Sinus. Hemispheric Cerebellar Veins (CB) entering the Transverse Sinus after short course in the tentorium. The Inferior Vermian Vein cannot be identified. There is a small, but recognizable, vein of the lateral recess of the IV ventricle (arrow), draining in the petrosal vein. (Taken from Bradac [4])

9.16 Evolution of the External Venous Drainage

The primordial evolution of the extracranial venous drainage has been already described in the previous section 9.3 (Figs. 9.4 and 9.5). Toward the embryo of 60–80 mm another important structure develops. This is the Pterygoid plexus (PP), appearing in the pterygoid region, receiving the blood of the region of the Maxillary process and Pterygoid muscle. To the PP converge several venous channels. Connections develop between the PP and the Inferior Ophthalmic vein (remnant of the Primary Maxillary vein) and with the Anterior Facial vein to a channel called *Deep Facial Vein.*

Other tributaries of the PP can be the Superficial Middle Cerebral Vein, the Uncal Vein and the Middle Meningeal Vein when these vessels take the drainage through the foramina of the middle cranial fossa (*Foramen spinosum* and *Foramen ovale*) reaching the PP. Sometimes a channel connects the Cavernous Sinus with the PP. This is the Vesalius Vein, passing through the foramen of Vesalius, described by the anatomist in the 1543 [72]. The foramen, located anteriorly to the foramen ovale, is not always present. It is however not so rare, as reported in more recent studies [18, 37].

The last channel appearing in the external venous drainage is the External Jugular Vein (EJV). It develops later receiving the blood of the developed occipital and the posterior auricular vein, draining the scalp of the occipital region and of the pinna. The scalp of temporo-parietal region drains in the Superficial Temporal vein, draining to the connection described above, in the IJV. The frontal region drains the scalp by the way of the Frontal vein, connected posteriorly with the branches of the Superficial Temporal vein and antero-inferiorly through two channels (supraorbital and supratrochlear vein) with the angular vein, running in the medial angle of the nose. This latter has connections with the Superior Ophthalmic vein, entering the Cavernous Sinus, and with the Anterior Facial vein, draining in the IJV.

In conclusion, only part of the Superficial Venous drainage is directed to the EJV (Fig. 9.5). Most of the scalp, as well as the Superficial and Deep venous of facial cranial area, drain in the Internal jugular Vein(IJV).

The phases of this complex evolution are shown in the diagram in Figs. 9.4 and 9.5c.

9.17 The Cranio-Cervical Region

The region deserves a few special considerations. As described in many studies [1, 2, 14, 30, 58], the region is a crossing point of several venous channels. One of these, almost constant is the so-called Anterior Condylar Confluences (ACC), which has been identified earlier by the French pathologist Trolard [67]. This is a venous pouch located in front of the Hypoglossal Foramen, extra-cranially, medially to the Jugular vein, a light caudal to the junction of the Inferior petrosal sinus with the Jugular bulb. The ACC is connected on one side with the Jugular bulb and on the other with the Anterior Condylar vein. This latter runs through the Hypoglossal canal, joining the Anterior Internal Vertebral Plexus. This is an epidural plexus connected cranially with the Clival venous plexus and the Marginal Sinus, and laterally joins a plexus surrounding the horizontal portion of the Vertebral Artery. This configuration has been called by Arnautowich "Sub-occipital Cavernous Sinus." There are connections between the horizontal portion of the plexus and the Deep cervical vein draining the deep cervico-occipital region. The plexus accompanies the Vertebral Artery in its cervical course.

Other connections are those between the ACC and the Lateral Condylar vein joining the horizontal portion of the venous surrounding the VA, and those with the Inferior Petrosal Sinus and those with the Petro-occipital sinus also called Inferior petro-occipital vein (IOPV). This latter Channel runs parallel to the IPS extra-cranially, joining the intracranial plexus surrounding the petrous segment of ICA (Rektorzik plexus) or directly the cavernous sinus.

Another venous channel in the area is the Posterior Condylar vein. The vein takes its origin from Jugular bulb or sometimes from the distal part of the Sigmoid sinus. It joins the horizontal plexus surrounding the VA.

As far as it concerns the Inferior Petrosal sinus, many studies have been devoted to it showing its typical as well as atypical configuration [2, 14, 41, 58, 60]. The IPS is commonly formed by a unique channel, but occasionally by a plexus of veins. It usually enters the jugular bulb, but can also run extra-cranially joining then IJV 3–4 cm below the cranial base. It has connection with the ACC and sometimes can end in it, having in this case no connections with the IJV. In extremely rare cases it can be absent.

This very complex venous configuration is shown in the diagram (Fig. 9.22).

As many studies have demonstrated, the venous drainage on the brain can change with a flow directed prevalently in the IJV in the supine position or directed in the vertebral sector (AV-VA) in the upright position [9, 10, 58, 71]. *As described above, these changes of venous drainage develop earlier in growing children passing from the horizontal to the upright position.*

This condition can be an important collateral way if the flow in the IJV is impaired. Furthermore, the awareness of this anatomy can be very useful in diagnosis and treatment of pathological conditions especially DAVF (Fig. 9.23).

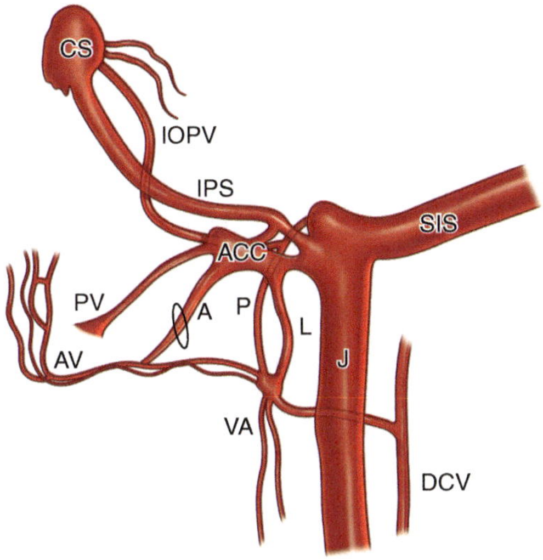

ACC	- Anterior condylar confluence	PCS	- Paracavernous sinus
A	- Anterior condylar vein running through the hypoglossal canal	IOPV	- Inferior petro occipital vein
L	- Lateral condylar vein connecting ACC with the LA	J	- Jugular vein
P	- Posterior condylar vein connecting jugular bulb with the VA and the DCV	SIS	- Sigmoid sinus
IPS	- Inferior petrosal sinus	AV	- Anterior epidural vertebral plexus with some connection with the clival venous plexus
CS	- Cavernous sinus	VA	- Vertebral artery venous plexus
		PV	- Prevertebral venous plexus
		DCV	- Deep cervical vein

Fig. 9.22 Drawing showing the venous drainage in the cranio-cervical region, AP view. Anterior condylar confluence (ACC), anterior condylar vein running through the hypoglossal canal, reaching the AV (A), lateral condylar vein connecting the ACC with the VA (L), posterior condylar vein connecting jugular bulb with the VA and the DCV (P), inferior petrosal sinus (IPS), cavernous sinus (CS), Inferior Petro Occipital Vein (IOPV), Jugular vein (J), Sigmoid Sinus (SIS), anterior epidural vertebral plexus with some connection with the clival venous plexus (AV), vertebral artery venous plexus (VA), prevertebral venous plexus (PV), deep cervical vein (DCV) (modified from [58])

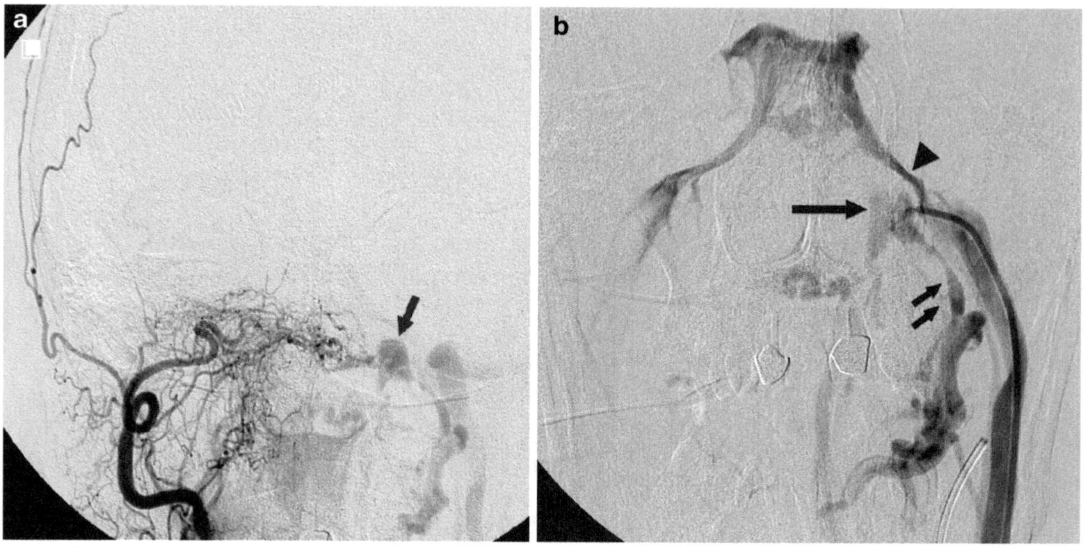

Fig. 9.23 Patient with DAVF involving the left ACC. Many supplying arteries were involved, especially both Ascending Pharyngeal Arteries. Particularly useful to localize the shunt was the right ECA angiogram. (**a**) Showing the involving of the right AphA (arrows). The artery supplied the DAVF through its clival branches. Early injection of the ACC (great arrow). Venous drainage continuing in the Lateral condylar vein. (**b**) Selective venous venogram with catheter in the Anterior Condylar confluence. Lateral condylar vein (arrows). IPS (arrowhead). Coils were placed in the ACC with occlusion of the fistula. (Taken from Bradac [4])

9.18 The Emissary and Diploic Veins

The emissary veins connect the intracranial with the extracranial venous sector. They are not constant, but when present they have a typical location.

- There are emissary veins related to the SSS connecting the Sinus with the veins of the nasal cavity, passing through the Foramen Cecum. Other veins connect the SSS with veins of the scalp in the parietal region.
- Sometimes there is an emissary vein connecting the small Petro-Squamous Sinus, remnant of the Pro-Otic Sinus, with the Deep Temporal veins.
- Others are located at the level of the Torcular Herophili and the Transverse Sinus, among them the most frequent is the Mastoid vein, connecting the Transverse Sinus with the Occipital or Posterior Parietal Auricular Vein, passing through the Mastoid Foramen.
- A few emissary veins are present in the cranio-Cervical region, as described more in detail above. The most important Venous structure in the area is the Anterior Condylar Confluence (ACC) receiving the blood from the IPS ad Sigmoid Sinus. The ACC drains further the blood in the Anterior Epidural Venous plexus and in the Vertebral Artery venous plexus. This latter, receives also the blood from the posterior condylar vein, arising from the jugular bulb.
- Other emissary veins can be the Superficial Middle Cerebral Veins and the Uncal Veins, draining in the pterygoid plexus, through the foramina of the middle cranial fossa, as well as the Middle meningeal vein, when the vein caudally has a connection with the PP becoming an emissary vein.
- As far as it concerns the Cavernous Sinus, it is connected through an emissary venous channel (Vesalius Vein) with the Pterygoid Plexus and with the ACC through the Petro-Occipital Sinus.

The diploic veins are frequently large venous channels, running in the diploic space of the calvarium, having connection with the Meningeal Veins and with the veins of the scalp.

References

1. Arnautović KI, Al-Mefty O, Pait TG, Krisht AF, Husain MM. The suboccipital cavernous sinus. J Neurosurg. 1997;86(2):252–62.
2. Benndorf G, Campi A. Aberrant inferior petrosal sinus: unusual transvenous approach to the cavernous sinus. Neuroradiology. 2002;44:158–63.
3. Bradač GB. The ponto-mesencephalic veins (radioanatomical study). Neuroradiology. 1970;1:52–7.
4. Bradač GB. Applied cerebral angiography: normal anatomy and vascular pathology. Cham: Springer; 2017. https://doi.org/10.1007/978-3-319-57228-4. 497 pages, ISBN 978-3-319-57227-7.
5. Cai CQ, Zhang QJ, Yang WD, Wang CX, Shen CH. Neuroimages of persistent falcine sinus in children. World J Pediatr. 2009;5:63–4.
6. Chaloupka JC, Huddle DC. Classification of vascular malformations of the central nervous system. Neuroimaging Clin N Am. 1998;8(2):295–321.
7. Doyon D, Aron-Rosa D, Ramee A. Orbital veins and cavernous sinus. Chap. 76. In: Radiology of the skull and brain, vol. 2. St Louis: Mosby; 1974.
8. Duvernoy HM, Vannson JL, Bonneville JF, Cabanis EA, Cattin F, Guyot J, et al. The human brain stem and cerebellum: surface, structure, vascularization, and three-dimensional sectional anatomy, with MRI [Internet]. Vienna: Springer; 2012. Disponibile su: https://books.google.it/books?id=GB_-CAAAQBAJ.
9. Eckenhoff JE. The physiologic significance of the vertebral venous plexus. Surg Gynecol Obstet. 1970;131(1):72–8.
10. Epstein HM, Linde HW, Crompton AR, Cine IS, Eckenholf JJ. The vertebral venous plexus as a major cerebral venous outflow tract. J Am Soc Anesthesiol. 1970;32(4):332–40.
11. Evans H. The development of the vascular system. Manual Human Embryol. 1912;2:570–669.
12. Falk D. Evolution of cranial blood drainage in hominids: enlarged occipital/marginal sinuses and emissary foramina. Am J Phys Anthropol. 1986;70(3):311–24.
13. Ferner H. Anatomische und phlebographische Studien der inneren Hirnvenen des Menschen. Z Anat Entwicklungsgesch. 1958;120:481–91.
14. Gailloud P, Fasel JH, Muster M, Desarzens F, Ruefenacht DA. Termination of the inferior petrosal sinus: an anatomical variant. Clin Anat. 1997;10(2):92–6.
15. Gailloud P, Ruíz DSM, Muster M, Murphy KJ, Fasel JH, Rüfenacht DA. Angiographic anatomy of the laterocavernous sinus. Am J Neuroradiol. 2000;21(10):1923–9.
16. Gailloud P, Muster M, Khaw N, Martin JB, Murphy KJ, Fasel JHD, et al. Anatomic relationship between arachnoid granulations in the transverse sinus and the termination of the vein of Labbe: an angiographic study. Neuroradiology. 2001;43:139–43.
17. Giudicelli G, Salamon G. Die Venen des Thalamus. Neuroradiology. 1970;1:92–8.
18. Görürgöz C, Paksoy CS. Morphology and morphometry of the foramen venosum: a radiographic study of CBCT images and literature review. Surg Radiol Anat. 2020;42:779–90.
19. Hacker H. Superficial supratentorial veins and dura sinuses. In: Newton T, Potts AG, editors. Angiography, Book 3. St Louis: Mosby; 1974.
20. Hanafee W, Rosen LM, Weidner W, Wilson GH. Venography of the cavernous sinus, orbital veins, and basal venous plexus. Radiology. 1965;84(4):751–3.
21. Harwood-Nash DC. Cerebral vessels in infants and children. Radiology of the skull and brain angiography. Section II. St Louis: Mosby; 1974. p. 1131–41.
22. Hochstetter F. Beiträge zur Entwicklungsgeschichte der Kraniozerebralen Topographie des Menschen: Vorgelegt in der Sitzung am 17. Dezember 1942. Springer-Verlag; 2013.
23. Huang YP, Wolf BS. Veins of the white matter of the cerebral hemispheres (the medullary veins). Am J Roentgenol Radium Therapy, Nucl Med. 1964;92:739–55.
24. Huang YP, Wolf BS. The veins of the posterior fossa—superior or galenic draining group. Am J Roentgenol. 1965;95(4):808–21.
25. Huang YP, Wolf BS. The basal vein and its tributaries. In: Radiology of the skull and brain, vol. 3. Great neck. St Louis: Mosby; 1974.
26. Huang YP, Wolf BS, Antin SP, Okudera T. The veins of the posterior fossa—anterior or petrosal draining group. Am J Roentgenol. 1968;104(1):36–56.
27. Huber P. Zerebrale Angiographie für Klinik und Praxis. Stuttgart: Thieme; 1979.
28. Johansson C. The central veins and deep dural sinuses of the brain. Acta Radiol. 1954:19541.
29. Kaplan HA, Ford DH. The brain vascular system. (No Title). New York: Elsevier; 1966.
30. Katsuta T, Rhoton AL Jr, Matsushima T. The jugular foramen: microsurgical anatomy and operative approaches. Neurosurgery. 1997;41(1):149–202.
31. Kim H, Su H, Weinsheimer S, Pawlikowska L, Young WL. Brain arteriovenous malformation pathogenesis: a response-to-injury paradigm. In: Zhang J, Colohan A, editors. Intracerebral hemorrhage research: from bench to bedside. Vienna: Springer; 2011. https://doi.org/10.1007/978-3-7091-0693-8_14.
32. König P. Zur Kenntnis des Verhaltens der äußeren Gehirnvenen zu den Hirnhäuten. Z Anat Entwicklungsgesch. 1950;114:605–10.
33. Lang J. Skull base and related structures: atlas of clinical anatomy. New York: Schattauer Verlag; 1995.
34. Lasjaunias P, Burrows P, Planet C. Developmental venous anomalies (DVA): the so-called venous angioma. Neurosurg Rev. 1986;9:233–42.
35. Leach JL, Jones BV, Tomsick TA, Stewart CA, Balko MG. Normal appearance of arachnoid granulations on contrast-enhanced CT and MR of the brain: differentiation from dural sinus disease. Am J Neuroradiol. 1996;17(8):1523–32.

36. Letteboer TG, Mager JJ, Snijder RJ, et al. Genotype-phenotype relationship in hereditary haemorrhagic telangiectasia. J Med Genet. 2006;43(4):371–7.
37. Maletin M, Vuković M, Marić D, Jeremić D, Petrović K. Foramen of Vesalius-constant or variable foramen. Srp Arh Celok Lek. 2020;148(11–12):689–94.
38. Markowski J. Entwicklung der Sinus durae matris und der Hirnvenen des Menschen. T. Tl. Bull internat Acad Polonaise Sci et Lettres No supplém. 1922.
39. Matsushima T, Rhoton AL, de Oliveira E, Peace D. Microsurgical anatomy of the veins of the posterior fossa. J Neurosurg. 1983;59(1):63–105.
40. McCormick WF. The pathology of vascular ("arteriovenous") malformations. J Neurosurg. 1966;24(4):807–16.
41. Miller DL, Doppman JL, Chang R. Anatomy of the junction of the inferior petrosal sinus and the internal jugular vein. Am J Neuroradiol. 1993;14(5):1075–83.
42. Mizutani T, Tanaka H, Aruga T. Total recanalization of a spontaneously thrombosed arteriovenous malformation: case report. J Neurosurg. 1995;82(3):506–8.
43. Oka K, Rhoton AL Jr, Barry M, Rodriguez R. Microsurgical anatomy of the superficial veins of the cerebrum. Neurosurgery. 1985;17(5):711–48.
44. Ono M, Rhoton AL Jr, Peace D, Rodriguez RJ. Microsurgical anatomy of the deep venous system of the brain. Neurosurgery. 1984;15(5):621–57.
45. Ostertun B, Solymosi L. Magnetic resonance angiography of cerebral developmental venous anomalies: its role in differential diagnosis. Neuroradiology. 1993;35:97–104.
46. Padget DH. The cranial venous system in man in reference to development, adult configuration, and relation to the arteries. Am J Anat. 1956;98(3):307–55.
47. Padget DH. The development of the cranial venous system in man, from the viewpoint of comparative anatomy. Contribut Embryol. 1957:81.
48. Parkinson D. Comments on the so-called cavernous sinus. Neurosurgery. 1982;11:716.
49. Raybaud CA, Strother CM, Hald JK. Aneurysms of the vein of Galen: embryonic considerations and anatomical features relating to the pathogenesis of the malformation. Neuroradiology. 1989;31:109–28.
50. Rosa M, Viale GL. Diagnostic value of vertebral phlebogram. Neuroradiology. 1970;1(3):147–50.
51. Rosenthal F. De intimis cerebri venis seu de venae magnae galena ramis. Nova acta physico-medica Academie Caesareae Leopoldino-Carolinae. Naturae Curiosorum. 1824;12:302–12.
52. Russell DS, Rubinstein LJ. Pathology of tumours of the nervous system. Baltimore: Williams & Wilkins; 1971. p. 250–64.
53. Ryu CW. Persistent falcine sinus: is it really rare? Am J Neuroradiol. 2010;31(2):367–9.
54. Sabin FR. Origin and development of the primitive vessels of the chick and of the pig. Contrib Embryol Carnegie Inst. 1917;6:61–124.
55. Saito Y, Kobayashi N. Cerebral venous angiomas: clinical evaluation and possible etiology. Radiology. 1981;139(1):87–94.
56. Salamon G, Huang YP. Radiologic anatomy of the brain. Berlin: Springer; 2012.
57. San Millán Ruiz D, Gailloud P, Angeles De Miquel Miquel M, Muster M, Dolenc VV, Rufenacht DA, et al. Laterocavernous sinus. Anat Record. 1999;254(1):7–12.
58. San Millán Ruíz D, Gailloud P, Rüfenacht DA, Delavelle J, Henry F, Fasel JH. The craniocervical venous system in relation to cerebral venous drainage. Am J Neuroradiol. 2002;23(9):1500–8.
59. Sandalcioglu IE, Wende D, Eggert A, et al. Vascular endothelial growth factor plasma levels are significantly elevated in patients with cerebral arteriovenous malformations. Cerebrovasc Dis. 2006;21(3):154–8.
60. Shiu PC, Hanafee WN, Wilson GH, Rand RW. Cavernous sinus venography. Am J Roentgenol. 1968;104(1):57–62.
61. Stein RL, Rosenbaum AE. Normal deep cerebral venous system. In: Radiology of the skull and brain, vol. 4; 1974. p. 1904–98.
62. Stephens RB, Stilwell DL. Arteries and veins of the human brain. (No Title). Springfield: Thomas; 1969.
63. Streeter GL. The developmental alterations in the vascular system of the brain of the human embryo. Contrib Embryol Carneg Inst. 1918;8:5–38.
64. Takahashi M, Okudera T. The choroid plexus and the choroid vein of the lateral ventricle: their angiographic appearance and clinical significance. Radiology. 1972;103(1):113–20.
65. Taptas JN. The so-called cavernous sinus: a review of the controversy and its implications for neurosurgeons. Neurosurgery. 1982;11(5):712–7.
66. Tobias PV, Clark WE. The cranium and maxillary dentition of Australopithecus (Zinjanthropus) boisei. (No Title). 1967.
67. Trolard P. De l'appareil veineux des artères encephaliques. J Anat Phisyol. 1890.
68. Truwit C. Embryology of the cerebral vasculature. Neuroimaging Clin N Am. 1994;4(4):663–89.
69. Tubbs RS, Ammar K, Liechty P, Wellons JC, Blount JP, Salter EG, et al. The marginal sinus. J Neurosurg. 2006;104(3):429–31.
70. Uranishi R, Baev NI, Ng PY, Kim JH, Awad IA. Expression of endothelial cell angiogenesis receptors in human cerebrovascular malformations. Neurosurgery. 2001;48(2):359–68.
71. Valdueza JM, von Münster T, Hoffman O, Schreiber S, Einhäupl KM. Postural dependency of the cerebral venous outflow. Lancet. 2000;355(9199):200–1.
72. Vesalius A. De humani corporis fabrica libri septem. 1543.
73. Virchow R. Die krankhaften Geschwülste: dreissig Vorlesungen gehalten während des Wintersemesters 1862–1863 an der Universität zu Berlin. Vol. 4. A. Hirschwald; 1867.
74. Von Rokitansky C, von Rokitansky KF. Handbuch der pathologischen Anatomie, vol. 1. Braumüller & Seidel; 1846.
75. Widjaja E, Griffiths PD. Intracranial MR venography in children: normal anatomy and variations. Am J Neuroradiol. 2004;25(9):1557–62.
76. Wolf BS, Newman CM, Schlesinger B. The diagnostic value of the deep cerebral veins in cerebral angiography. Radiology. 1955;64(2):161–77.

GPSR Compliance

The European Union's (EU) General Product Safety Regulation (GPSR) is a set of rules that requires consumer products to be safe and our obligations to ensure this.

If you have any concerns about our products, you can contact us on ProductSafety@springernature.com

In case Publisher is established outside the EU, the EU authorized representative is:

Springer Nature Customer Service Center GmbH
Europaplatz 3
69115 Heidelberg, Germany

Batch number: 10732801

Printed by Printforce, the Netherlands